The Inner World of American Psychiatry,

1 8 9 0 – 1 9 4 0

The Inner World of American Psychiatry,
1 8 9 0 – 1 9 4 0

Selected Correspondence

GERALD N. GROB

Rutgers University Press   *New Brunswick, New Jersey*

Library of Congress Cataloging in Publication Data

Grob, Gerald N., 1931–

The inner world of American psychiatry, 1890–1940.

Includes index.

1. Psychiatry—United States—History—20th century.

2. Mentally ill—Care and treatment—United States—

History—20th Century.   3. Psychiatry—United States—

History—19th century.   4. Mentally ill—Care and

treatment—United States—History—19th century.

5. Psychiatrists—United States—Correspondence.

I. Title.   [DNLM: 1. Psychiatry/United States—corres-

pondence.   WZ 112.5.P6 G873i]

RC438.G75   1985   150'.973   84-17692

ISBN 0–8135–1081–3

For Roger Bibace

CONTENTS

Acknowledgments ix

A Note to the Reader xi

Abbreviations xiii

ONE
The Emergence of American Psychiatry, 1820–1940
1

TWO
Human Behavior and Mental Illness
19

THREE
Mental Hospitals
56

FOUR
Psychiatric Therapies
102

FIVE
Mental Hygiene
138

SIX
The Boundaries of Psychiatry
185

SEVEN
The Demand for Autonomy
229

EIGHT
Psychiatry and Society
266

Index 297

ACKNOWLEDGMENTS

The following individuals and organizations graciously granted me permission to reprint materials:

Mrs. Julia Meyer Asher and The Johns Hopkins Medical Institutions (Adolf Meyer Papers).

Saint Elizabeths Hospital and the National Archives (William A. White Papers).

James K. Hall, III, and the Southern Historical Collection, University of North Carolina, Chapel Hill (J. K. Hall Papers).

Mr. Carel Goldschmidt and the Library of Congress (Smith Ely Jelliffe Papers).

Dr. Eric T. Carlson and the New York Hospital–Cornell Medical Center (American Foundation for Mental Hygiene and Clifford W. Beers Papers).

Rockefeller Foundation Archives (Rockefeller Foundation Papers).

American Psychiatric Association (Clarence B. Farrar and John C. Whitehorn Papers).

University of Alabama Library (William D. Partlow Papers).

Dr. Frances H. Gitelson and the Library of Congress (Maxwell Gitelson Papers).

Clark University Archives (G. Stanley Hall Papers).

Betty Gonzales and the Association for Voluntary Sterilization (Association for Voluntary Sterilization Papers).

Joseph Wortis (Joseph Wortis, "Observations of a Psychiatric Intern").

The materials for this volume were gathered over a period of years, during which time a number of organizations provided assistance. I am deeply indebted to the National Institute of Mental Health and the National Library of Medicine (both of which are part of the Public Health Service, U.S. Department of Health & Human Services), which supported my work with generous research grants (MH 39030 and LM 2306), and the National Endowment for the Humanities and the John Simon Guggenheim Memorial Foundation, which gave me fellowships to pursue my work. A number of friends and scholars—including George A. Billias, Nancy Tomes, and Jacques Quen—offered me the benefit of their insights, and Marlie Wasserman provided very helpful suggestions. Muriel Clawans gave indispensable assistance by transcribing the letters and preparing the final copy of this book.

Gerald N. Grob
Rutgers University
New Brunswick, New Jersey
May 1984

A NOTE TO THE READER

In recent years the private papers of leading psychiatrists and others prominent in the mental health professions have become available to scholars. The purpose of this collection, simply put, is to provide a cross-section of psychiatric correspondence and thereby to illuminate the varied concerns of those involved with the care and treatment of the mentally ill. Privately, people tend to be less reticent and constrained, and psychiatrists are no exception. Their correspondence reveals a much more varied universe as well as the presence of haunting doubts and uncertainties. Historians and social scientists who have portrayed the specialty as monolithic have often ignored manuscript sources, and their work has suffered correspondingly. Admittedly, the letters in this collection represent only a minute fraction of the total. I hope, however, that this selection will stimulate others to make greater use of the wealth of materials that have become available.

Since this edition is not intended as a definitive one, I have omitted much of the annotation characteristic of projects that seek comprehensiveness. In the introductions and headnotes I have identified the major issues and participants, as well as the specific collection in which the item is to be found. I have not, on the other hand, attempted to identify every person mentioned in the letters. The index, however, includes (with a few isolated exceptions) the complete name of every person, which should enable the reader to gather additional biographical information. The letters themselves correspond exactly with the originals; I have corrected misspellings or typing errors and occasionally added commas and other punctuation to enhance readability. In a few letters, the names of individual patients and attendants have been replaced by the initial of the last name to maintain confidentiality.

ABBREVIATIONS

USED IN TEXT

AAPSW   American Association of Psychiatric Social Workers

AMA   American Medical Association

AMPA   American Medico-Psychological Association

APA   American Psychiatric Association

NCMH   National Committee for Mental Hygiene

LOCATIONS OF MANUSCRIPT COLLECTIONS

AAPSWP   American Association of Psychiatric Social Workers Papers, Social Welfare History Archives, University of Minnesota, Minneapolis, Minn.

AFMHP   American Foundation for Mental Hygiene Papers, Archives of Psychiatry, New York Hospital–Cornell Medical Center, New York, N.Y.

AMP   Adolf Meyer Papers, Alan Mason Chesney Medical Archives, Johns Hopkins Medical Institutions, Baltimore, Md.

AVSP   Association for Voluntary Sterilization Papers, Social Welfare History Archives, University of Minnesota, Minneapolis, Minn.

CBFP   Clarence B. Farrar Papers, American Psychiatric Association Archives, Washington, D.C.

GSHP   G. Stanley Hall Papers, Clark University Archives, Worcester, Mass.

JCWP   John C. Whitehorn Papers, American Psychiatric Association Archives, Washington, D.C.

JKHP   J. K. Hall Papers, Southern Historical Collection, University of North Carolina, Chapel Hill, N.C.

MGP   Maxwell Gitelson Papers, Library of Congress, Washington, D.C.

RFP   Rockefeller Foundation Papers (Record Group 1.1, Series 200), Rockefeller Foundation Archive Center, Pocantico Hills, North Tarrytown, N.Y.

SEJP   Smith Ely Jelliffe Papers, Library of Congress, Washington, D.C.

USVAP   U.S. Veterans Administration Papers (Social Work Service Papers, 1921-1963), Social Welfare History Archives, University of Minnesota, Minneapolis, Minn.

WAWP   William Alanson White Papers, in Records of Saint Elizabeths Hospital, Record Group 418, National Archives, Washington, D.C.

WDPP   William D. Partlow Papers, University of Alabama Library, University, Ala.

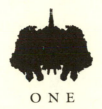

ONE

The Emergence of American Psychiatry, 1820-1940

In recent decades American psychiatrists have come under sharp attack. They have been accused of a variety of transgressions: of rationalizing deviant behavior in medical terms, thus facilitating the incarceration of persons in mental hospitals; of demanding legitimacy for a specialty that lacked a foundation in medical science; of insisting on an ability to cure and to prevent mental illness that had no justification in practice; and of advancing claims for autonomy that disregarded any liability for accountability. Indeed, in the 1970s and 1980s psychiatry remained a marginal specialty that was increasingly ignored by new medical graduates applying for residencies.

In one sense many of the charges directed against psychiatrists were justified, but in a larger sense many of the critics were attacking an image that bore little relation to reality. Public debates, of course, are rarely intended to enlighten, and the debate about the nature of psychiatry and mental illness was no exception. For psychiatry, like other medical and nonmedical specialties, was not unified or cohesive; diversity rather than unity was characteristic. Indeed, in their private correspondence psychiatrists presented a self-portrait that differed sharply from the more popular and conventional image. Popular perceptions to the contrary, psychiatrists—including such eminent figures as Adolf Meyer, William A. White, J. K. Hall, Smith Ely Jelliffe, and others—disagreed among themselves as frequently as they agreed. Differences of opinion persisted on virtually every issue, including the very definitions of mental illness, therapy, public policy, and mental hygiene. The purpose of this collection, therefore, is to shed light on the inner world of American psychiatry from 1890 to 1940 and also to encourage scholars to make far greater use of a growing body of manuscript material. Although the first half of the twentieth century may seem remote from the turbulent years of the post–World War II era, many of the underlying issues have their contemporary counterparts. What emerges from a careful analysis of this earlier era is a far more complex and ambiguous reality. To understand these decades, it is first necessary to describe the origins of American psychiatry, the status of mental hospitals, and the structure of public policy in the nineteenth and early twentieth centuries.

During the first half of the nineteenth century, Americans created an extensive network of public mental hospitals. Whereas before 1820 only one state had made provision for cases of mental illness, by 1875 there were more than sixty public institutions in thirty-two states; the average number of resident patients in each hovered around the five hundred mark. These institutions had two different but related functions. First, they were structured to provide restorative therapy for curable cases. Second, they offered care (food, clothing, and shelter) for those who for one reason or another failed to respond to therapy and who lacked either financial resources or a family able and willing to provide for their survival.[1]

One of the by-products of the founding of mental hospitals was the creation of the specialty of psychiatry. This fact is of crucial significance, for it means that psychiatric thought and practice were not dominant in shaping the structure and function of these institutions. Instead the reverse was true. Psychiatry, for the most part, was shaped by the institutional setting within which it was born and grew to maturity. Many of the dominant characteristics of psychiatric thought were but rationalizations of existing conditions within mental hospitals and coincided with popular attitudes. In its formative years the mental hospital was an institution created by society to deal with mentally ill patients, many of whom were unable to survive without assistance. The result was that psychiatry—despite its insistence that it was a scientific discipline—reflected the role assigned to it by society. This is not to imply that psychiatrists deliberately or consciously attempted either to define their discipline within such a context or to jus-

1. Many of the generalizations in this and subsequent chapters are based on my previous books, *Mental Institutions in America: Social Policy to 1875* (New York, 1973), *Mental Illness and American Society, 1875–1940* (Princeton, N.J., 1983), and *The State and the Mentally Ill: A History of Worcester State Hospital in Massachusetts, 1830–1920* (Chapel Hill, N.C., 1966). Readers interested in pursuing the sources of the data and generalizations can consult the extensive bibliographies and footnotes in these volumes.

tify institutionalization on other than medical grounds. It is only to say that psychiatry, like most professions and institutions, was influenced by its peculiar origins. Having developed professionally within an institutional framework created by society in response to perceived needs, psychiatrists inevitably absorbed the validity of these needs into their view and understanding of their speciality.

The newly emerging specialty in many ways reflected broader social and cultural values. Psychiatric theory and practice, for example, were not simply derivatives of European experiences or of seemingly disinterested scientific analysis. On the contrary, theory and practice evolved within a much broader context. Although psychiatrists preferred to conceive of the mental hospital as a strictly medical institution, their analysis of the nature and etiology of mental illness as well as modes of care and treatment were in some ways derived from the values of the larger society.

Superficially, the concepts of mental illness held by American psychiatrists seemed neutral. Mental illness in their eyes was a somatic disease that involved lesions of the brain (the organ of the mind). Disease followed the violation of the natural laws that governed human behavior. In other words, mental illness (like organic illness), though somatic in nature, could have psychological, hereditary, or physical origins. Thus the abnormal behavior of the individual (who possessed free will) could be the primary cause of insanity, leading as it did to the impairment of the brain. Mental illness, therefore, was to some extent self-inflicted; by ignoring the laws governing human behavior, people placed themselves on the road to disease (a belief that dated from antiquity).

Without doubt, most psychiatrists were far more interested in the moral (i.e., psychological) causes of mental illness, partly because of their own commitment to prevention and partly because these seemed to account for the largest proportion of cases. As firm believers in the tenets of Protestant Christianity, they felt much freer in their discussions of morality than they did in their observations on pathology. The moral causes of insanity included—to cite only a few examples—intemperance, overwork, domestic difficulties, excessive ambition, faulty education, personal disappointments, jealousy, pride, and above all, the pressures of an urban, industrial, and commercial civilization. Mental illness, in other words, was the inevitable consequence of behavior that represented a departure from accepted social norms.

Despite their belief that mental illness was largely a function of individual and structural defects, psychiatrists did not draw pessimistic conclusions. As a group, they were persuaded that insanity was as curable, if not more curable, than most somatic illnesses. If derangements of the brain and nervous system were the consequences of environmental pressures that led people to violate the natural laws governing human behavior (thus leading to lesions of the brain), it followed that a change in the environment could lead to a reversal of improper physical development. Treatment thus began with institutionalization.

Heirs to a holistic medical tradition, early nineteenth-century psychiatrists elaborated what became known as "moral treatment" or "moral management." By manipulating the environment and the patient, the psychiatrist could overcome past associations that had led to disease and create an atmosphere in which the natural restorative elements could reassert themselves. By providing a balanced diet and using tonics, laxatives, and drugs to restrain moderate abnormal behavior (excessive energy and lassitude), the hospital ministered to the patient's physical needs. Simultaneously the psychiatrist oversaw the institutional environment that acted upon the deranged mind. Moral treatment, while susceptible to many interpretations, meant kind, individualized care in a small hospital; resort to occupational therapy, religious exercises, amusements, and games; repudiation in large measure of all threats of physical violence; and only infrequent application of mechanical restraints. In effect, the patient would be reeducated within a proper moral atmosphere.

During the 1840s and 1850s superintendents claimed striking successes in curing mental illness, especially in cases where a person had been ill for less than twelve months. Although some of the claims were undoubtedly exaggerated, there is some evidence that early nineteenth-century mental hospitals achieved some striking successes. A follow-up study in the late nineteenth century at Worcester State Lunatic Hospital in Massachusetts, for example, found that nearly 58 percent of more than eleven hundred patients discharged as recovered in the mid-nineteenth century were never again institutionalized. It is therefore possible to infer that the character and internal environment of many early mental hospitals, together with the charismatic personalities of first generation superintendents, had a beneficial impact on patients.

Admittedly, some patients did not respond to moral treatment. For them the hospital served a largely custodial function by providing the basic necessities of life. Most mid-nineteenth-century psychiatrists found nothing wrong in accepting a dual role that gave them responsibilities both for acute yet curable patients and for chronic patients for whom the future appeared bleak. A combination of medical, ethical, and religious considerations weighed heavily against rejecting a custodial role. As Thomas S. Kirkbride noted in his famous and influential treatise on mental hospitals in 1854:

> The first grand objection to such a separation is, that no one can say with entire certainty who is incurable; and to condemn any one to an institution for this particular class is like dooming him to utter hopelessness. . . . When patients cannot be cured, they should still be considered under treatment, as long as life lasts; if not with the hope of restoring them to health, to do what is next in importance, to promote their comfort and happiness, and to keep them from sinking still lower in the scale of humanity. Fortunately, almost precisely the same class of means are generally required for the best management and treatment of the curable and incurable, and almost as much skill may be shown in caring judiciously for the latter as for the former. When the incurable are in the same institution as the curable, there is little danger in their being neglected; but when once consigned to receptacles specially provided for them, all experience leads us to believe that but little time will elapse before they will be found gradually sinking, mentally and physically, their care entrusted to persons actuated only by selfish motives—the grand object being to ascertain at how little cost per week soul and body can be kept together—and, sooner or later, cruelty, neglect and suffering are pretty sure to be the results of every such experiment.

When Kirkbride published a second edition of his book a quarter of a century later, his views had not changed. "What is best for the recent," he insisted, "is best for the chronic."[2]

The fortuitous circumstances that had created the conditions for therapeutic successes proved, however, to be short-lived. By the third quarter of the nineteenth century the structure and functions of mental hospitals—and therefore of the specialty of psychiatry—had begun to undergo a gradual transformation. At the time of their founding, mental hospitals were presumed to be providing restorative therapy; yet from the very beginnings they retained large numbers of patients who failed to show any

2. Thomas S. Kirkbride, *On the Construction, Organization, and General Arrangements of Hospitals for the Insane* (Philadelphia, 1854), 59; second edition (Philadelphia, 1880), 248.

improvement. The retention of chronic cases, in turn, restricted efforts to offer therapy to the remaining patients. In their early days, hospitals had also been designed for small numbers of patients to encourage close relationships deemed necessary for sound treatment. Later they grew in size because states either placed higher ceilings on the number of patients or did not take steps to build new facilities. In theory, all patients were supposed to receive the same quality of care; in practice, class, race, and ethnicity promoted a different quality of care for different patients. Superintendents were supposed to function in a medical capacity; they became, in fact, hospital administrators immersed in managerial problems, and considerations of order and efficiency sometimes overshadowed therapeutic concerns.

Regarded as a self-contained medical institution, the mental hospital was, however, unable to retain any significant degree of isolation from the larger society in which it existed. Public policy remained a legislative responsibility, and hospital officials found their autonomy significantly limited by the general legal, administrative, and fiscal environment in which they functioned. The decentralized and prebureaucratic nature of mid-nineteenth-century American society inhibited the formulation of consistent and coherent policies; mental hospitals were often caught up in the vortex of change and confusion and saw their goals transformed by circumstances beyond the control of their officials. Nor did local governments bring any measure of stability or continuity to policy issues; community control and participation—at least as far as the mentally ill were concerned—were inversely related to quality of care and level of funding. The fact that problems arising out of mental illness were inseparable from the broader issues of dependency also had major implications. When many states began to centralize and rationalize their welfare systems during the last third of the nineteenth century, mental hospitals became further enmeshed in an ambiguous welfare system. Under these circumstances the goals of mental hospitals were constantly shifting as psychiatrists were forced to respond to changes in the larger environment.

"It is fair to say," E. C. Seguin, a distinguished American neurologist, wrote in 1880, "that in the present state of psychiatry in America, to be pronounced insane by physicians, by a judge, or by a jury, means imprisonment for months, for years, or for life. To put it another way, there is a disease which reduces its victims to a level with persons accused of crime, and exposes them to loss of liberty, property and [to] unhappiness."[3] The moral was clear: the mental hospital was nothing more than a prison for mentally ill patients.

In so sharply criticizing his psychiatric colleagues, Seguin was not alone. On the contrary, during the 1870s and 1880s psychiatrists found themselves under attack from a variety of individuals and groups, including other physicians, social activists, lawyers, state regulatory agencies, and former patients. On occasion it appeared that critics were determined to undermine the very legitimacy of institutional psychiatry that an earlier generation had forged. Such hostility posed a serious threat to the continued vitality of the specialty.

In reaction to widespread criticisms, psychiatrists began to redefine the foundations of their specialty. Between 1890 and 1940 they began to look beyond the institutions in which their specialty had been conceived and to which it had been wedded for more than half a century. Influenced by the theoretical and institutional changes in medical science as well as by those social and intellectual currents that gave rise to efforts to transform American society, they redefined not only concepts of mental disease and treatment but the very context of the specialty. In so doing, psychiatrists implicitly posited a conflict between the traditional mental hospital and its function of providing custodial care for large numbers of chronic patients on the one hand and the imperatives of modern psychiatry on the other. Although the majority of psychiatrists before World War II continued to be affiliated with mental hospitals, the thrust of their specialty was increasingly away from institutional practice. That the internal ferment did not necessarily conclude in theoretical innovation or demonstrably effective therapies was little noticed. When the process of change had run its course, psychiatry and mental hospitals were no longer synonymous terms.

By the 1880s the transformation of American psychiatry was under way. In 1885 the Association of Medical Superintendents of American Institutions for the Insane (founded in 1844) modified its membership requirements and permitted assistant physicians to become ex officio members. Seven years later it changed its name to the American Medico-Psychological Association (AMPA). These changes, which culminated in 1921 when the AMPA became the American Psychiatric Association (APA), represented

3. E.C. Seguin, "The Right of the Insane to Liberty," in Conference of Charities and Correction, *Proceedings*, 7 (1880): 166.

a fundamental shift in focus. Nineteenth-century psychiatrists had emphasized managerial and administrative issues because they had made the care of institutionalized patients their primary responsibility. Their late nineteenth- and early twentieth-century successors, by way of contrast, were as much concerned with disease as they were with individuals, and slowly the former replaced the latter as the primary focus as psychiatrists attempted to integrate themselves into the structure of scientific medicine.

The psychiatric emphasis on pathology reflected the general orientation of medicine, which was altering the social role of physicians in the late nineteenth century. As medicine became identified with bacteriology and other biological and physical sciences, its practitioners created a new doctor–patient relationship. More and more patients assumed a passive role, especially as physicians justified their dominant role in terms of special training and knowledge. Imbued with the ideals of European—and especially German—science, American physicians created a new institutional complex that placed the modern general hospital and an increasingly elaborate technology at the center of medical practice. To those entering psychiatry, it appeared that the specialty had to change its ways if it was not to become a backwater.

By the turn of the century, American psychiatrists were looking beyond the institutions that had been linked for so long with their specialty. Some explored the physiological and biological roots of mental disease; some developed a more analytic psychiatry that incorporated Freudian insights; some attempted to integrate psychological and physiological phenomena to illuminate the inner workings of abnormal minds; some experimented with novel therapeutic approaches; and others reached beyond the boundaries of medicine to create a mental hygiene movement that sought to demonstrate the social utility and relevance of modern psychiatry. "I regard the future of mental medicine as filled with golden promise," Charles G. Wagner informed his colleagues in his presidential address before the AMPA in 1917. "Serious, thoughtful students of psychiatry are busily at work on problems of vital importance, and I venture to predict that within the period of a decade or two their labors will result in a much better understanding of the etiology, pathology, diagnosis and treatment of mental diseases than we now possess."[4]

4. Charles G. Wagner, "Recent Trends in Psychiatry," *American Journal of Insanity*, 74 (1917): 14.

The ferment within psychiatry in the early twentieth century was also marked by institutional change. By the turn of the century, two innovations had appeared: the research institute and the psychopathic hospital. The creation of such institutions was related to changes in medicine in general. To many, it seemed that medical science was standing on the threshold of a new era. The specific germ theory of disease suggested an explanation that was empirically verifiable and that seemed to point the way toward specific therapies.

Scientific and technological innovation also created conditions that made possible the emergence of the hospital in its modern form. Before 1880 the small number of general hospitals that existed offered care for poor and socially marginal groups. After 1880 the hospital began to embody the scientific and technological imperatives that legitimated a changing profession, and it commenced serving a more affluent clientele. Consciously or unconsciously, psychiatrists began once again to find in general medicine an appropriate model to follow.[5]

Perhaps the most visible symbol of change was the mental hygiene movement begun after 1900. Reflecting a commitment to science, mental hygienists viewed disease as a product of environmental, hereditary, and individual deficiencies whose eradication required a fusion of scientific and administrative action. As members of a profession that they believed was destined to play an increasingly central role in the creation of a new social order, psychiatrists began to redefine their role. The new emphases on scientific research rather than care or custody, on disease rather than patients, and on alternatives to the traditional mental hospital were merely a beginning. More compelling was the utopian idea of a society structured to maximize health and minimize disease. In 1917 Thomas W. Salmon, a key figure in the reorientation of psychiatry, spoke about the future of the specialty. The new psychiatry, he insisted, had to reach beyond institutional walls and play a crucial part "in the great movements for social betterment." Psychiatrists could no longer limit their activities and responsibilities to the institutionalized mentally ill. On the contrary, they had to lead the way in research and policy formulation; to implement methods in such

5. See Charles E. Rosenberg, "Inward Vision and Outward Glance: The Shaping of the American Hospital, 1880–1914," *Bulletin of the History of Medicine*, 53 (1979): 346–91, and Morris J. Vogel, *The Invention of the Modern Hospital: Boston, 1870–1930* (Chicago, 1980).

areas as mental hygiene, care of the feebleminded, eugenics, control of alcoholism, management of abnormal children, treatment of criminals; and to help in the prevention of crime, prostitution, and dependency.[6]

One of the major by-products of the mental hygiene movement, oddly enough, was a growing preoccupation with internal professional issues rather than issues that related directly to patient welfare. Before 1930 psychiatrists had not only helped to popularize the concept of prevention but had invited a number of nonmedical groups to join them. By the 1920s, however, conflict between psychiatrists and these older groups seeking recognition and status was not uncommon. The friction between psychiatrists, on the one hand, and psychiatric social workers, clinical psychologists, psychiatric nurses, and occupational therapists, on the other hand, was also in part a conflict over gender roles; psychiatry was a male-dominated specialty, whereas before 1940 the others were largely female. The American Association of Psychiatric Social Workers (AAPSW), for example, had a virtually exclusive female membership. Similarly, the main register of the American Occupational Therapy Association revealed that in 1932, 408 out of 419 members were female.[7] Concern with the claims of these emerging mental health occupations led the APA in the 1930s to direct its energies toward the development of mechanisms to safeguard its professional territoriality. In 1934 it succeeded in creating the American Board of Psychiatry and Neurology, thus setting the stage for board certification.

The creation of a specialty board also reflected a faith that the content of psychiatry had reached a level susceptible to fairly precise measurement. In a larger sense, such beliefs were characteristic of other occupational groups that defined themselves in professional terms and were persuaded that they possessed the ability to control events within their respective spheres of competence. In a more limited sense, however, the emphasis on certification was an attempt to secure reinforcements from the field of medicine to support the legitimacy of the psychiatric claim to overarching competence in contrast to the various would-be usurpers of the nonmedical professions. The effort to shift the foundations of psychiatric practice seemed appropriate in view of the widespread, if not always accurate, belief that

6. Thomas W. Salmon, "Some New Fields in Neurology and Psychiatry," *Journal of Nervous and Mental Disease,* 46 (1917): 90–99.

7. American Occupational Therapy Association, *1933 Directory of Qualified Occupational Therapists Enrolled during 1932 in the National Register* (New York, n.d. [c. 1933]).

scientific medicine was responsible for the decline in mortality from infectious diseases and the increase in life expectancy at birth. By identifying with the field of medicine, psychiatric practice increasingly shifted from mental hospitals to outpatient clinics, child guidance clinics, and private practice.

As the locus of practice changed, the careers of psychiatrists were less and less bound up with the hundreds of thousands of patients in mental institutions whose conditions seemed to be beyond effective intervention. Indeed, by mid-century the role of state hospital psychiatrists in the APA was sharply reduced. In 1895 virtually all members had been in hospital practice. By 1956 only about 17 percent of the ten thousand or so members of the APA were employed in state mental hospitals or Veterans Administration facilities; the remainder were either in private practice or employed in various government and educational institutions, including community clinics. As psychiatrists succeeded in identifying themselves with the larger medical profession, they were less and less prone to act—as their nineteenth-century predecessors had acted—as the representatives of the institutionalized mentally ill.

At the same time that psychiatrists were altering the nature of their specialty, the mentally ill population in institutions was undergoing profound changes. In simple terms, the bulk of patients in mental hospitals increasingly fell into the chronic category. For them, meaningful therapy was not available; they required certain basic essentials without which life was impossible. The needs of such patients were, however, far removed from the concerns of psychiatrists. Having absorbed a new vision of a "scientific" specialty, psychiatrists slowly but surely began to ignore and reject—if not explicitly, then implicitly—the custodial or caring responsibilities accepted by their nineteenth century predecessors.

In the half century following 1900, the nature of mental hospitals was transformed by a series of demographic and functional changes. Before 1880, patient populations at public hospitals were made up of large numbers of acute cases institutionalized for less than twelve months. Although national data are lacking, a sample of individual institutions reveals that their custodial function had not yet become paramount. The experiences of Worcester State Hospital, the oldest and most influential institution in Massachusetts, are instructive. In 1842, a decade after its opening, 46.4 percent of its patients had been hospitalized for less than a year; only 13.2 percent had been in the hospital for five or more years. In 1870 the comparable figures were 49.6 and 13.9 percent. Nor was Worcester atypical. In 1850 41.1 percent of patients at the Virginia Western Lunatic Asylum had been institutionalized for less than a year and 29.6 percent for five years or more; the respective figures for the California Insane Asylum in 1860 were 40.2 and 0.1 percent.[8] Although exceptions were by no means uncommon, most hospitals before 1890 included large numbers of patients who were admitted and discharged in less than a year.

By the turn of the century the pattern began to be reversed as the number of short-term cases fell and long-term increased. In 1904, 27.8 percent of the total patient population in the United States had been confined for less than twelve months. By 1910 this percentage had fallen to 12.7, although it rose to 17.4 percent in 1923. The greatest change came among patients institutionalized for five years or more. In 1904, 39.2 percent of patients fell into this category; in 1910 and 1923 the respective percentages were 52.0 and 54.0. Although data for the United States as a whole were unavailable after 1923, the experiences of Massachusetts were perhaps typical. By the 1930s nearly 80 percent of the available beds in state hospitals were occupied by chronic patients.[9]

The shift toward a predominantly custodial institution whose inmate population was made up of long-term chronic cases reflected other broad social changes. The growing number of aged people in mental hospitals is a case in point. Before 1890 relatively few older people (over sixty) were confined in mental hospitals. Where the aged were destitute or without families willing or able to provide care, they were generally sent to local almshouses. Throughout much of the nineteenth century, almshouses served as undifferentiated welfare institutions; one of their primary functions was the care of aged dependent people, many of whom were undoubtedly senile or frail.

Between 1880 and 1920, however, the almshouse declined in significance as a public institution. Admissions fell from 99.5 to 58.4 per 100,000 be-

8. Worcester State Lunatic Hospital, *Annual Report*, 10 (1842): 17–27, 38 (1870): 38–60; Virginia Western Lunatic Asylum, *Annual Report*, 23 (1850): 14–23; California Insane Asylum, *Annual Report*, 8 (1860): 16–32.

9. U.S. Bureau of the Census, *Insane and Feeble-Minded in Hospitals and Institutions 1904* (Washington, D.C., 1906), 37; *idem, Insane and Feeble-Minded in Institutions 1910* (Washington, D.C., 1914), 59; *idem, Patients in Hospitals for Mental Disease 1923* (Washington, D.C., 1926), 36; Neil A. Dayton, *New Facts on Mental Disorders: Study of 89,190 Cases* (Springfield, Ill., 1940), 414–29.

tween 1904 and 1922. The decline in the number of the mentally ill aged sixty and over was even sharper; by 1923 only 5.6 percent of the almshouse population fell into this category. The decline, nevertheless, was more apparent than real, for the number of aged mentally ill committed to mental hospitals was rising steadily.[10] What occurred was not a deinstitutionalization movement but, rather, a transfer between types of institutions. The shift was less a function of medical or humanitarian concerns (although these were by no means absent) than a consequence of financial considerations. As states moved to accept fiscal responsibility for all insane people in the late nineteenth and early twentieth centuries, local public officials seized upon the fiscal advantage inherent in redefining senility in psychiatric terms. If the senile were cared for in state hospitals rather than local or county almshouses, the burden of support would be transferred to the state. To many families, confinement in a mental hospital may have been preferable to almshouse care. Not only did hospitals provide better care, but paradoxically, the stigma of insanity—especially if an aged person was involved—may have seemed less than that of pauperism.

Between 1890 and 1940, the proportion of aged people in mental hospitals mounted rapidly. In New York, to offer a specific illustration, 18 percent of all first admissions to state mental hospitals in 1920 were diagnosed as psychotic because of senility or arteriosclerosis. By 1940 this category accounted for nearly 31 percent of all first admissions. In 1950, 40 percent of all first admissions were aged sixty and over, as compared with only 13.2 percent of New York State's total population. Nor was New York unique in this respect; the data for such states as Pennsylvania, Massachusetts, and Illinois exhibit similar patterns.[11]

10. U.S. Bureau of the Census, *Paupers in Almshouses 1904* (Washington, D.C., 1906), 182, 184; *idem, Paupers in Almshouses 1910* (Washington, D.C., 1915), 42–43; *idem, Paupers in Almshouses 1923* (Washington, D.C., 1925), 5, 8, 33; *idem, Insane and Feeble-Minded in Hospitals and Institutions 1904,* 29; *idem, Patients in Hospitals for Mental Disease 1923,* 27.

11. Benjamin Malzberg, "A Statistical Analysis of the Ages of First Admissions to Hospitals for Mental Disease in New York State," *Psychiatric Quarterly,* 23 (1949): 344–66; *idem,* "A Comparison of First Admissions to the New York Civil State Hospitals During 1919–1921 and 1949–1951," *Psychiatric Quarterly,* 28 (1954): 312–19; New York State Department of Mental Hygiene, *Annual Report,* 52 (1939–1940): 174–175; U.S. Bureau of the Census, *Census of Population: 1950,* vol. II, *Characteristics of the Population,* pt. 32 (Washington, D.C., 1952), 58; Mor-

Not only did the number of aged patients in mental hospitals increase, but age-specific admission rates for older people rose markedly compared with those for younger people as institutions such as almshouses declined. In their classic study of rates of institutionalization covering more than a century, Goldhamer and Marshall found that the greatest increase occurred in the category of those aged sixty and over. In 1885 the age-specific first admission rate per 100,000 in Massachusetts for people aged sixty and over was 70.4 for men and 65.5 for women. By the beginning of World War II, the corresponding figures were 279.5 and 223.0.[12]

In addition to the aged, mental hospitals cared for large numbers of people whose behavioral peculiarities were related to an underlying somatic etiology, for example, paresis (the tertiary stage of syphilis). Between 1911 and 1919 about 20 percent of all first admissions to New York State mental hospitals were cases of general paresis. Given the nature of the disease, few households were willing or prepared to cope with paretic cases. Despite the relative absence of aged people among paretic patients, its prognosis was decidedly negative. In 1920, for example, 825 such cases were admitted for the first time to New York State mental hospitals. Of this number, 322 (39 percent) died in less than six months, 113 (13.7 percent) in six to eleven months, and most of the remainder in one to four years after admission. Between 1913 and 1922, 87.7 percent of all first admission paretics in the state died during their confinement.[13]

Generally speaking, at least one-third and probably one-half or more of all first admissions to state mental hospitals were cases with behavioral symptoms probably of known somatic origins. In 1922, 52,472 people were admitted to state mental hospitals for the first time. Of this number, 3,356 were without evidence of any psychoses; they were admitted be-

---

ton Kramer et al., *A Historical Study of the Disposition of First Admissions to a State Mental Hospital: Experiences of the Warren State Hospital During the Period 1916–50,* U.S. Public Health Service Publication No. 445 (Washington, D.C., 1955), 10; Carney Landis and Jane E. Farwell, "A Trend Analysis of Age at First-Admission, Age at Death, and Years of Residence for State Mental Hospitals: 1913–1941," *Journal of Abnormal and Social Psychology,* 39 (1944): 3–23.

12. Herbert Goldhamer and Andrew W. Marshall, *Psychosis and Civilization: Two Studies in the Frequency of Mental Disease* (Glencoe, Ill., 1953), 54, 91.

13. Horatio M. Pollock, *Mental Disease and Social Welfare* (Utica, N.Y., 1941), 93–109; New York State Department of Mental Hygiene, *Annual Report,* 52 (1939–1940): 176.

cause of epilepsy, alcoholism, drug addiction, psychopathic personality, or mental deficiency. Of the remaining 49,116 first admissions, 16,407 suffered from a variety of identifiable somatic conditions, including senility, cerebral arteriosclerosis, general paresis, Huntington's chorea, pellagra, and brain tumors. Between 1922 and 1940, the proportion of patients admitted for the first time with such somatic conditions increased from 33.4 to 42.4 percent.

Assuming that many people in the functional-psychosis categories also suffered from a variety of conditions with a somatic origin—an assumption that may be warranted from other present-day data—it is evident that mental hospitals provided care for a patient population with severe physical as well as mental problems. The fact that the somatic group had a higher death rate than the functional-psychosis group suggests that the diagnoses were not inaccurate. In 1940, for example, the somatic group accounted for 19,357 deaths out of a total of 31,417, or 61.6 percent.[14]

A significant proportion of the total institutionalized population were, in other words, suffering from physical disabilities that also involved behavioral symptoms. Whether or not the mental hospital was the appropriate place for them was beside the point; most required some form of comprehensive care. It is true that it was theoretically possible to care for such people in a home environment, but such a solution was not always feasible. In many cases, home care proved disruptive; in others, no home existed. Ultimately many families accepted hospitalization as an unwelcome but necessary last resort.

What about the thousands of other mental patients who apparently did not suffer from known somatic diseases? Who were they and why were they institutionalized? Of those identified as psychotic but not suffering from identifiable or known physical disabilities, the overwhelming majority were diagnosed as manic depressive, schizophrenic (dementia praecox), or alcoholic. In 1922 these three groups accounted for 44.4 percent of all first admissions; by 1940 the percentage had declined to 39.2 percent. These categories present obvious problems, partly because of their etiological and descriptive vagueness. Certainly it is possible to delineate the demographic characteristics of these groups. Nevertheless, it is by no

14. The statistics in this and the previous paragraph have been compiled from U.S. Bureau of the Census, *Patients in Hospitals for Mental Disease 1923* (Washington, D.C., 1930), *Mental Patients in State Hospitals 1926 and 1927* (Washington, D.C., 1930), and *Patients in Mental Hospitals 1940* (Washington, D.C., 1943).

means certain that such characteristics were linked to the nature of the disease or condition of the patients.[15]

The nature of the patient population in mental hospitals, however, is not a completely unknown entity. Although it is impossible to determine the precise reasons for the institutionalization of patients or to categorize the nature of their condition with any degree of accuracy, it is possible, by using available data, to make some reasonably informed guesses. Specifically, discharge and retention rates and mortality indicate that hospitals were caring for two distinct groups. The smaller group was composed of those who appeared to benefit from brief periods of confinement and were thereafter able to return to their communities and resume their lives. The larger group included those with severe mental and physical difficulties who required continuing assistance.

Several studies published in the 1930s gave some indication of the kinds of patients hospitalized during the second and third decades of the twentieth century. In 1931 Raymond G. Fuller and Mary Johnston conducted a retrospective study of all first admissions to New York state hospitals in terms of outcomes. They selected three periods for intensive analysis: 1909–1911, 1914–1916, and 1919–1921. They then followed the history of every person admitted during each of these periods until mid-1928. Between 1909 and 1911, 2,481 patients admitted for the first time were schizophrenics; 1,579 were manic depressives; and 1,104 were alcoholics. The medical history of each of these groups was dissimilar. The manic depressives and alcoholics had a much more favorable prognosis; 59.7 percent of the former and 62.7 percent of the latter spent less than a year in hospitals, whereas the comparable figure for the schizophrenics was 27.4 percent. The schizophrenics also remained in hospitals for far longer periods. For those patients who did not improve or recover within six months of admission, the prognosis grew steadily bleaker. No less than 722 out of the 2,481 schizophrenics admitted between 1909 and 1911 remained in the hospital for the full sixteen years covered by the study.[16]

Fuller and Johnston calculated that of every 100 first admissions, about 35 were discharged as recovered or improved, 7 remained unimproved, 42 died in the hospital, and 16 were in the hospital when the study ended. Of those institutionalized for less than a year, about half were discharged

15. *Ibid.*

16. Raymond G. Fuller and Mary Johnston, "The Duration of Hospital Life for Mental Patients," *Psychiatric Quarterly,* 5 (1931): 341–52, 552–82.

as recovered or improved, three-eighths died, and one-eighth were discharged but declared unimproved. Although the average duration of hospital confinement was 49.2 months, the median was only 11.4 months. Of those who were below the median, the average confinement was only 3.7 months; the other half averaged a stay of 99.6 months. Using some of the same and additional data, Benjamin Malzberg also found that the mentally ill had far higher mortality than the general population.[17]

The character of patient populations was a critical variable for mental hospitals. Although psychiatrists and public officials tended to emphasize the prime importance of therapy, the fact of the matter was that hospitals were fulfilling a quite different function. Simply put, they were providing custodial care for dependent people. Indeed, the debate as to whether certain groups, such as the aged senile, belonged in mental hospitals was beside the point; some form of care for such patients was required irrespective of the setting in which it was provided.

In 1940 the mental hospital seemed central to the care of the mentally ill. Diversity was the rule; hospitals varied both qualitatively and quantitatively. Despite such variations, the hospital was the only institution in society structured to provide basic care for those whose mental conditions, whatever the origins of their illness, had rendered them dependent on others for their survival. That the hospital had numerous defects and shortcomings went without saying: the quality of care left much to be desired; staff–patient relations were often disruptive; internal regimens rested in part on coercion; and the institutional environment was often antihumanistic. Yet these shortcomings were not limited to mental hospitals; they mirrored the imperfection and limitation of human beings in general. For patients, the choice was not between institutional forms of care and other alternatives; the choice was between institutional care and no care at all.

Paradoxically, the role of the mental hospital in providing care for thousands of people was largely ignored. Even before 1940, psychiatrists were caught up in enthusiasm for new therapies, an enthusiasm that reflected a commitment to medical science and disease rather than to patient care. Such concerns helped to resolve the traditional tensions within psychiatry between therapy and custody in favor of the former. This is not to imply that psychiatrists were unconcerned about the fate of chronic patients, for

17. *Ibid.;* Benjamin Malzberg, *Mortality among Patients with Mental Disease* (Utica, N.Y., 1934).

such was not the case. It is only to note that their attention as professionals tended to be focused on patients for whom interventionist therapies would presumably make a difference. Psychiatrists who continued to be employed at institutions were preoccupied with new therapies; others simply left institutional employment and practiced in different settings. Whatever the case, it is clear that between 1890 and 1940 the intimate relationships between mental hospitals and psychiatry had begun to disappear, and the latter took a new form.

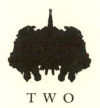

T W O

Human Behavior and Mental Illness

Early twentieth-century American psychiatrists looked forward to a time when the puzzle of mental disease would be solved, yet their optimism was not accompanied by a shared consensus about the nature of mental disease. If anything, they divided into a bewildering variety of groups, each with its own assumptions and beliefs. Conflict, not harmony, was the norm. Although friction was sharpest within psychoanalysis and between psychoanalysis and the more traditional psychiatry, it was by no means absent from the latter alone.

By the turn of the century the older psychiatric somaticism was under attack. Somaticism, of course, was never completely rejected; to do so might have transferred medical concepts to the realm of metaphysics. Critics of the older somatic style could, however, present strong counterarguments: the absence of evidence demonstrating a relationship between lesions and abnormal behavior; a classification system that was both rigid and vague; an etiological scheme based on personal and superficial observations rather than on biological findings; an approach that ruled out the study and analysis of mental phenomena; the neglect of therapeutics that arose from a belief that many insane people fell into the chronic category; and the failure to pursue systematic neuropathological and laboratory research.

The criticisms of traditional somaticism, however, did not reflect theoretical clarity, nor were they based on the kind of empirical data that might be used to construct a new synthesis. American psychiatry remained a heterogenous specialty, and a variety of different and often unrelated concepts appealed to different practitioners. Those psychiatrists who to one degree or another assimilated Freudian concepts into their thought generally had few links with public mental hospitals, where the overwhelming bulk of patients were concentrated; analytic and psychoanalytic psychiatry had its greatest influence in smaller private hospitals and private practice.

The disunity of early twentieth-century psychiatric thought was not due simply to the lack of a tradition of basic research or to the relative weaknesses of American medical schools compared with European ones, although both elements played a role. More important was the fact that the very concept of mental disease was inseparable from the deeper and more profound problem of explaining the nature of human beings in general and their behavior in particular. At one extreme were certain deterministic systems that reduced behavior to physiological mechanisms and ruled out independent thought or actions that did not have specific causal antecedents. More widely accepted, however, were eclectic models that posited a link between mental and biological factors. But the nature of such links remained shrouded in mystery, and the very concept of mental phenomena posed seemingly unresolvable theoretical difficulties.

In general medicine, the demonstration of a relationship between the presence of certain symptoms and a specific bacterial organism had led to the development of a new classification based on etiology rather than on symptomatology, at least for most infectious diseases. The inability to pursue a parallel course left psychiatry with a classification system based on external behavioral signs that tended to vary in the extreme. Conclusive evidence that paresis (general paralysis of the insane) was actually the tertiary stage of a disease that began with a prior syphilitic infection offered an attractive model for psychiatric diseases. Nevertheless, neither psychiatrists nor pathologists were able to identify other comparable specific psychiatric disease entities.

The formidable divisions among psychiatrists did not, however, lead to a generalized or paralyzing pessimism. Few shared the belief of Simon Flexner, director of the prestigious Rockefeller Institute for Medical Research (now the Rockefeller University), that it might be impossible to undertake meaningful neuropsychiatric research, given the state of medical science and the absence of a certain kind of medical technology. Indeed, Flexner went so far as to argue that "there were no problems in a fit state for work." Like physicians generally, psychiatrists advanced explanations that appeared to embody the latest available knowledge. The reasons are not difficult to grasp. Unlike those outside the specialty, psychiatrists were responsible for thousands of patients in mental hospitals. Their existential involvement with such a large and varied group precluded consideration of the claim that mental disease could neither be understood nor treated. Evidence did exist, after all, that certain patients clearly benefitted from interventionist therapy. Moreover, the training and education of psychiatrists—which did not differ from that of other physicians—rendered untenable any abandonment or modification of the traditional therapeutic role. Such a role, of course, required some sort of theoretical justification. Had psychiatrists rejected an effort to explain mental disease, they might have impaired their professional legitimacy and prepared the way for other groups willing to fill an existing void and meet perceived social needs.

The effort to provide theoretical explanations for extraordinarily complex phenomena may in retrospect appear both immature and futile. But to argue in such terms is to neglect the intellectual and social milieu in which all humans live and to suggest that our predecessors should have known what we know (or what we hope to know in some remote future). A more plausible approach involves, at the very least, an effort to understand how psychiatrists could interpret mental illness in the terms they did. To make such an effort requires a sympathetic understanding of what was known as well as an appreciation of the limitations—scientific, technological, philosophical, and social—that barred efforts to arrive at a fuller comprehension of the foundations of an etiology of mental illness.

Adolf Meyer (1866–1950) was one of the most influential American psychiatrists of the early twentieth century. Born and educated in Switzerland, he migrated to the United States in 1892. After a brief career in Illinois and Massachusetts, he served successively as the director of the Pathological Institute of the New York State Hospitals and the Henry Phipps Psychiatric Clinic of the Johns Hopkins Medical School. "Psychobiology"—the name he gave to his understanding of psychiatry—involved the integration of the life experiences of the individual with physiological and biological data. Influenced by Darwinian biology and the concept of adaptation, Meyer stressed the interaction between organism and environment. In his eyes, mental illness was largely a behavioral disorder involving defective habits; certain early experiences produced inefficient adaptation in adulthood. Although never rejecting a somatic etiology or the role of constitutional and genetic influences, Meyer tended to emphasize psychogenic factors. In the following exchange, Meyer and August Hoch (1868–1919) discussed de-

mentia praecox, a term associated with Emil Kraepelin (a German psychiatrist who helped to lay the foundation of modern clinical psychiatry).

August Hoch to Adolf Meyer, December 29, 1904 (AMP, Series II).
I see that the spirit moved us both about the same time, and I was very glad to hear from you.

I do not know about my coming to New York to that meeting and I do not know just what I would have to say, but if it is best for me to come and if the time agrees with the time at which we should meet for the sake of the book I will get up something.

I have been thinking a good deal about dementia praecox, and have come to the conclusion that we might call the disease or whatever name we may give to it a process of dissociation for which we have analogies in dream, delirium, and hysteria. Dream and delirium especially are states of rapid, extreme dissociation, in which, (of course this holds only for deliria,) the picture of the outside world is much disorganized. If such a dissociative process is more limited, then the general picture of the outside world does not suffer, but what we have then is symptoms which are also present in dreams and deliria, viz. arising impressions and notions not connected with the situation, or autochthonous ideas representing the same thing in a less extensive way, or hallucinations, symptoms which also occur in the deliria and dreams, as do, for example, the paramnesias. We may therefore say that these symptoms are symptoms of dissociation, and we are then only confronted with the fact that hallucinations occur also at the melancholic states (I don't mean depressive deliria) but here we have also in a way dissociation, only it is secondary, and due to the undue emphatization [*sic*] of certain contents of consciousness. The same may be said about the delusion of reference, or the feeling of reference. This is too slight a symptom to establish any analogy in the deliria, but we know from experience that it is a very important symptom in dementia praecox, and is probably related to the autochthonous ideas. It also is found in melancholy states, probably for the same reason.

Another difficulty is the alcoholic hallucinosis, which is not delirium, but we may say that this forms a milder dissociation process, whereas the delirium is a much more extensive, and active, and acute form.

I do not see why the catatonic phenomena may not be regarded from the same point of view.

The idea of a general dissociation is then of course supported by the outcome in a confused dementia.

Now there is of course the transition to the paranoias, not to all, but to certain ones which are based on the reference as well as those which simply begin with a hallucinosis. These are cases who are older, and it seems that the older cases not only show less extensive dissociative processes, but they show in the general course a greater resistance towards dissociating influences, being as they are more well formed personalities.

When Stransky speaks of his ataxia and his dissociation between intellectual, will, and emotional side, he evidently means something similar, but the comparison with the deliria as the dissociative process par excellence seems to me very important, as does also the laying stress on the various symptoms as dissociation symptoms, and consequently their relation among each other aside of the practical diagnostic value which such a course has.

The trouble is how to explain the milder apathetic states which often pass into the dissociative complex.

This is very crude and I don't know just what you will think about it. Of course you will recognize your own ideas in some of these things. If we are able to bring some harmony into this difficult question, to show why some hallucinosis, for example, is related to a case with a lot of queer notions, etc., etc. we have at least gained something, and some such view as the above seems to be borne out by my cases.

I shall be interested to hear from you. In the meantime, I wish you a Happy New Year.

Adolf Meyer to August Hoch, December 30, 1904 (AMP, Series II).
Thanks for your letters, especially for the last one. I think it is a very good thing to discuss matters of this sort promptly when the spirit moves.

The concept of dissociation is very much in the air at present; it is, however, so strongly used in the somewhat prejudicial studies of Sidis, Janet and others, that I should dislike using it instead of the much more positive concept of habit disorder. To bring in delirium and the whole complex in which there is essentially an allopsychic disorder with a very crude affection of the habit adjustment, creates difficulties. With hysteria we have to be very cautious; it is one type of habit disorganization in which we must demand the demonstration of the dominant interference of an emotional affect with its characteristic results of narrowing of the field of attention; tendency to suggestion, automatism, etc, nota bene, a very definite type of dissociation not essentially based on dissociation of habits of activity. The majority of hystericals can have quite a useful sphere of activity in their limited field of attention, and above all things most of the accidents can be directly influenced by proper management of the digestion of ordinary emotional disorder. I realize that this is somewhat dogmatic, but it is something per se unless there comes to it the necessary disorganization of activities, volition and tendencies and the insufficiency in the adjustment to actuality. There we have analogies with dreams, even more marked than in hysteria.

I realize fully that in my purely empirical scheme of speaking of a delirium paranoia series, and on the other hand, a series of essentially dissociation of activities, we meet plenty of cases in whom both factors are to be reckoned with; that is a point which would never come up unless it was for the classification notion, and if we wish to make much of the delirium part we must make it plainly understood that in the cases of dementia praecox the important feature is the extending and prevalent reaction type of the personality, which is not able to cope with the more general and more frequent occurrences of delirium. An acute hallucinosis or delirious episode in melancholia, or in other diseases, are therefore something essentially different. They are conditions in which the most general form of dissociation gets a fairly prominent position in the general picture, whereas in dementia praecox types the habit-disorder is in the center.

Now what is this habit-disorder? You might call it affective personality, deficiency of those leading instincts which direct the interests and adapt them to the necessary interrelation with things as they go and are, which seem to be as much needed for healthy life as oxygen. This is not very luminous yet and I shall have to avoid the last metaphor, but as I see the cases the point holds, and it agrees very well with what you say about the paranoiac states, that they mark more complete personalities, whereas in cases in which phantastic trends establish themselves, in the form of hallucinosis or delirium, and the personality is only involved transitorily and incidentally, you have evidently a different situation.

I amused myself yesterday with a tabulation of about one-half of my dementia praecox cases to see about the onset of the first plain symptoms, and the time of admission; it is really remarkable how many cases had long premonitory stages, and it will be our duty to single out the cases of supposedly acute onset; their number grows smaller as one looks up the facts more carefully, and where the trouble seems to have arisen suddenly, the frequency of the difficulty of coping with some actual situation, such as sexual interests, is very striking. That is what I call difficulties of practical adaptation compared with which the hysterical difficulties of adjustment are far less upsetting.

I feel that I am simply thinking aloud and do not furnish much digestive matter; I shall, however, let you have what I get up for next Wednesday, and I hope you will "think" aloud just as frankly, and let me have your views no matter whether they will be wholly digested or not.

You need not consider yourself refuted by the above. I should, however, strongly advise you to read in Janet's last book the chapter on the hierarchies, and to read over Sidis' chapters on dissociation, and I hope especially the latter will convince you that it will be best to keep aloof of the term wherever one can help it.

Around the turn of the century, southern mental hospitals began to receive cases of pellagra and insanity. It was not then recognized that pellagra was a disease caused by a dietary deficiency. In some instances it gave rise to some of the behavioral signs associated with mental illness. In 1911 Meyer and E. M. Green, a psychiatrist at the Georgia State Sanitarium in Milledgeville, corresponded about the proper classification of such cases, thus illuminating the difficulty of employing external behavioral signs to designate a particular disease entity.

E. M. Green to Adolf Meyer, October 5, 1911 (AMP, Series I).
I write to ask your advice in a matter which is of considerable importance to the Medical Staff of this institution. While I appreciate the fact that your time is so fully occupied that you cannot afford to respond in every case where your advice is asked, I will be grateful if you can find time to set us straight in this particular.

Our Staff is divided on the question of classification of the many cases of pellagra which come to us.

My position is that *at this time* we cannot make a separate group of "Pellagrous Insanity"; that the cases of this disease which present symptoms of infective-exhaustive states should be grouped with the "Infective-exhaustive Psychoses"; those presenting the picture of dementia praecox should be classified as "Dementia Praecox"; those showing the different combinations of elation–depression, flight–retardation, psychomotor activity–slowness, should be considered to be "Manic-depressive Psychosis".

The question of infection or intoxication as the cause of the disease being still undetermined, we incline to the former theory.

Some members of our Staff believe that all cases of pellagra, without regard to the mental symptoms manifested should be grouped as "Infective-exhaustive Psychosis," while others take the position that "Pellagrous Insanity" is an entity and that these cases should be so classified, distinguishing the following subdivisions according to the mental manifestations:

Infective-exhaustive type
Dementia praecox type
Manic-depressive type
Demented type
Paretic type

Our idea is not to provide a label for every case, the tendency to which you so justly criticise, but to find a correct working basis for the consideration of these cases.

I am sure that your opinion will be of interest and value to each one of us and will help us to view these cases in the proper light.

Adolf Meyer to E. M. Green, October 9, 1911 (AMP, Series I).
Your letter touches a very fundamental difficulty of psychiatry in which I find it hard to advise you. I feel myself that it is best to let the issue be decided according to what appears most important at a certain time and to a special staff. There is no doubt that to-day pellagra is quite in the centre of attention and, therefore, might well be a focus of classification, with sub-heads as to indicate the five types specified. Under all circumstances I should urge that *both* issues be attended to in any group. There will always be some features due to the external cause and others to the individual make-up of the patient, but, inasmuch as the question whether a condition implies pellagra or not, is the most burning issue at the present time. I should yield by speaking of pellagra, and give the types as indicated by you.

I am very sorry that I have, as yet, very little experience with pellagra, most of which was obtained in Italy many years ago—it undoubtedly is a very serious problem in which the alienist has to delve into matters of general hygiene, submerging the interest of the psychopathology problem.

I was much interested in the account of the medical work of your institution sent me last Spring. It is quite easy to see your hand in the general organisation of the work, and I hope the methods from Wards Island proved stimulating. You may know, of course, that for a number of years we have been very anxious to push the problem of deeper analysis of dynamic factors, as you can see in the July 1910 number of the *American Journal of Psychology*, and the August number of the *Psychological Bulletin*, 1908. . . .

E. M. Green to Adolf Meyer, October 13, 1911 (AMP, Series I).
Your letter of Oct. 9th received. I thank you very much indeed for the advice it contained and will read my letter and your reply to the Staff at our meeting tomorrow. I have been quite undecided for some time about these cases, the increasing number of which presents so serious a problem. In future we will group all of our cases in which pellagra seems to be the cause of the psychosis under the term "Pellagrous Psychoses," indicating the type, which I did not intend to limit to the five mentioned.

I thank you too, for your kind mention of my work here. We are trying to obtain a better insight into Psychiatry, but I feel keenly my unpreparedness for the position I hold and my lack of training under those who could give me a better knowledge of the work.

The few weeks I spent at Ward's Island revolutionized my former ideas and methods, while Dr. Kirby's instruction is wholly responsible for our improved methods here.

Mrs. Green and I would feel honored to have you and Mrs. Meyer as guests at any time you might find it convenient to spend a time in the South and I am sure that a visit from you would stimulate the interest of every member of our Staff.

During World War I the American Medico-Psychological Association and the National Committee for Mental Hygiene (NCMH) developed the first standardized classification of mental diseases. Although the purpose of this early effort was to facilitate the collection of statistical data to illuminate the etiology, nature, and course of mental illness, the attempt to standardize nomenclature quickly outgrew that original purpose. The debate over nosology was attended by considerable controversy, if only because the vagueness of psychiatric categories reflected the basic theoretical problems facing the specialty. In the following exchange, E. E. Southard (1876–1920), who played a major role in public policy in Massachusetts and served as the first head of the Boston Psychopathic Hospital; Albert M. Barrett (1871–1936), head of the Psychopathic Hospital at the Uni-

versity of Michigan, president of the AMPA, and a former student of Meyer; and Meyer himself debated the wisdom and propriety of the effort to arrive at a standard classification of mental disease.

    E. E. Southard to Adolf Meyer, December 11, 1918 (AMP, Series II).
Being president of the A.M.-P.A., I hardly know whether it is quite *au fait* to precipitate any very lively discussion of the classification question. I have read carefully your little paper on the Aims and Meaning of Psychiatric Diagnosis and sympathize especially with the plan of attack you there advocate, proceeding from the more general impression to the final particular diagnosis. Stripped of its verbiage, my own recent stuff on diagnosis by exclusion in order seems to me to be logically identical with your own general plan of attack. Perhaps you would not think I did away quite so absolutely with the objectionable "one person, one diagnosis" difficulty.

    At all events, do you not think that certain additions might be made to the list of allowable diagnoses prepared by the committee? Take one example: a psychiatrist might not be willing for himself to admit the existence of let us say anxiety neurosis; another psychiatrist might object to paraphrenia, but why should anybody legislate against the employment of any terms that have fairly good scientific backing, as that of Freud or Kraepelin?

    As for the nomenclature question, that is surely subordinate. The statistical committee could give as synonyms such names as it chose to regard as synonyms for the leading names of its list. Let any psychiatrist, however, use what name he chooses. If I do not believe that paraphrenias exist, all I need do is go to the institution which announces in its annual report that it has four or five cases and investigate its records by permission to learn whether I think these cases belong in this new entity or not. If, on the contrary, the statistical committee does not permit me to state that I think a case is one of paraphrenia, what am I to do? It seems to me that any new light is going to be hidden under the bushel of this classification as it is now hardening into form.

    By the way, I was much interested in your list of reaction-complexes as given in the penultimate paragraph of the article on Aims and Meaning. Some of the young men here are asking me what groups of mental diseases, if any, you there intimate; for example, does the affective reaction-complex mean something on the order of the manic-depressive psychosis and what exactly do you mean by the benign and malignant substitutive process? Do you include epilepsy under constitutional defect or under perversion?

Have you anywhere written out this matter of the reaction-complexes so that we may study your plan of attack on diagnosis?

Meantime, do you recommend my inducing a small controversy at the next meeting of the Association or since the war is over, do you counsel against it?

Adolf Meyer to E. E. Southard, December 16, 1918 (AMP, Series II).
Somehow several times in these last few weeks I have been on the point of writing to you to ask you whether you could not send me the section material of a few of your cases of dementia praecox, so that I might, at some leisure, go over the facts, and I am therefore glad to have your letter about the so-called classification question. I do not think that there need be any fear about individual freedom and I therefore take with equanimity even the official declaration of the Association. The main point of difference is, I think, this, that I have no use for the essentially "one person, one disease" view; that I prefer to speak of an individual *presenting* certain facts that we can do something with in the way of definite demonstration, and if possible, in the way of some prediction of a type of lesion, and along the lines of attack in the way of some therapeutic activity, and also along the lines of prognosis. Whether a person has a dozen such facts or only one, is to be a matter of demonstration and not of legislation. The answers to your questions about the reaction types will, I hope, soon get into a formulation in which the matter can be brought to a wider discussion. With regard to the question of introducing a controversy at the next meeting of the Association, I can naturally not say very much because I personally have little tendency to treat the matter as controversy. It is after all a question of personal work and I do not think that debates are especially fruitful, to judge by even the results of one's reading a paper before an association. The time will, I hope, come when those who work seriously come together for the comparing of facts and interpretations, rather than for defensive argumentations.

As I said at the outset, I should very much appreciate representative section material of a few of your cases, so that I might get firsthand contact with the facts and a firsthand basis for conclusions.

Albert M. Barrett to Adolf Meyer, November 4, 1921 (AMP, Series II).
Dr. Haviland has recently sent to me a letter in which you express your conviction that it is advisable for you not to continue as member of the Committee on Statistics for the American Psychiatric Association.

I wish you might appreciate how deeply I regret your taking this course and I am writing to you in the hope that I may be able to change your decision.

My regrets are partly because, as President of the Association for this year, I will greatly appreciate your valuable experience and interest in making the work of the year successful, and also because I feel that your position in psychiatry in this country is such that any work the Committee might do would be embarrassed if we did not have your co-operation.

I appreciate clearly the reasons that seem to impel you to withdraw and personally I find my own attitude is much in sympathy with yours as to the desirability of getting away from too precise and formal designations of psychiatric problems in our patients. I, however, cannot get away from the conviction that a nosological approach to the handling of the medical activities of a psychiatric hospital, such as the ordinary state hospital for mental disorders, is perhaps the most useful method that can be followed at the present period. There is a stimulus to the medical interest and activity of the hospital physicians that comes from this, that were it to be dropped would lead to a deterioration of medical work. Such a stimulus is less needed in the clinical services such as exists in university clinics and research centers. Whether this is the right or wrong way to approach our problems, to give up interest in the differential diagnostic problems that are essentially involved in following a scheme of classification would work harm in most of our state hospitals.

I am also convinced that some uniformity of compilation of records of medical and administrative activities of hospitals for mental disorders in this country is essential. The value of this in its bearing upon public health problems and economic and social aspects of national life has been amply shown. If this is so, then the directions that these compilations should take should be determined by some central agency such as the committee that has been appointed by the American Psychiatric Association and the National Committee for Mental Hygiene. I have had the impression that your objections have largely concerned the principle of emphasizing in psychiatric approach the method of formal diagnosis and that the schemes that have been supported by the Committee emphasized this aspect. I, however, cannot believe that you feel that no efforts at a statistical compilation should be undertaken. If there are better schemes and more acceptable designations than those that the Committee has suggested, I am sure that we would all be most grateful to you for aiding us in finding these. Could this not be best done by the influence you will be able to exert upon other members of the Committee as it makes its deliberations?

Can I not prevail upon you to reconsider your intention of withdrawal from the Committee, and allow us to have the benefit of your rich psychiatric experience in meeting the problems that the Association has assigned to this Committee?

I have recently received from Dr. Pollock a resume of what has been accomplished thus far by the work of the Committee and I take the liberty of enclosing a copy of this.

Enclosure, "The Value of the Uniform System of Records and Statistics of the American Psychiatric Association," with letter from Albert M. Barrett to Adolf Meyer, November 4, 1921 (AMP, Series II).

In 1917 when the American Medico-Psychological Association voted to adopt a classification of mental diseases and a uniform system of statistical reports, there was no generally recognized classification of mental diseases in this country. Certain states had adopted classifications for use within their own borders but no two states were using exactly the same classification and in some states there was no official classification.

There was also no standardization of terms used in reporting financial data and information concerning the movement of patients. It was utterly impossible to collect accurate comparative data concerning cost of maintenance, additions and permanent improvements, first admissions, readmissions, recoveries, etc.

The elaborate attempt made by the Federal Census Department to collect statistics from State Hospitals for the insane in 1910 proved almost a failure because it was found impossible to secure reliable data concerning the mental diseases of admissions or of the patient population of the hospitals and first admissions could not be separated from readmissions.

All of the State hospitals of the country were making records of patients and compiling and publishing annual or biennial reports but, as the hospitals of each state were working in their own way without reference to what other hospitals were doing, the records and statistics gathered were almost worthless.

The plan adopted in 1917 substituted system for chaos. It substituted standardized for meaningless terms. It established uniformity in the place of diversity and irregularity in statistical records and reports. It made possible the combination and comparison of data compiled in different hospitals and different states. In other words the new system substituted uniform scientific procedure for the irregular, impractical, unscientific methods previously in vogue.

The new system while adopted at the meeting of the American Medico-Psychological Association in 1917 did not become operative in many states until the beginning of the following fiscal year. Some states waited two years before falling in line, and unfortunately a few scattering hospitals have yet to adopt the new system. The statistics that the Bureau of Statistics of the National Committee for Mental Hygiene has been able to compile under the new system, although incomplete, threw more light on the problem of mental disease in the United States than any study prior to 1917, although the Bureau obtained all its data through correspondence and relied entirely on the voluntary cooperation of the superintendents of hospitals in the various states. Had it been possible to send paid workers to obtain data from the hospitals in 1920, as the Census Bureau did in 1910, a very comprehensive review of mental disease in the United States might have been compiled.

The hospitals are now collecting data along the right lines and these data will be found useful for comparison with data compiled 10, 20 and 30 years hence; while going backward from the present time we find no data concerning mental disease to be compared with our present statistics.

The uniform system has therefore accomplished two fundamental statistical objects; first, it has made possible the combination and comparison of data collected in different places at the same time; second, it has established a basis for the comparison of statistics now being compiled with those that will be compiled in coming years.

In addition to these fundamental accomplishments the new system has given the hospitals of the country a much better classification than was previously in use. This classification has been made elastic and provision has been made for its revision every five years. This will serve to keep the classification in line with the developments in psychiatry. The new system, requiring as it does the compilation of considerable data concerning patients, has caused more thorough study of the history of patients and the keeping of better case records. By the use of this system every hospital will have at hand more definite data concerning its patients than it previously had and all persons interested in psychiatry and the care and treatment of the insane will be able to procure specific information concerning many matters that were formerly entirely unknown.

The introduction of the uniform system of statistics in state hospitals was really the beginning of a new era in institution statistics in this country. The marked improvement in the statistical reports of the hospitals for the insane have caused the institutions for the feebleminded, those for criminals and delinquents, and those for children to seek a like standardized system.

The American Medico-Psychological Association planned wisely when it placed a group of leading psychiatrists on its statistical committee. These insure wise guidance in the introduction of the new system and are also a guarantee that the classification will be kept in harmony with the demands of modern psychiatry.

The uniform system of course is not perfect but it is so much in advance of anything previously done along this line in this country and so much better than that in use in any other country that no one acquainted with the facts could think of abandoning it. Let us perfect the classification from time to time as new facts are discovered and modify the system when necessary but let us not regress to the unhappy conditions of former days.

Adolf Meyer to Albert M. Barrett, November 10, 1921 (AMP, Series II).
It always hurts me to have to refuse the request of a friend. But it also goes very much against my grain to go on insisting on a hearing and to impose my views on others if they are persistently turned down. My action is determined by the experience at the round-table in Boston, where I asked in vain for a positive expression of attitude of those present and finally had to pocket a very uncomplimentary comment from Solomon that we older members had spoiled the evening. If nothing constructive could come from such a discussion, it is best to go home and work until one has something more acceptable to offer. It is true, it was all improvised. I had no idea that I was to bear the burden of the discussion; yet I saw no evidence that even a well prepared discussion would have overcome the indifference or the difference of opinion. Hence my determination to work quietly until I might have something more acceptable to present. My 1906 report was shorn of very essential safeguards by I do not know whom. My requests for modification were not heeded and I cannot go on repeating old stories. In two or three years I hope to know what my own material dictates to me. Till then I prefer to leave myself and others undisturbed.

Let us pick out the facts on which we can agree and feel sure about, and among these especially the facts important for action or at least recommendations to the workers and the public. A mass of other facts had best be given in an unpretentious way for what they are worth, not under the form of a pernicious nosological dogma. Are not the traditional nosological entities largely killing this purpose? I am not opposed to what is worth calling diagnosis, but to a farce which estranges the physician from developing an interest in the facts at work. It is the fact that there have been no deliberations or moves to use the appeals that makes me superfluous on the committee. If one single item had been picked up from my discussions and brought under consideration, I should have felt justified in coming forth again. But as things stand, I can see neither need nor justification.

Hence the policy not to interfere but also not to make a nuisance of myself by insistence or to go on feeling very uncomfortable on account of being forced to subscribe to what I do not approve of. Why should I not be let alone? If my suggestions could not be used, why should I have it rubbed in by having to sign as champion and supporter of that which I did not approve of?

Pollock's statement is reasonable enough but devoid of insight into the issues. He is the compiler but not in touch with the actual material. I have helped him where I could and some good work has come forth that might well make us tired of being an annex to the imperial German sphere now even largely given up by its own author!

I am afraid this inability to accede to your wish is not a good occasion to renew a personal request for a few sample sections of the large-celled encephalitis type and of the dementia material. Will you show me that you forbear with me?

Along with Adolf Meyer, William A. White (1870–1937) was among the most influential American psychiatrists of the early twentieth century. He served for nearly thirty-five years as the superintendent of the influential Saint Elizabeths Hospital, a large federal facility in the District of Columbia. Extraordinarily broad in his interests, White played a major role within the speciality of psychiatry and also helped to disseminate psychoanalytic concepts. He wrote extensively on a variety of issues, including children and crime and, in partnership with Smith Ely Jelliffe, owned a firm that published many important monographs as well as the Psychoanalytic Review. *In the following exchange with Meyer, White discussed his interpretation of behavior and thought.*

William A. White to Adolf Meyer, November 5, 1919 (AMP, Series I).
I have your letter of the 29th ult. I am afraid that the history of the concept

of symbolization as used in my book would be a pretty difficult thing to get. It is the result of innumerable thrashing out of the subject between Jelliffe and myself extending over a period of several years, in which I believe Jelliffe largely furnished the material suggested in a way which I elaborated in my mind along the lines that I have presented in my "Mechanisms of Character Formation." The French article that you have in mind I believe is probably the exposition of Le Chatelier's theorem. There is a foot-note reference to this on page 64. I never read the original exposition in French, but got my idea from an address by Prof. Bancroft before the Cosmos Club here in Washington and subsequently wrote him and got a reprint of his paper, to which my foot-note refers. Prof. Bancroft was, and I think still is, professor of chemistry at Cornell University, and if you will write him I am sure he will be glad to send you a reprint. I have tried to find my copy of his reprint, thinking that I could send it to you, but I cannot put my hands upon it.

I am minded in this connection to mention another aspect of the subject which seems to me fundamental, and which Jelliffe and I have discussed briefly on one or two occasions with reference to the concrete arrangement of the matter in our text book. You will recall that the book is divided into three parts,—the first part dealing with the physico-chemical level, devoted to a consideration of the vegetative nervous system, and the endocrinopathies, and the second part made up of what is ordinarily called neurology, namely dealing with the central nervous system and peripheral ramifications, and which taken together we call the sensory motor level, and the third part dealing with psychiatry under the caption of the symbolic level. We have tried to present the subject from the standpoint of these three separate levels. Now each of us have thought for a long time that it would be a good plan to reverse the order and present the symbolic level as part one of the book, leaving the sensory motor level naturally as part 2, and the physico-chemical coming at the end as part 3. Both of us are, I believe, constitutionally disposed to look at the human machine from the psychological standpoint as opposed to the usual method of looking at it from the physiological standpoint. For this attitude of mind I think there is very good philosophical justification, at least I have recently run across what seems to support my natural bent. I have been reading Schiller's "Riddles of the Sphinx," and he sets forth, it seems to me, quite plainly that we must look upon the processes of nature from a teleological standpoint. The difficulty of being teleological in the past has been that the wrong variety of teleology has been used, namely a teleology that was anthropocentric. Eliminate the anthropocentric aspect and realize solely that natural processes are tending toward certain goals, and I think we must all agree. Now if this is true, and it seems to me that it certainly is in the biological sciences, it must necessarily also be true that we can only understand the whole meaning of the individual at the end of this process after the goal has been attained and by looking backward over the successive steps from the knowledge gained by an understanding of where the individual was headed. In other words, the greater must contain the lesser, but not vice versa. In the finished product we must be able to see the explanation of all of the processes that have led up to its unfolding, but in the original protoplasm we by no means can find the explanation for what is coming after in the process of development. We can posit its existence perhaps, but that is purely hypothetical. It is therefore, in my mind, much more logical to undertake to seek the explanation of the processes that go on within the human individual by reasoning from the psyche backward than it is to undertake to explain for example psychological processes by chemistry and physics.

This attitude of mind, which I trust I have made clear in the preceding paragraph, but fear that I have not, is also responsible in part at least for considering the symbol as an energy carrier. The whole process of development and evolution may be considered from the standpoint of the rearrangement and redistribution of energy, and the symbol looked at from the teleological standpoint must be conceived to contain all of those factors which have been operative in its production.

Dr. Timme, as you may know, is violently opposed to this conception of the symbol, and he has tried to make me see his standpoint, which is simply that the symbol is only a releaser of energy and he would find his energy in the various chemical unions and physical states of the body, and he would further explain the enormous amount of energy which the human machine can release by the recent disclosures of colloid chemistry which have shown the tremendous amount of energy which is bound up in such states as surface tension and various other forces that bind the chemical and physical parts of the body together. I believe that this is another example of reasoning in the wrong direction, endeavoring to make the lesser explain the greater. I find myself in considerable harmony with Jung's attempt at defining a social consciousness, although I confess I have not read his paper fully. I believe, in other words, that when we think of a group of units as being associated we are too much inclined to think that their association is the mathematical sum of what each of them individually represents, but I believe this to be a very gross error. Society is composed of individuals, the smallest society conceivable would be composed of two individuals, but there is another element that enters that is of great importance and that is the relationship between the two individuals, and that relationship is a higher state than either one of the individuals alone and contains possibilities which are not resident in either one. For example it would be just as absurd to speak of the body as being made up of the mathematical sum of the characteristics of so many million cells. The relationship of these cells to each other is of fundamental importance and it is their relation and their action and harmony and dominance and subordination and all the rest of it which has made possible the whole individual. Now I look upon the group as containing higher possibilities than the individual, and the symbol as being, so to speak, the instrument of this higher association and the means for effecting energy redistributions. You know my concept of the individual, or at least you know that I do not think that there is any such thing as an individual in the ordinary sense, that the individual as we ordinarily think of him is a pure abstraction, the individual merely merges into his environment, and is part and parcel of it. In this way, therefore, the union of individuals in societies becomes a still further development, a still higher power of the great creative energy.

Adolf Meyer to William A. White, November 8, 1919 (AMP, Series I).
Many thanks for your interesting letter of November 5. It gives me a very interesting picture which in the main I am in complete accord with. The arrangement of the material in the book naturally is one determined by didactic as much as by philosophical considerations. I hope to see the third edition soon and shall be interested in the transformation.

The discussion between you and Timme naturally touches the very center of the problem of integration. Timme evidently is one of those who have to think of the symbol as detached rather than as imminent. Hence the aversion. Your emphasis on the social consciousness shows exactly where one might be tempted to withdraw from making integrative units, because in the end we would hardly want to speak of a group soul except in a metaphorical sense. It is always activity of some leaders and the following of the rest.

I am very glad indeed that I troubled you with my inquiry. I feel it was well worth while to get this clearing of ideas.

In 1920 Dr. R. S. Woodward, president of the Carnegie Institution of Washington, asked William A. White to review a manuscript dealing with epileptics. White's negative reply provides insights into early twentieth-century behavioral and psychiatric research.

    R. S. Woodward to William A. White, January 27, 1920 (WAWP).
The Institution has had submitted to it the manuscript of "One Thousand Epileptics with Their Family Histories; A Study in Heredity," by David Fairchild Weeks, M.D., and Dr. Lucille Field Brown. This manuscript has been forwarded to us by Dr. Charles B. Davenport, Director of the Department of Experimental Evolution and in charge also of the Eugenics Record Office recently turned over to the Institution by Mrs. E. H. Harriman.

    The question we raise with regard to this manuscript is whether it is sufficiently well done to be up to the standard which should be attained by a research establishment. Our Trustee, Dr. Stewart Paton, assures us that you are one of the experts of work in the field of epilepsy and suggests that we get an expression of opinion from you concerning this manuscript if practicable. I write, therefore, to learn whether you could take the time to look at the paper, which embraces about two hundred pages of typewritten material and about the same amount of tabular records. What we want to know are, first, whether the observational work has been done in a trustworthy manner; and, secondly, whether it is presented in such a form as to be clearly intelligible; and, finally, whether the conclusions reached are justified.

    If you can undertake the work I will bring the manuscript to your office or to any place you may designate and call for it when you have finished with it.

    The Institution will expect, of course, to pay you a reasonable honorarium for this work.

    William A. White to R. S. Woodward, February 10, 1920 (WAWP).
I have your letter of the 27th ult. and the Mss. "One Thousand Epileptics with Their Family Histories.—A Study in Heredity," by David Fairchild Weeks, and Dr. Lucille Field Brown. I have looked this Mss. over carefully and with a view to arriving at a conclusion as to its value as a contribution to our knowledge of epilepsy and with respect to the specific inquiries you make. I may say for your information that appreciating the great amount of

work that the preparation of this Mss. has involved and being personally acquainted with its particular author, Dr. Weeks, I have been loathe to voice my original opinion, and have carefully reviewed the evidence. As a result, however, I am constrained to the conclusion that the result of all this work is practically nil as far as contributing any new information to the subject of epilepsy is concerned.

In order that you may have some idea of the grounds upon which I base my conclusions I will briefly review the more important ones. In the first place the character of the material studied has not been defined with sufficient accuracy. While the authors appreciate that epilepsy is not a unitary concept, but that there are many different types of epilepsy, in fact quite different diseases are included under this general term, still no effort is made to distinguish these various types in the material studied. For example (p. 15) a physician's diagnosis has been considered sufficient for including a patient in the group studied. Such a method of procedure is clearly the method of the social worker who gets a lot of information by hearsay and rumor and general reputation and who deals in terms that from the scientific point of view are ill defined. And this comment applies to the entire material. Even such terms as "feeble-minded," "insane," "alcoholic," "migrainous," "criminalistic," are definitely such terms, while such descriptive terms as are used in the histories to designate character traits, as "irritability," "bad tempered," "incorrigible," "unconquerable," "immoral," and the like are quite as indefinite for such purposes as this type of investigation. The net result of dealing in such generalities is that the character of material which has been studied and which is included in these thousands of cases must of necessity represent the widest varieties and which have only one trait in common,—the fact that they have convulsive seizures. This single trait is by no means sufficient to warrant grouping of individuals who have it together in an hereditary study unless some means is taken for differentiation, the narrowing down of sub groups by elimination or some such method for reducing a heterogeneous mixture to smaller and more definite groups. No such method is employed in this presentation.

Quite gratuitous assumptions have been made in many instances which evidently control the viewpoint of the author, but which do not appear to show up specifically in the results of the investigation. For example, certain definite characteristics of epilepsy are considered as sufficiently well defined to constitute what might be called bio-types, although that term is not commonly used. Of this, periodicity is one, and then the desirability immediately appears of including in the study all of the pathological conditions which manifest themselves periodically. For instance migraine or sick headache is one. This disease has for a long time been considered to have some relation to epilepsy but there have never been any adequate reasons advanced for this relationship other than such a superficial analogy as periodicity which would apply to a great number of things, malaria perhaps more prominently than any other. Whereas migraine figures in the statistical tables, nothing seems to be demonstrated regarding it one way or another. In fact the conclusions with regard to each group are meagre and often practically nil. Of course negative evidence, or evidence which definitely disproves a more or less generally accepted theory would be valuable, but the same criticism against the evidence from its positive aspects holds good for this negative type of evidence, and therefore I do not consider that anything has been contributed.

With reference to your specific query, therefore, I can say that I do not think that the observational work has been done with sufficient accuracy to warrant its utilization for scientific purposes. Secondly, I do not think it is presented in such form as to make it clearly intelligible as to what conclusions may or may not be reached from it. And thirdly, such conclusions as are implied in the course of the article in many instances I do not believe justifiable. I may add a hurriedly practical conclusion with reference to which you have not asked my opinion, and that is that the great size of the Mss., considering the immense amount of tabulated material and the very great expense which I know would necessarily be incurred in setting this matter up, is altogether out of proportion to the scientific value of the Mss. as a whole. The very detailed tables probably belong to that great group of such productions that never would be studied by any one. Such tables would undoubtedly be eagerly studied if the text warranted the expectation of finding there material of great value, but inasmuch as it does not, the tables I think would never be examined. I believe that all that is valuable in this paper could easily be reduced to a simple printed communication of not more than 100 pages, and probably 50 pages, leaving out all of the complicated tables, and perhaps only printing an occasional illustrated chart or putting an illustrative family history here and there.

I trust I have made myself sufficiently clear. If not I should be glad to respond further to any inquiries you may choose to make. I am holding the Mss. and can either send it to the Institute by the regular hospital team or if you prefer to send your messenger for it we will deliver it to him any time he calls, provided he comes during the regular office hours.

I should be pleased to receive such honorarium as the Institute is accustomed to offering for similar service.

James King Hall (1875–1948) was one of the more important southern psychiatrists during the interwar period. He played an important role in public policy toward the mentally ill in Virginia, North Carolina, and South Carolina; served as associate editor of the influential Southern Medicine and Surgery; *and was elected to the presidency of the American Psychiatric Association in 1941. In the following letter to his uncle Albert Anderson (the superintendent of the state mental hospital in Raleigh, North Carolina), Hall wrote about the absence of knowledge about dementia praecox (schizophrenia).*

J. K. Hall to Albert Anderson, October 29, 1923 (JKHP).

I am obliged for the good words you had to say about my paper. It was quite imperfectly, because very hastily, written, and I am going to place it in a little more finished form.

I presume that dementia praecox constitutes probably the greatest single health problem in this country, and perhaps in the world. So far as I am able to ascertain nobody knows what it is; no progress is being made in the study of it, and we are doing nothing with the disease and we are only keeping alive, mostly through the aid of the state, those who are disabled by it. The number of praecox patients is steadily increasing, I suppose, and I wonder how long the state will be able to totter along under such an increasing burden. I have an idea that North Carolina alone is spending on praecox patients confined in State Hospitals more than half a million dollars annually, and the state is losing on account of disability of these citizens perhaps two or three millions of dollars each year in the way of productiveness.

I am wondering if you do not think it is time for the state of North Carolina to set on foot some plans looking to the investigation of this problem. We hear much each day about the ravages of tuberculosis and of cancer, but nothing at all in the general press or in the talk of people about dementia praecox. I wish you would seriously contemplate the establishment in your institution of a bureau of research. Ask for a generous appropriation for its establishment and maintenance, and put good scientific men in charge of it. I have often wondered what splendid work a man like Bill MacNider would do in such a bureau. Before much progress can be made in the study of the disease, however, it would become necessary to insure the workers an adequate number of postmortems. I believe that the backward condition of medical teaching in the South is due more largely to lack of postmortem material than to any other single fact. Such an investigating bureau as I have in mind would need certainly a good clinical psychiatrist, a good pathologist, and a good laboratory man who could examine all the fluids and other constituents of the body. I wish you would give the matter serious thought. You occupy a very important and dominant place in the medical and economic life of the state, and your attitude in such a matter would carry with it very great weight. The establishment of such a bureau in your institution would be a feather in your cap, too, because it would be the first thing of the kind in the South, so far as I know. Boiled down to absolute facts and stripped of all hot air, the truth is that we are doing nothing with dementia praecox in the South except to take care of the patients who have it. Our talk about it all has reference to the curious behavior of these people, and we hardly think further and deeper than their behavior. Such writing is practically nothing but a waste of words and of paper.

The problem of classifying mental diseases remained a perennial and seemingly unresolvable issue. In the early 1930s Meyer had a lengthy correspondence with Dr. H. B. Logie, the executive secretary of the National Conference on Nomenclature of Disease, the result of which was the highlighting of the extraordinary problems involved in any effort to develop a uniform classification system for psychiatric diseases.

H. B. Logie to Adolf Meyer, December 5, 1930 (AMP, Series II).
Your kind letter of November 29 arrived when I was out of town, and I hasten to forward to you enough of our schema of classification to illustrate its application to mental diseases. The covering notes which I enclose may be read as generally applicable to mental diseases, with certain reservations and modifications.

It is clear that we can have no anatomical site for mental diseases. It is equally clear that, if we assign them to some intangible mechanism such as the psyche, we shall have difficulty speaking of infection, degeneration and other tangible pathological processes in connection with the psyche. In order to get over this difficulty the term psycho-biological unit was adopted to afford a name for a mechanism which could be injured by tangible means. Without becoming involved in the question of the somatic (e.g. endocrine) cause of all psychoses, it did appear reasonable to consider that the psychoses associated with infection, structural degeneration, and so on, might be allocated in part to a tangible structure. It was likewise thought that mental diseases which have no known tangible cause and produce no evident structural change might be assigned simply to the psyche. As you will observe from the enclosed copy of System O, the psycho-biological unit was divided to show structures and mechanisms in various groupings as these are affected by known mental diseases, including, besides the psychoses proper, mental deficiency simple and in association with degenerative structural changes in the central nervous system.

It is thought that the eleven etiological categories are almost all applicable to mental disease. However difficult it may be to define schizophrenia, manic depressive psychosis, and paranoia in terms of etiology or symptomatology, there would appear to be no difficulty in segregating the mental diseases which result from congenital defect, infection, intoxication, trauma, disturbance of circulation, disturbance of nutrition, new growths, and chronic degenerative processes. Even if it is true that the majority of cases of mental disease are still left for Category X, it is equally true that the minority of diagnoses will come under this Category.

I hope you will have grasped from the "Explanatory Notes" that every somatic disease is classified both topographically and etiologically, and that, if a uniform system is to be followed throughout all diseases, mental diseases too must be classified on a dual basis. The criticism which I expect is that we have no justification in assigning one mental disease to the psyche proper and another to the psyche and any particular organic structure. What I hope will meet with your approval is the attempt to segregate the psychoses associated with organic changes and known cause from those characterized by symptoms only. When the latter important group is thus set off by itself, each morbid entity within it can be defined in terms of symptomatology and psychology; for this is the decision in regard to Category X (speaking generally) that it shall be divided and subdivided to suit the distinctions in each of the groups of diseases which come within its scope. The differences between the so-called functional diseases of the heart will be defined in terms of cardiac symptomatology, and similar diseases of any other system will be defined in terms suitable to that system. This is because distinctions based on symptoms cannot be worded in general terms.

It is because of the difficulty of describing on paper our attempt to classify mental diseases that I have hoped for an opportunity to do so in person. Furthermore I am sure I could profit better by your criticisms and suggestions if you could spare the time to talk to me about this plan.

Adolf Meyer to H. B. Logie, March 18, 1931 (AMP, Series II).
I am afraid you may become impatient with us, even when I let you have the notes given me by my associate, Dr. Diethelm. He referred to my 1906 report of the Pathological Institute of N.Y. State Hospital, when I launched the foundation for the present statistics in New York State.

Somehow, I feel we cannot have universally useful schemes for statistics of disease. Certainly when we come to mental disorders, there are so many aspects to the cases that need consideration from different angles, that we must make our groupings according to what we want and need. If it is for life (i.e., death) statistics, it may be one thing; if for an understanding for needs in treatment, it may be very different. Almost any generally valid compromise becomes distorted if we stretch it on the Procrustes bed of traditional pathology. Neither heredity, nor infection, nor intoxications, nor trauma, nor circulation, nor convulsions, nor new growth, nor organic changes and involution stand as clear units. It is nearly always a more or less with various possibilities. (Hence my simple reaction-type scheme). And 00—X becomes a bewildering group, certainly very difficult to read off from the figures.

I feel a little as I do with legal classifications of our cases. From your angle you probably see most use in a uniform general pattern. But it may in the end be relatively unimportant whether one of the chapters has to suffer. Psychiatry certainly does not get any stimulating help this way except that which comes from revolt against inappropriate systems. Which are the fields of medicine that *do*?

I may be more able to see the helpfulness of the scheme when I see the most tangible items and begin to read the rank and file of your numbers with some practice.

I truly regret not being of more help to you. I am grateful to you for the stimulus in the direction of taking up the question anew, and while it may be on too individualistic a line, perhaps with some prospect of getting further in the direction of definition. If something useful comes of it, I shall be glad to send it to you.

Smith Ely Jelliffe (1866–1945) began his career as a neurologist and finished as a major figure in psychoanalysis and a close collaborator with William A. White. Roy G. Hoskins (1880–1964) was an eminent endocrinologist who served as the director of the Memorial Foundation for Neuro-Endocrine Research in Boston and headed a famous study of schizophrenia during this period. In 1932 the two figures discussed the age-old problem of the relationship between mind and body (psychological/somatic dualism).

Roy G. Hoskins to Smith Ely Jelliffe, April 21, 1932 (SEJP).

I am much interested in the information regarding your personal observations of identical twins in relation to schizophrenia. I wonder if the material has been published? I wonder, too, whether you have seen any cases of double incidence of schizophrenia in identical twins as a check on the three cases in which it did not occur? I know personally of only one instance, that of a pair in the McLean Hospital. I am rather impressed with Lange's series in which the identical twins were controlled with non-identical. Quoting from memory, Lange reported ten cases of the same psychosis and four of somewhat dissimilar psychoses in seventeen cases of identical twins, whereas there was no instance of double incidence in the ordinary fraternal twins. Of course the number available are not sufficient to constitute an experimentum crucis but even as they stand, are, to my mind, the most cogent evidence we have of the importance of an organic liability factor.

I aim as far as is humanly possible to avoid a doctrinaire position, but I like to play with organic factors and there seems to be abundant room for research on these. It seems to me that the most convincing proof of the operation of dynamic factors in the production of schizophrenia would leave the question still open as to whether they do or do not operate only in specially prepared soil.

The fundamental philosophy is about the same I judge for either the dynamic psychiatrist or the organicist. In case of any given manifestation one has to test for consistency of concomitance, then for causality. We certainly agree with you that "mere enumeration" of traits will not get any one below the descriptive level. On the other hand, no one but a biologist would attempt to quantitate or rationalize a situation that had not been decently qualitated.

I am not sure as to whether we shall get reprints of our recent paper before the Boston Society. If we do, it will be a pleasure to send you one.

Smith Ely Jelliffe to Roy G. Hoskins, May 6, 1932 (SEJP).
My cases have not been published. They were observed before I knew much about the possibilities of the twin situation and hence my data are grossly incomplete.

There are, however, as you probably know, other studies which negative [*sic*] the too dogmatic statement to which I called attention. You probably know Luxenburger's numerous papers and the classic of Siemens on Twin Pathology. The literature in Luxenburger's papers is quite up to date. I think Lange is a bit too doctrinaire also and as already noted no human experiment is known to me where monozygotic twins were separated at birth and grew up in environments which nominally had different parental images.

This opens up the large discipline of ecology and here, in the botanical field, with which I am in partial contact, one gets clues that point to the belief that much more intensive study of ecological factors is needed to correct the one sided "heredity" conclusions.

When it comes to such a complex assortment of personality images, as in the large schizophrenic medley, there are still lacking enough careful case studies.

Although I began as a sincere believer in working from the bottom up, I have come to an entirely opposite position and believe that interpretation, as of functional value, can only come from above down.

Naturally, from the description point of view, all three general fields, matter, life, and mind have their respective claims to validity, but only from the field of mind as a holistic synthesis of the other fields will come complete understanding of the dynamic meaning in behavior. This is my present credo.

Roy G. Hoskins to Smith Ely Jelliffe, June 30, 1932 (SEJP).
Your letter of May sixth was read with much interest.

I doubt if our viewpoints are nearly so far apart as superficial consideration might suggest.

Whether one regard the organic or "psychologic" aspects as of greater significance smacks to me of the "hen and egg" situation. Pragmatically, one seems to come out about the same way in either case.

Even granted that one might ultimately find some of the essential causal factors of schizophrenia in a test tube, the real problem would still remain—How are phenomena of test tube order translated into personality deviations?

Furthermore, no amount of ratiocination will suffice to settle problems of concomitance vs causality. As soon as one gets below the descriptive level the entire strategy shifts.

As remarked before, the chief necessity on all sides—it seems to me— is for controlled evidence, an easy formulation most difficult to follow out. The most significant aspect of the research problem perhaps is, what line of attack is most likely to yield usable, significant data.

> *Smith Ely Jelliffe to Roy G. Hoskins, July 7, 1932 (SEJP).*

I was much interested in your chicken–egg comparison but I wonder how valid it is in re. the structural–functional situation. I cannot persuade myself that the matter is as simple for is it not probably more true that function *precedes* and makes structure? To use Semon's conception "experience is written into protoplasm" (engraphy) and thus new structures (i.e. organs) arise. Is not Maudsley's phrase—I think he first used it— an organ is a bit of structuralized experience—a useful one in the survey of the organic–psychological play of activities? Psychological is here made synonymous with the purposeful patterning of an entire organismic response—in the more simple terms—"a wish not implying by this that which is present in consciousness as such, but the expression of inner drives—instinctual or tropistic if one will—unconscious.["]

So it is not immaterial in the chicken–egg sense at all as to the primary instigator of reaction formulae, some of which we envisage as diseases.

I agree with you most heartily as to the "probable value of the mode of attack" in which connection I have been enjoying what seems to me an excellent presentation of the psychological mode of approach. It is E. Glover's paper in the *Brit. Jl. Med. Psychology*—Vol. 9.

Mankind has been trying all kinds of substance magical [*sic*] forms of approach (i.e. organic) for some thousands of years. Now that psychological magic is being refined, as it were, i.e. grown up out of its magic to science—which in the thought of M. D. Eder, *Brit. Jl. Med. Psychol.,* Vol. 10, p. 175—"Psychology and Value"—i.e. has become more scientific in reality than the so-called physical sciences—"where the belief in 'significant data' has at times illusional if not delusion value," is it not about time to give it a run?

I hope you don't mind these intrusions. I am in the country, the gnats and midges are ubiquitous, and by contagious magic maybe I take on some of their annoying patterning.

Born in Scotland, C. Macfie Campbell (1876–1943) came to the United States in 1904, taught in the Department of Psychiatry at Johns Hopkins from 1913 to 1920, and then served as the director of Boston Psychopathic Hospital and professor of psychiatry at the Harvard Medical School. In the following letter to C. M. Hincks, the general director of the National Committee for Mental Hygiene, Campbell discussed the bedeviling problem of explaining schizophrenia.

C. Macfie Campbell to C. M. Hincks, December 14, 1934 (AMP, Series II).
I started more than two weeks ago to submit a brief memorandum to you on schizophrenia, but it threatened to develop into a monograph so I dropped it.

I am somewhat hampered in presenting the topic because in one way I do not believe that there is such a thing as schizophrenia, and on the other hand I think it is the most important topic for investigation in our field. To put it another way, I do not think that there is a *disease* schizophrenia, but, on the other hand, it is useful at this period to have some group term for an extremely large number of cases of mental disorder of the more serious type.

From the point of view of one who is angling for money to support his work, it is a great advantage to believe in a specific disease. He can then give figures with regard to its morbidity, he can specify the general group of forces within which the real cause is to be found like the nigger in the woodpile, he can budget the funds necessary for the investigation and even suggest certain time limits within which the nigger will be discovered, the woodpile will be safe, schizophrenia will be eliminated, the taxpayers' burden will be alleviated.

The philanthropist who may have little knowledge of detailed biochemical or bacteriological problems will thus feel that recondite studies are going to bring about a practical social result. He will have the comfort of seeing a specific piece of work going on, well delimited, with clean-cut formulations and with steady output of scientific facts which at least will be useful by-products even if the nigger is not found. He may be willing to accept the comparison of the needle in the haystack, and realize that he must think in generous terms of time, money and personnel. The main thing is that he is working with a definite disease, that the general concepts are those already familiar to medical science and to philanthropy, and that schizophrenia may be put in the same group as yellow fever and those other scourges of humanity which have been brought within control.

To one who looks at schizophrenia in a somewhat different way and who sees it just as a useful term embracing a very heterogeneous group of mentally sick people, angling for funds is a somewhat more disheartening process. He can, of course, use the same bait as the person who believes in the nigger theory of schizophrenia, but that may go against his conscience. He may have to tell the philanthropist that he does not believe there is such a thing, that the schizophrenic patients whom he has studied most thoroughly seem to represent people of very varied physique and personality, brought up in the most varied circumstances, exposed to a great variety of life situations and who break down in many complicated ways which are perhaps a combination of their physical status, their personal difficulties and the social and cultural situation in which they are enmeshed. He may have to tell the philanthropist that the topic of schizophrenia is almost as broad as the topic of human nature, in fact the chief value of its investigation may be that it is the clearest and most striking demonstration of the real facts of human nature, facts of human nature which are concealed by the ordinary conventional repressions of the socalled [*sic*] normal man. The normal man is the person who so adapts himself to social regimentation that he manages to conceal the underlying crudities of human nature so that practically nothing about them can be learned from a study of him.

A research into human nature would naturally send a chill down the spine of a practical philanthropist who wishes to budget for definite projects and who would like to see, if possible, some return for his money. He may suspect the person who rejects the nigger-in-the woodpile theory as being a somewhat loose thinker, fond of generalizations, unable to give precision to his problems, with no definite lead as to the further course of his investigations, and with no promise that his investigations will have any practical value. Here, of course, is a challenge for us to take up. I should accept the challenge of ignorance with regard to the schizophrenic field, but emphasize my interest in it. I should say that the first procedure in dealing with such a problem is to know what we are talking about, to go directly to the source material, to make the most accurate observations with regard to that source material, and, in close contact with the material, to formulate those factors which seem to be of most importance and in regard to which systematic investigation requires to be carried on.

That has essentially been our program of investigation at the Boston Psychopathic Hospital for the last ten years, and a group of reprints of statistical studies, which you will shortly receive, will give you some indication as to the application of merely one method to the study of the schizophrenic problem. To the non-mathematical statistical studies always seem somewhat dreary and devoid of life. To the person interested in the fullness of the living individual a skeleton is a somewhat cheerless presentation. On the other hand, familiarity with a skeleton may be a very essential condition of adequate knowledge of the living individual.

The statistical method was utilized by us as in 1925 [when] there was the possibility of getting some support for a study of this whole field, with some bearing upon broader social factors and of some value from the point of view of the study of scientific method. We did not emphasize the statistical method because it was the one which appealed to us most or which we were most competent to handle, but statistical studies could be financially supported, while laboratory studies had to be carried on with the most meagre facilities.

The cost of production of the individual volume which you will receive was about five hundred dollars, although I have no doubt you will be willing to sell your copy for less, and its market price may be negligible.

One of the first results of our statistical review of a very large number of schizophrenic patients (over one thousand) was to show us that any thorough investigation of the subject, even for the purpose of preliminary classification, required a much more accurate observation of the original material. We thereupon settled down to accumulate a chosen body of material, paying attention to those factors which have not been adequately recorded in the earlier group of over one thousand patients. We thus cumulated a chosen group of one hundred and fifty cases in which there was a fair review of the physical status, of the personality of the patient, of the symptomatology and course of the disorder, of environmental factors both those which had moulded the individual earlier and those which might have served to precipitate the psychosis. The scrutiny of this material enables us to separate the heterogeneous group of schizophrenic patients into several smaller and more homogeneous groups, in regard to which further lines of investigation seem distinctly indicated.

The precipitate of my ruminations over the schizophrenic problem was presented in the Salmon Lectures of last winter.

As to further lines of investigation, they may be divided under the two heads of (a) research into impersonal processes (b) research into personality factors and environmental influences.

In every case of schizophrenia the total clinical picture is the result of a great many component forces. The psychosis, after all, is merely one section of a life experience. In every case one has to attribute its respective value to bodily functions, personality components, environmental influences. In no case can one safely limit one's formulation to merely one or other of these three fields. On the other hand, in individual cases the influence of one or other of these fields seems to be the predominant factor and to be of the greatest practical importance. In the various sub-groups into which one can reasonably divide the schizophrenic group there are clear indications for specialized investigations.

(a) Thus in a group that may roughly be referred to as that of deterioration without marked trends and in another group of more definitely stuporous cases one feels that it would be profitable to make a very much more searching review of the fundamental physiological mechanisms than has hitherto been done. In cases of stupor the reaction of patients to CO_2 and other drugs has also stimulated us to make a searching investigation of the underlying biochemical processes which play a part in these conditions. The complexity of any investigation of fundamental underlying processes may be illustrated by a piece of work which was carried on at the Boston Psychopathic Hospital with regard to the possible influence of gastro-intestinal intoxication upon mental disorders of this type. The ordinary type of investigation of such a problem has been of a most superficial nature, and in order to take up this problem in a satisfactory way Dr. Agnes Goldman Sanborn for a period of under two years and with funds collected with difficulty from various sources carried on an investigation on the fecal flora of adults, with particular attention to individual differences and their relationship to the effects of various diets (see *Journal of Infectious Diseases,* volumes 48 and 49). Lack of funds and the magnitude of the undertaking prevented the continuation of this investigation.

The observations made in the stuporous patients, however, led to a very consistent effort to study the underlying biological processes, and this investigation has now been followed consistently for several years by Dr. d'Elseaux who has at present a useful organization for carrying on systematically further investigations along these lines.

It is, however, not only along these lines that one would wish to make an intensive study of this chosen group of patients, but one would also like to have the opportunity for, at the same time in the same patients, making a satisfactory study of their endocrine functions. The principles underlying such an investigation and the actual nature of the investigation may be indicated by the following extract from the annual report of the Boston Psychopathic Hospital for 1934.

Dr. d'Elseaux has continued his activity in studying the psychoses at a physiological level. As a result of his work there has been a gradual growth in the research laboratory which has finally culminated this spring and summer in the building of a rather ideal arrangement of laboratories and experimental rooms, with ample space and good equipment, concentrating previously scattered facilities into a single unit. The additional space permits the work of a larger personnel to carry out the complex time-consuming experiments necessary to work up the problems which have grown out of the original CO_2 studies. The problems which have grown out of the original CO_2 problem fall into three major groups; (1) the acid–base balance of the blood, brain, and muscles and the inter-relations of this balance in each of these tissues; (2) the regulation of respiration; (3) cardio-vascular activity in its relation to respiration. . . . . Through this work there has been gained a detailed and exact knowledge of the functioning of the systems, which offers opportunity not only of comparison of the normal with the psychotic in regard to the activities of these systems, but also offers an opportunity of studying the control exerted over these systems by the autonomic endocrine and humoral systems by virtue of the precision and ease of observation of these systems. Through such studies of the changes in systems such as the respiratory system the autonomic system may be studied.

Seven papers dealing with this material are about ready for publication. From the point of view of the impersonal processes involved in the schizophrenic psychoses intensive histopathological studies should be undertaken, and it has been a great regret of mine that facilities for such studies at the Boston Psychopathic Hospital have not been provided during the past ten years.

(b) It is only the incubus of the disease concept and a certain doctrinaire attitude supported by very respectable authority that encourages many workers to see in all cases of so-called schizophrenia nothing but the same processes which in these previous groups may very well play a predominant role. If one comes to the actual material of one's patients with a willingness to consider the whole situation, there is very little in a large group to suggest that the key to the trouble is to be found in even the most intensive study of biochemical and physiological processes. We do not study the mentality of the Christian Scientist, of the aggressive pacifist, of the communist, of the spiritualist, of the mediaevalist, of the poet, of the extra devout by biochemical methods. We study these manifestations in the light of the special needs and endowment of the individual, of the special experiences through which he has gone, of the culture in which he is steeped, of the actual situation in which he finds himself. There are many cases called schizophrenic whose mal-adaptation to life seems, to a large extent, to be determined by the same factors which determine the unusual careers of many other somewhat aberrant types who, however, are tolerated by the community and who manage to float owing to some native resources or to some fortunate combination of circumstances. It is true that the more severe deviations from the conventional norm which we call schizophrenic seem unintelligible in the light of what is conventionally understood as human nature, even that human nature which is studied by the psychologist. One has to realize, however, that the conventional presentation of human nature pays little attention to those real facts of human nature which are visible in the psychotic but which are repressed and ignored in the ordinary relations of human life, although there, too, they exist and exert a continuous influence.

In a large number of our schizophrenic patients, therefore, the problem is how human nature in certain individual cases fails in its adaptation to the demands made upon it and finally develops a mode of behaviour or belief so seriously divergent from the norm that the individual can no longer be left to his own devices but has to be put in the care of physicians.

While in this group of patients physical anomalies may contribute their quota and a thorough study of the physical status is of course obligatory, the main problem consists of an intensive analysis of the personality of the individual and a painstaking and detailed review of the whole evolution of his life and an evaluation of the environmental factors which have, on the one hand, moulded the personality and, on the other hand, involved a positive strain or lack of essential supporting elements. In some of these cases the difficulties and deficits of real life give rise to compensatory wish-fulfilling phantasies. In other cases intolerable elements of the personality which cannot be ignored are projected on to the environment. In other cases the morbid ideas and behaviour of an individual are not easy at once to reduce to such formulae but present difficult problems in interpretation.

Starting from these views one therefore would wish to plan out a very comprehensive systematic and detailed investigation which would cover various topics (a) the genetic equipment of individuals; (b) different types of personality with an analysis of the dynamic components of these types; (c) the special role of the sex factor in the evolution of the individual case;

(d) the influence on the evolution of the sex life of the family and social atmosphere with its conditioning codes and influences; (e) the influence on the individual of the bond between child and parent; (f) the role played by the intelligence endowment and by the facility of imagination; (g) the influence of suitable occupational outlets, of satisfaction from actual skills, or recognition for constructive activity; (h) evasive and substitutive types of reaction, their onset, evolution and resistance to corrective influences; (i) social factors and community organization which favor the development of various types of mal-adaptation; (j) the detailed symptomatology and course of the individual case, variation in evolution and in outcome, and a study of the factors which modify the same, the response of the individual case to therapeutic influences.

I personally believe that the slow accumulation and careful digestion of such a material, with clear realization of the factors involved, would make an important contribution to our total knowledge of these disorders. I also believe that the results of such an investigation would have a much wider bearing than mere knowledge of a certain group of handicapped people. It would be a most valuable contribution to general psychology, it would throw a great deal of light upon the mechanisms of human nature in general, it would tend to dissolve the rigid mediaeval view of the insane as so completely alien from the so-called normal, it would supply a valuable body of data with regard to the actualities of the sex life in our present culture, it would throw useful light upon the structure of the family, it would help us to analyze the community from the standpoint of a sound mental hygiene.

It is with this point of view that I have for long tried to organize a satisfactory service in which these problems could be satisfactorily worked at. The busy routine of a Psychopathic Hospital with two thousand admissions and with a very limited staff obviously makes it impossible without additional resources from external sources to carry on such an investigation in a satisfactory way. I have tried to keep these problems before the staff in their busy clinical activity so that in the interstices of their routine work they might think about these problems, and also so that in their routine work the spirit of scientific curiosity might be kept awake.

For the last nine years the Rockefeller grants, which unfortunately have now come to an end, enabled us to carry on the special investigations, the reprints from which are being sent to you.

I personally believe that with the rich clinical material available at this hospital, with its situation and close contact with a large medical centre, not only could our laboratories be utilized for the intensive investigation of the problems which have been referred to above, but a special research clinical service could be developed which would enable one to contribute a good deal to our knowledge of those disorders grouped together under the term schizophrenia and also of many important problems involved in human relations in general.

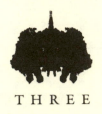

THREE

Mental Hospitals

Although the mental hospital was an established and seemingly secure institution in the late nineteenth century, its functions, structure, and at times its legitimacy came under sharp attack by critics. An extreme but not atypical example was Dorman B. Eaton's "Despotism in Lunatic Asylums," published in the influential *North American Review* in 1881. Eaton bitterly condemned the closed nature of asylum management and emphasized the opposition of medical officers to "inspection and publicity." In asserting the rights of the public insofar as the mentally ill were concerned, he was implicitly calling medical authority and legitimacy into question. The most famous attack on institutional psychiatry came from S. Weir Mitchell, the eminent neurologist. In an address before the American Medico-Psychological Association in 1894, Mitchell compared psychiatry with other medical specialties and found it wanting. Psychiatry, he observed, remained isolated from medical science. "You were the first of the specialists," he added, "and you have never come back into line. It is easy to see how this came about. You soon began to live apart, and you still do so. Your hospitals are not our hospitals; your ways are not our ways. You live out of range of critical shot; you are not preceded and followed in your ward by clever rivals, or watched by able residents fresh with the learning of the schools." Mitchell went on to deplore the absence of a spirit of scientific inquiry in mental hospitals; the widespread distrust of asylum therapeutics; the psychiatric disregard of any responsibility to educate the public about the dangers of insanity and its treatment; and the role played by political considerations in hospital management and administration.[1]

1. Dorman B. Eaton, "Despotism in Lunatic Asylums," *North American Review*, 132 (1881): 263–75; S. Weir Mitchell, "Address before the Fiftieth Annual Meet-

In addition to external attacks, implicit criticisms came from within the ranks of institutional psychiatry. The founding generation of American psychiatrists had accepted the dual responsibility of providing both care and treatment and had formulated standards of institutional management and administration. Their views, however, were increasingly ignored by a younger generation of physicians imbued with a vision of a new scientific and biologically oriented medicine. These younger figures were eager to transform the institution that had given birth to their specialty by applying the insights of medical science to psychiatry and by reintegrating psychiatry and scientific medicine.

To transform the mental hospital was easier in theory than in practice. A variety of impediments had to be overcome. First, and perhaps least understood or recognized, was the nature and behavior of the patient population, which was anything but pliable and malleable. Although psychiatrists assumed that their authoritative decisions on governance, care, and treatment were decisive, the character of hospitals was more often than not shaped by patient behavior and the nature of staff–patient relations. To establish institutional goals and to mandate change was relatively simple. To control events with any degree of precision proved far more difficult, if not impossible. Most psychiatrists found that there was a fundamental distinction between their authority to issue directives and their power to ensure implementation, if only because patients often responded by modifying their own behavior and thus altering the actual effects of new policies. Few psychiatrists recognized that there was at best a precarious balance between institutional order and stability on the one hand and patient behavior that appeared arbitrary, unsettling, and unpredictable on the other.

More important, the mental hospital did not function in a political or social vacuum. More than 90 percent of all mentally ill patients were in public hospitals subject to policies established by legislatures and various public regulatory agencies. The financing of hospitals, the authority of physicians, and even the process of commitment were all determined by external agencies. The perceptions and concerns of legislators and public officials, on the one hand, often differed in the extreme from those of psychiatrists on the other, and neither group made a concerted effort to learn and understand the concerns of the other. The thrust toward centralization

ing of the American Medico-Psychological Association . . . 1894," *Journal of Nervous and Mental Disease*, 21 (1894): 413–37.

and rationalization of welfare at the state level that began in the late nineteenth century only increased the possibility of a clash between the psychiatric objective of autonomy and governmental insistence on accountability. Above all, there was no *national* policy regarding mental illness, for the nation's decentralized political structures and culture gave regional and local interests a paramount role.

Last of all, psychiatrists themselves never agreed on a single set of priorities or the ideal shape of public policy. They were unable to forge a consensus and disagreed on a variety of crucial issues: the proper size of mental hospitals; the appropriate structure that ought to govern public institutions; the relationship, if any, between custodial and therapeutic functions; the paradigm of mental illness; or the mechanisms that would assure accountability and prevent abuses. Diversity rather than unity was characteristic of both psychiatry and mental hospitals.

Yet psychiatrists were both physicians and administrators who confronted the daily problems of managing large and complex institutions, many of which held thousands of patients. Their perceptions and responses, particularly as expressed in their private correspondence, shed light on their activities and also suggest the presence of a wide gap between psychiatrists and mental hospitals as the public perceived them and as they actually were.

Shortly after his arrival in the United States from Switzerland in 1892, Adolf Meyer accepted a position as pathologist at the Illinois Eastern Hospital for the Insane at Kankakee. Opened in 1880, Kankakee was designed as an innovative institution. It had a number of small buildings, which were intended to maximize patient comfort and freedom. The promise of the segregate system (in contrast to the older congregate hospital that centralized patients in a single large structure) was never realized in practice, however, in part because of unplanned growth, inadequate construction, and the involvement of the institution in the vortex of state politics. Meyer's experiences during his three years at Kankakee were generally unhappy. When offered a comparable position at Worcester State Lunatic Hospital in Massachusetts (one of the oldest and most influential public institutions in the nation), he leaped at the opportunity in the hope of creating a new kind of institution. Yet a variety of factors frustrated his dreams. In the first letter, written to G. Stanley Hall, president of Clark University and one of the founders of American psychology, Meyer spelled out in detail his unhappy experi-

ences at Kankakee and his hopes for the future. The second letter, to Hosea M. Quinby (superintendent of the Worcester hospital), detailed Meyer's frustration after three or four years.

Adolf Meyer to G. Stanley Hall, December 7, 1895 (GSHP).
In compliance with your note of Dec. 6 [?], 1895, I beg to submit to you the following notes on the reforms to be suggested at the Worcester Lunatic Hospital, it being understood that this communication is personal.

My aim in coming to Worcester was the organization of a clinic for mental diseases, not primarily for teaching purposes, but as a source of study and investigation. The propositions made to me by Dr. Quinby were, that I should be free of routine duty, "a guide, philosopher and friend" to the assistants and employing my time so as not to feel as if I were frittering it away. He did not suggest a definite plan of work, but left this to me. The encouragement that Dr. Cowles had given me and the assurance that you and other members of the University would help me prepare the conditions for work induced me to leave the West and to believe that this hospital offered the first and best chance for my plans.

My first connection with an American institution for the insane taught me the fact that there is a desire for scientific work but that the best friends of scientific work in that Asylum were not trained in its methods and did not know the simplest requirements. I was appointed "pathologist," with the understanding that I should study the nervous system and the changes underlying insanity. Microscope and microtomes I could get; material more than enough for 4 men; with books the difficulty began because back numbers of journals, esp. of foreign journal[s] did not seem to be worth buying on ground of the ultra-wise dictum that in medicine a work is antiquated within 2 years; and also because neither superintendent nor physicians could read them. But the worst and fatal defect was that I was expected to examine brains of people who never had been submitted to an examination; the notes which were available would be full of reports of queer and "interesting" delusions, of logic terms like "disturbed," "noisy," "unable to get about," "untidy"; but whether there had been delirium or other psycho-pathological symptom-complexes, or a paralysis at the bottom of the "unable to go about," or paralysis of the sphincters—nobody could tell. The information was usually given in that pseudo-medical jargon which a physician may use with lay men in order to make the necessary impression, but which is the death of medical work if carried into medical discussion.

The first task was to try and interest the physicians in something better. The idea used to be that the autopsy should be made in order to show the cause of death. The clinical diagnosis would be exhaustion and the pathologist had then to find out the rest. The demonstration that in most cases of "exhaustion" the physician should have known of an existing pneumonia and peritonitis, in other words, that the lack of a diagnosis was a carelessness and something unworthy of a physician of ordinary standing, began to call for better reports. I never failed to show that by some method of examination many of the conditions could have been found before death and used as a guide for treatment. A certain plan of record was to be followed in which the methods were indicated and finally the discouraging defense of laziness and ignorance: What is that good for anyhow? began to withdraw from the daily conversation. The lectures on neurology and on mental diseases delivered two evenings a week in winter and in a summer course even one hour every afternoon—roused some interest and finally when I began to examine the new patients myself—always in the presence of the staff, after dinner—the desire to follow the methods and the studies became quite general and with it the feeling that the few physicians were not doing the 2100 patients justice. The superintendent who had not gone through all this drilling was not easily convinced of this and used to brag with the fact that in 1875 he had 300 patients to look after and kept his notes well etc. Undoubtedly they were good for the standard of that day in that special hospital; but to-day it is an impossibility to look after more than 100 patients or 150 at the outside and to do all that should be done for the patient and for the profession. Kraepelin has altogether 150 patients and 4 assistants for them!

The Superintendent and the 3 Trustees (a brewer, a station-agent and a small country banker) could not be moved well enough. But the State Board of Charities, whose president, Dr. Bettman, showed much interest in my efforts, induced Governor Altgeld to ask the Superintendents to appoint internes who should help the regular assistants. The plan suggested was that of a competitive examination, the only means to undo party-influence and, what is quite as bad, the nepotism of the superintendents and trustees customary in that state. Notwithstanding the most childish stratagems on the side of the Superintendents, who claimed that they could get along without internes and sent articles to the journals intended to scare away applicants and delayed the announcement of the whole matter till about 3 or 4 days before the examination—12 candidates appeared and 5 were chosen.

3 months later, our Superintendent told me, he was sorry that he had not more internes; he never had been so agreeably disappointed. It began to dawn upon him that my policy had been a benefit to the hospital and he entered upon my plans shortly before I left. The chief reasons of my leaving were the fact that I found it impossible to supervise the work of 2100 patients and that the tendency of the Superintendent towards show and bragging display and his position to the physicians did not give the best prospects for quiet patient and honest work. These external developments helped me to formulate the plans for the Worcester Hospital. There are between 900 and 1000 patients and 4 physicians who have never had any special training. They are rooted in the old-fashioned asylum-practice, ready to ask "what is that good for" wherever a new duty is spoken of; they spend an hour in the morning and a small hour in the evening on the wards; for the rest of the time they have to put up their own medicines, write the records (in the office, away from the patients) and write the letters to the patient's friends. There is neither druggist nor stenographer for them. You know the quality of the records; I may say that to me they seem charming illustrations of the "good old" times, if anything, a little worse than those which I found in Kankakee.

Thus I stand again before the task of educating my superiors and associates to the point where they recognize the necessity of all the innovations. They must be: Requiring from the physician to educate himself in order to be able to keep satisfactory observations and records—in return the clerical and drug work must be reduced to a minimum by the appointment of a druggist who would at the same time be able to make chemical analyses and by employing one or two stenographers. There used to be a 5th physician here. His salary should be taken to be divided among 4 internes or 5, one for each physician; they should receive about $20 a month (by all means!); otherwise many able men who have to pay for their own clothes etc. would be excluded from the competition. The reorganisation of the work should be carefully prepared, but carried out completely, because half-measures are discouraging and paralysing. The expense of the innovation is small; the salary of the internes would be $1000 altogether, that of the druggist $600 and the stenographer $20 a month. There is evidently perfect willingness to make expenses for laboratory and library, but the question of salaries is always a bug-bear in these institutions: the number of employees is always kept below the limit and the "administration" believes that this is economy!

My work here is promising if I get the assurance that I can choose good men. I do not know how Dr. Quinby stands to the question of appointments. So far he would ask the trustees whether he could "go ahead"; then he would pick from his acquaintances or from the acquaintance of his friends and equals a person sufficiently recommended to him—and this settled the appointment. If he appoints men or women who would do under his regime, they would probably not do for what work I want from them. The trouble is that our Superintendents are acquainted among themselves only, but not with the best younger clinicians of this country against whom they have a prejudice and—of whom they are somewhat afraid. Dr. Cowles is free from that because he belongs to one of the best general Hospitals; but those who do not, have nothing to do with the rising generation of clinicians, such as Prof. Osler. Recommendations are a dreary thing to go by for appointments. The best plan would be to announce in the best medical schools of the country each medical vacancy and to choose the applicants according to the purpose for which they take up the candidature and their fitness for work as established by a practical examination. Only in exceptional cases recommendations alone should suffice.

As general rules we should put down the following:

1. Every interne or assistant must recognize the necessity of doing the work so that it can be used for clinical investigation; this holds especially for the examinations and records; and he must be able to acquire the training necessary for good work. (Reading knowledge of German and French! at any rate for the assistant-phys.) (At present we are apt to get men who ask all the time "what is that good for?" etc.; I maintain that there are in this country enough men who have high enough intentions and ideals to accept positions where that question is considered as settled and where the doubt of laziness has made place to the determination for work. Positions in insane Hospitals are despised now because they are known as clerical positions, breeding places for inaccuracy, laziness etc. which would disqualify young men for future work in active competition).

2. Every interne or assistant must enter upon the work with the determination of using every opportunity for self instruction and of contributing to a system of mutual instruction.

3. A man who has not the ability and ambition to contribute some time and energy for the further working out of the medical and pathological observations, is not fit for the position.

(This latter condition is very essential. I avoid the word original research, because it has been misused and does not suggest the right thing).

Dr. Quinby's letter to me contains the remark that I should not have to get acquainted with all the cases, but perhaps follow the more interesting and acute cases. This plan rests on a great fallacy. Frequently those who seem least promising on admission prove to be most important later on; such was at least my experience at the post-mortem Table. Therefore, we cannot decide whether a case is interesting or not without looking at it closely, i.e. without looking at all cases equally well. The best thing to do is to try to get the same examination of each case. History of the family, of the patient (which takes about 1 hour altogether, correspondence included); status praesens (on the average 2 hours, often more), records as often as needed, written on the spot in sight of the patient when the findings are made (the physician dictates to the interne, or for practice the reverse is done). The same holds for post-mortems. Records which are not written to dictation while everything is seen by several people, are not worth the paper and should not be recognised as a basis for further work. We *must* exclude the fallacies of memory and have a certain degree of control given by such cooperation.

These are rules which have made the German Hospitals what they are, although they have and spend so little money. Here positions in insane asylums are nothing but an easy way to become old enough for practice and to save enough money to go abroad or into practice. This is what the men tell me themselves; and this is why they cannot understand why a position here should be "worth" as much as another better salaried one in a place without a future. —A few words on the work itself: If I have all the help, we can arrange systematic courses and mutual instruction in methods of examination, of diagnosis; we must make a study of groups of our cases and compare them with the classical pictures of the literature; find out the differences and the problems suggested by them; the methods of treatment, of psychological and medical observation should always be arranged so that they could be confronted with the present standing of the knowledge in that field and assimilated, or where they show something new we should become conscious of it and recognize the relative value of new observations.

If our expectations of giving trained psychologists a field of work in the hospital shall ever be realized, we must be able to furnish the student all the data of the clinical record; he can not get them himself because it takes much time and practice. If somebody wants to work on heredity, let him go through the histories which wherever possible shall contain a pedigree and a record of signs and causes of degeneration. If someone wants to work on paranoia, let him study the histories of all the cases observed, not only a few "interesting" cases but the whole array—then he will see things in their natural connections.

For this purpose each history must be recorded in an index catalogue for diagnosis, symptoms, causes, treatment etc. This may seem pedantic; but Prof. Osler told me that they carried out this whole system to perfection in old merry England, in Guy's Hospital and that he himself has used it, and undoubtedly owes much of his success to it.

This hasty sketch will, I hope, give an idea of the needs and of the feasibility of the organisation. It is not a question of money but a question of work, and it has the greatest difficulty in the fact that everybody will have to do about twice the amount of work. But then, instead of merely earning a little money each year, the men will be able to carry out something into the community which only Johns Hopkins, McLean and a few other chosen places do now.

Adolf Meyer to Hosea M. Quinby, undated, written between 1899 and 1900 (AMP, Series I).

In view of the fact that a conversation on the matter we spoke of is very unsatisfactory because the points are easily confused, I take the liberty to put before you the following statement of things:

When I started into psychiatry I was partly aware of the difficulties in my way, but I trusted in the cooperation of those with whom I might throw my lot. I cannot say that this was a wise plan. It is a fundamental mistake to undertake anything in this country in which one is dependent on others concerning the means with which the work is to be done. I made plans in which I have a good enough believe [*sic*] in; but they go to pieces over matters in which I have nothing to say. Therefore, I become more and more convinced of the verdict—psychiatry is not a feasible problem in this country and to save myself further worry and disappointment, I must give it up.

I put all my hope on this hospital. There are so many things which really justified my doing so. It is true, Kraepelin never concealed his skepticism. He felt sure that under the existing arrangement, where I have no power of action nor any possibility to even oversee the chances of the hospital as a whole, nor stated funds to control and no touch with the general policy—

a sort of side-show merely—, I should fail to carry out the very difficult enterprise. I refused this view, because I hoped you would not make things unnecessarily difficult.

The habit of cooperation is, however, a more difficult thing to acquire than I had imagined. You say you consulted the supervisors on the new buildings; but you will not remember ever having asked me for what would seem desirable to carry out for what we need for our plan of work. This I should call a fundamental mistake from my point of view, although it is quite justified from your old point of view as superintendent, who alone has responsibility and therefore the only [?] in a State Hospital.

You must not misunderstand these rather harsh words. I know that you have far more than ever before or than many other superintendents would, endorsed suggestions coming from me and allowed me to have full control of many matters. These features are however counterbalanced by the absence of a plain summary of the problems of the hospital as an entity and as long as that is absent much of the judicious attitude which you certainly take, is overshadowed by difficulties under which the whole suffers. The new additions were made exactly as they would have been made 4 years ago. And yet, we can say without overestimating things, we stand in our medical efforts and plans on a wholly different ground to-day. There is no proportion in our efforts and all we are doing is therefore patch work—not subservient to one recognized entity.

The business-administration of this hospital has probably never been changed since it was started. I am sure I could not handle it even if I had years of experience in the complicated way it is managed to-day.

I don't see that there is any possibility now to state at any given time what tasks are before each department. Therefore, when something new comes up its importance can never be measured except by the guess-method. Then, when the day's work is planned, only that is considered which is in one's mind at the time and other matters drift into oblivion.

The problem of housing etc. is settled on a priori negation. This building is, of course, of very poor construction for what it is needed for now; but nothing would be easier than to find some way out of the blockade. If we are unable now to make provisions we always shall be until the regime is changed.

Looking over matters as well as one can now, the conditions do not appear unmanageable, except for personal reasons. These are however such that I propose the following alternative:

I limit my work to the summing up of what has been done these two years, and to the laboratory. Since no steps are taken to make the necessary improvements in the therapeutic and clinical department, I let that go in order not to "fritter away my time" on work half done. In the meantime I shall take the liberty of looking around for neurological work on other ground.

Or—a careful plan of what is planned to be done in the near future and estimate of the time and labor and money needed for them is to be made and the work to be planned accordingly.

There were days when I favored division of medical work and management of business. I am getting away from this view and see that they had best be handled as one, and under one head for ultimate decisions, but in well organized departments. As things are, I see no opportunity to try anything for myself; I must remain a subordinate part of a whole if I want to stay in psychiatry. Owing to the fact that my work is looked upon as a laboratory-department, I see no chance of ever getting beyond that in a reasonable time; I am therefore compelled should I stick to psychiatry, to look upon this hospital and the position I hold now as a final one for many years to come. The lesson I was taught last winter shows me that I do not stand it unless causes of continual aggravation are removed.

It is no use to move in general phrases in this matter. I allow myself therefore to state plainly the principle [*sic*] difficulties I have found.

I am averse to asking for favors. What I ask for is usually of a character that amounts to a requisition of something necessary beyond much question. Before I ask I think things over and find out whether the request will meet any opposition which I had not thought of. When I first came here, I inquired for many things which I thought were granted without question, and I was given the answer by those long associated with you, that this request had been refused before—so I let it go. This holds for requests concerning the Table—Dr. Jones had been refused a change from oatmeal; I never asked for one for that reason although I was disgusted by the uniformity, until, lately, Miss Gordon arranged a change for me. Now I get a sort of special diet. How easy it would be to make things pleasant for everybody and to have Miss Gordon observe similar matters in others! There is plenty; yet many things are hardly touched; and whether any improvements were possible, is never looked into under the present regime.

Dr. Mooers made what seems to me a legitimate request concerning the keeping of a horse. She was refused and I did not care to ask for the same "impossibility." Apart from the business managers nobody has a chance to avail himself of any vehicle. When I was ill, I had to ask for being taken down town, and once had to walk, and the only outing I got was given me by friends out-side. Friends have to walk from and to the station even in bad weather. Unless there is a positive understanding the first step to an offer lies in your hands.

At night all the lights in the halls are put out and the people must grope around because it has always been so. A small-flame burner would have been easily put into the place of some other business and the sudden order that all lights should be turned at 11 would have lost something of its abruptness. You asked me whether you had ever declined to talk with me concerning anything—you seem not to remember the entire episode concerning my rooms, which ruined my entire winter; or the remarks with which you answered some suggestions of mine before that also concerning the room—questions, amounting to about: Come to me whenever you want to and have your say; those things are all settled anyhow.

When you said this morning: Do you mean you were not enough consulted concerning the new wards? characterizes the situation beautifully. It looks as if you thought my feelings had been hurt because I might have been slighted. All I contend is that the buildings and all the innovations were made without any special consideration for the needs which after all are very closely connected with our clinical problems. Only in as much as I feel somewhat responsible for these—there was not a step made before I came—am I inclined to think that I should have liked to see them better in harmony with what needs was bound to come. When you showed me the finished plans, the whole was already accepted by the Trustees and in the hands of the State Board. My plans had been quite different and based on the conviction which could not as I thought at first be assimilated with the new enterprise. The new wards are certainly a valuable addition, but only a partial solution of the problem. I believe now I have the general plan so arranged though that they will fit in well enough; but for a long time I was at the utmost loss to see what could be done.

Then the fact that I fail to see any indication for a change in the dining-room question in the present plan convinces me that we must be able to make more of the present rooms at some time. Why should we not be able to do that now. I am willing to stay away from Table and give a place to a druggist.

As to the working-place for the latter: I do not worry for his place so much as for the work. The work is at best more difficult now, and for the fabrication of tinctures etc. we may find a basement-room for the man.

Finally the Trustees. I repeat what I said before. Whoever approaches a board of trustees with a full knowledge of what is wanted and how it is to be obtained, and with the conviction that the demand is reasonable in the eyes of any well informed man, meets with very little difficulty. Of course, there is the burden of evidence; but I feel that I need not bring to the Trustees any more evidence to convince them than I need for myself to convince myself of the justification of the request. But just for this purpose it is absolutely necessary to have the facts always ready for them to look into them; we cannot have everything beautiful all the year round and then come and say that we need much more. They believe we have a model-institution; if pains were taken to show them a little what Western Hospitals do, they would be heartily with us.

You know as well as I do that the whole plan of psychiatry which I mapped out makes it necessary that the same material should be followed for years. This is one reason why I cannot wander from one place to another without breaking up my entire plan. And since I do not see in any near future a chance to start on a clinic of my own, I have either to follow up this, or give up my plan as a failure—and then the sooner the better.

If I thought that this were the only solution I should not think a moment of bothering you with matters which are just as painful to me as they may be to you. I always hope and hope and hate to give in to the general clamor that Lunatic Hospitals have nothing to do with Medicine. I know that open and free talk alone can make the grievance clear. Last spring, I allowed myself to do the same thing in a moment of unbearable annoyance and felt this and allowed you to feed me on a few kind words. To-day, I know that a serious question demands serious consideration; that I am not bringing up petty matters of a day, but a sober view and questions which must be faced. I do not believe that we must all sink into impotence because you do not know what I am worried about. I am simply answering your request to say what I mean by uncertainty etc.

I know how things were here under Dr. Eastman and Park and can understand that you felt like making front against the physicians. But you have other elements to deal with now, men who work hard, who are ready to work too much, but who do not stand the petty treatment and do not like to be passed by as after all unimportant ornaments.

Weeks pass by without you ever coming near me or into the laboratory or in the way of some friendly interest. Since I returned every interview was solicited by me. You never venture to relieve the feeling that you rather avoid me. And if something is asked for, one never has a written order— books or something tangible, whether something has been looked after or not. We must wait a few weeks to find out whether it really was forgotten or not.

There may be some help for this. We saw one another once a week and I should gladly go to the trouble of keeping an easily accessible summary of things before you. If other departments would do the same—have books for work done and work to be done, we might learn to estimate what time is needed for a job and what labor and the whole matter could be kept open to inspection by anyone who thinks we are living here for our pleasure.

You spoke once of a training school for assistant-physicians; every good hospital cannot help being one. But where could a man get any knowledge here of what training is really needed to hold together an institution like this and at the same time promote its inner growth? Everything here is so personal, so uncontrollable, that nobody ever can learn anything. As a matter of fact, this constitutes the back-bone in a hospital like this and an assistant who realizes nothing of its importance is a reed in the wind of his own little schemes.

Believe me, that not a word of this comes from any other desire than to try and make further cooperation possible. I cannot give up without having tried to find a way further. If I do it in a clumsy way and perhaps injudiciously, I excuse myself by saying that I had tried other less outspoken ways in vain. I hate to try a line of work practically under the eyes of the whole profession at least in our specialty; everybody thinking that I am working in a paradise of opportunities and advantages, and then in the end break down. I surely know what I owe you gratitude for and means to do what my feeble powers permit to justify the confidence that has been put on me; but I owe myself and my family the avoidance of continued worry which would in a short time make me a burden for them instead of a support.

Hospital superintendents often expressed anger with the executive and legislative authorities of their respective states. Concerned with the welfare of their own institutions, they were frustrated by the seeming lack of understanding manifested by public officials and by an inability to retain a large degree of independence from the vortex of politics. In the following letter Dr. Charles H. Clark, super-intendent of the Cleveland State Hospital, expressed his views to William A. White.

Charles H. Clark to William A. White, February 23, 1909 (WAWP).
I desire to express to you the gratitude of this hospital for the volume "Gross Morbid Anatomy of the Brain in the Insane" by Dr. Blackburn, and published under your supervision and direction. You are to be congratulated for such a magnificent piece of work. It will be very instructive to physicians in hospitals of this character, who do not have the opportunity to witness many post-mortem examinations made by a skilled pathologist.

At a recent meeting of the superintendents of Ohio hospitals a committee was appointed to look up the subject of hospital dietaries and report at a special meeting to be held sometime next month. It is our object, if possible, to arrange a uniform diet for all of the state hospitals. I recall the fact that a man from the Agricultural Department spent some time at St. Elizabeth's studying the food proposition, and that you have a summary of his work published in your first annual report. If such is the case, please mail me a copy of this report.

The hospital has been running along quietly for sometime, nothing unusual has occurred to mar the even tenor of our way. Our admission rate has been unusually high of late, and we only have a few vacancies in the hospital with no prospect for immediate relief. I made a strong appeal to the finance committee for an appropriation of $125,000 for a new building. The general appropriation bill has passed the House and my recommendation was ignored. I have an appointment the latter part of this week with the Senate Finance Committee and hope to be able to influence them to make this appropriation. If we do not succeed in getting a new building this year the hospital will be in a very much overcrowded condition before we can obtain any relief, and I dread to see the wards crowded for it surely is not conducive to good discipline, good health, etc.

I have not met officially our new Governor; there is a naturally considerable apprehension among the hospital officials as to just what policy he will pursue. If you believe the newspaper stories that are constantly being published there will be a general housecleaning in all of the hospitals at a very early date. However, I am more conservative and feel that the new Governor will not make any changes unless a great deal of pressure is brought to bear upon him. I must say that it is quite discouraging when one is compelled to contemplate the probable loss of his position for no other cause than party affiliation. I hope the day will soon come when the Ohio hospitals will be under civil service rules.

We are having just now our annual agitation for a state board of control for all of the benevolent institutions of the state by the Legislative body. The Governor I believe favors such a Board and I suppose we will come to it sooner or later. One of the principal arguments used in favor of such a Board is that the institutions will be managed more economically, waste, excessive living, graft, etc. will be cut off. The gross per capita cost (including patients and all employees) of this hospital last year was 18 cents a day. If a state board of control would conduct an institution cheaper than this they would establish about a third rate county infirmary.

I hope to have the pleasure of seeing you at the meeting of the Association in Atlantic City. . . .

The use of restraint in mental hospitals was always a controversial subject. Critics generally emphasized its pervasiveness and charged that mental hospitals were dehumanizing institutions. Psychiatrists, in contrast, insisted that in certain instances restraint prevented patients from inflicting harm on themselves as well as others and that it was only infrequently used. In 1911 Dr. L. Vernon Briggs, a Massachusetts psychiatrist, launched a public crusade to transform mental hospitals and abolish by statute any kind of restraint. In so doing, he solicited the views of William A. White and gave the impression that he had the latter's support. In the following exchange with Dr. Henry R. Stedman, White clarified his views about restraint.

Henry R. Stedman to William A. White, March 26, 1911 (WAWP).
Dr. L. Vernon Briggs of Boston recently read at a hearing at the State House a letter from you regarding the use of restraint in hospitals for the insane which gave the impression that you advocate his bill providing for the abolition of mechanical or chemical restraint *by statute*. He is not a hospital man and although he seems sincere in his efforts to improve the condition of the insane, he is advocating measures to meet needs and abuses which do not exist. Three of our State hospitals for example do not use restraint and in another it has been reduced to a minimum. This public hearing has given an opening for attacks on hospital management and the treatment of the insane by a number of people who are ignorant of the real

condition of things in our hospitals, as well as former patients, who have enlarged on exceptional instances pointing to abusive treatment, some of which are greatly exaggerated and others which never happened. In short he is in a fair way to arouse by sensational means a public antagonism against our institutions at a time when by advanced and progressive work, general and in detail, chiefly through Dr. Copp of our Board of Insanity we were priding ourselves as having progressed in the care of the insane to a point where we were second to none in the country.

Dr. Tuttle, Dr. Channing and I therefore thought that you should know the whole story and wish especially to make sure whether you really advocate non-restraint by statute, because we doubt very much whether you would approve of the radical change of making obligatory by law the details of care and medical and other treatment in our hospitals in place of the present, usual and time honored practice of entrusting such matters to the humanity and discretion of our superintendents.

If you agree with us a speedy reply, if convenient, would be greatly appreciated and might do much good at the right time.

William A. White to Henry R. Stedman, March 29, 1911 (WAWP).
I am just in receipt of your letter of the 26th instant. In reply let me quote you exactly what I said in my letter to Dr. Briggs about the matter of restraint.

> As regards the restraint bill, I am in sympathy with the thing you are trying to do. I believe that a tremendous amount of suffering is still the lot of the insane person because he is misunderstood. Restraint usually is harmful. It is rarely valuable except in cases of severe accidents or surgical operations. I foresee, however, that if your bill becomes a law, that instead of using physical restraint, there will be an abundance of chemical restraint used, and in either case I see very little in the bill that controls the applications. The bill simply prohibits the using of certain things. It would be so much better if the law provided for the immediate transfer to hospitals for the insane of persons who are in penal institutions in any such condition as requires to be dealt with by such a bill. In the absence of the possibility of doing that, I think that all of the restraint and seclusion which is used should be reported at stated intervals to some official in control, should be in other words, quasi-public, and if it be shown that one institution is using vastly more restraint than another it will become

desirable at once to inquire why such a disparity exists. It will also stimulate the institutions that are not doing so well to try to measure up to the standard set in other institutions. I think by all means, that the reports of restraint and seclusion should be sent to a central of-fice,—to the Superintendent of Prisons, the Commissioner in Lu-nacy, or whoever the proper official may be in your State. I would sug-gest, also, that it would not be a bad plan to find out the quantity per capita of such drugs as hyosciamin that are used in the institutions, as whatever may be said to the contrary, such drugs are used almost en-tirely for restraint purposes rather than for therapeutic purposes.

You will note from the above that I did not make any specific recommen-dation that provision for the abolition of restraint should be made by stat-ute. As a matter of fact I believe that there are certain occasions where re-straint of some sort has to be used, and of these there are a certain number in which mechanical is preferable to chemical restraint. For example, I have a man in the criminal department who spends all his time in endeavoring to mutilate himself. This man is more or less continuously restrained by a pair of muffs, which do not hurt him or cause him discomfort in any way, and prevents him from injuring himself. Such cases are, fortunately, rare, but if one has to deal with the criminal insane one finds them more fre-quently. A criminal, for example, who has homicidal impulses, I might ad-vise that he be restrained by a simple leather belt and padded wristlets that put him in a position where he cannot hurt anybody, and which does not even discomfort him. In fact I have such a man in mind who asks for it. Then again there are certain highly delirious, disoriented patients who have such a high degree of confusion that their attention cannot be gained in any way. These are active conditions, and they may have to be restrained over a short period. During the month of February last in a total popula-tion of 2921 patients, we had seven cases of restraint for various reasons and for varying periods, but that was the total number for the month.

I am entirely opposed to the regulation of such a thing by statute in the way of a mandatory law absolutely abolishing its use, for such a thing would certainly work harm, for example, if it were not possible to restrain, for a brief period of time, cases that had to submit to major surgical pro-ceedings. The things that I suggested in my letter came to my mind as the result of a method of procedure which was put to use in New York State five years ago in which a special blank form was provided for reports of restraints and seclusions. The doctor in charge of each department made his report, and these reports were accumulated and forwarded to the Lunacy Commission. There a comparative study of the rules in the different hospitals in the state of restraints and seclusions could be made by a body eminently fitted to look over the situation from that standpoint and see whether there were any material discrepancies. You must know, of course, from time to time abuse crops up, not because of excessive indulgence in such easy methods, but where there should for any reason have been a laxity of oversight.

Believe me, I do not wish to be a party, in any sense, to any sort of agitation that will bring unjust criticism upon the hospitals. I have too much of that sort of thing myself to bear to wish any one else to have to put up with it.

Your letter is the first indication I have had that Dr. Briggs in his contention might be going too far or acting unwisely. I shall be cautious in my replies in future. The doctor, however, seems to be possessed of a great deal of energy and a vast amount of good intentions, which it would seem might be directed to good advantage.

Henry R. Stedman to William A. White, April 30, 1911 (WAWP).
I am glad to hear from you and wish in the first place to thank you for your effective letter bearing upon the Restraint Bill before our Legislature. I read to the Committee your views advising restraint in special cases and your decided opposition to the regulation of the details of care and treatment of patients in hospitals by statute. Your letter and those of Dr. Chapin and Dr. Ferris seemed to quite impress the Committee. The Bill has not, as you think, failed to pass, the Committee not having even reported it yet. Dr. Briggs has made so many changes in the way of exceptions in which restraint can be used that it now covers all conditions in which it is ever employed, thus not only defeating its own ends but making possible the indiscriminate use of restraint *by law!*

As to the popular lectures on insanity there are a number of "fallacies" left as it was impossible to crowd them into an hour's time. Several other popular lectures have been given on other aspects of insanity as you probably know. I made some suggestions in this line, in a paper of mine a while ago, as possibly you may remember, and am sending you a reprint of it to refresh your memory and in the hope that it may still further encourage you to inaugurate a series yourself.

The allegations by L. Vernon Briggs about the substandard care and treatment of the mentally ill in Massachusetts led to a heated debate. Many psychiatrists were offended at Briggs's charges and accused him of blatantly misrepresenting the actual state of affairs. The bitterness of the public controversy led the governor of Massachusetts to ask Adolf Meyer to prepare an independent evaluation of mental hospitals and public policy. In the following two letters, E. E. Southard spelled out the reasons for his dislike of Briggs, and Meyer indicated some of his own views about conditions in the Bay State.

E. E. Southard to Adolf Meyer, June 15, 1911 (AMP, Series II).
I have been mulling over our talk of the 10th inst. ever since. I know you said that, if you had to make a report on the insanity work of Massachusetts *it would not be a dangerous one!* And, for my part, I would not care how dangerous or alterative a report should be made to our governor, provided that the facts concerning our present conditions and tendencies are presented as such.

I am free to say, however, that Briggs has persistently misrepresented these conditions and tendencies in his public utterances to such an extent as to leave a number of erroneous impressions in the minds of some otherwise well-disposed persons. I enclose a statement published in the *Boston Traveller* by Briggs that speaks for itself. So far as the statement is accurate, it will be found to be culled from reports of the Board of Insanity, or to be an elaboration of the obvious, based upon no capable investigation of conditions.

A man who can draw conclusions like those in the last paragraph (to take one example) is a man for whose intellect I can have no respect. The innuendoes concerning reasons for Dr. Page's retirement and concerning Dr. Copp's responsibility for the idleness found by Frost at the Boston State Hospital stamp Briggs as distinctly unfair if not dishonest in his characterizations of our conditions. Briggs knows, if he knows anything, that Page left for no such reason and that Copp is responsible for the well-nigh magical improvement in conditions at the Boston State Hospital, conditions into which it had slumped under municipal control.

I think you will find that Briggs is distinctly biassed, if not deluded, in many of his statements. People ask me how Meyer can stand back of a man like Briggs, and I generally reply that Meyer does not have an intimate knowledge of present Massachusetts conditions and has probably taken Briggs at his face value. Everywhere I go I find that Briggs has been there, filling people's ears with inaccurate statements concerning Copp, the Board of Insanity, The Boston Society of Psychiatry (which he conceives has formed a sort of cabal against the great reformer Briggs), and the condition of the Massachusetts insane.

I have actually found not one local physician in whose judgment I have the least confidence who supports Briggs. And, as you know, Massachusetts is always distinguished for hyperconscientiousness.

Nobody believes Massachusetts conditions, or those of any other state, are perfect. But practically every defect to which Briggs adverts is one already discovered and in process of correction by our Board and the other boards, and taken bodily from their reports.

Of course you may say that your opinion has nothing to do with Briggs (whether in support of glycothymoline or anything else). But I am sorry to say that the names of Briggs, Meyer, Brush, and Cotton are being most frequently quoted as the authorities who have discovered Massachusetts evils and their remedies. Our governor has not seen fit to rely upon the Board of Insanity for his knowledge of conditions. Perhaps he agrees with Briggs that "we have to go outside of Massachusetts to other states and other countries to get the disinterested opinion of what we are really doing." What a reflection upon the character, intellectual and moral, of the men who have planned the colonization work, the boarding-out work, the psychopathic hospital, the reduction of restraint to a minimum, the establishment of hospital laboratories, the work on hospital hygiene and epidemics, the work of the institution for feeble-minded and for epileptic, the occupational work of many institutions spreading rapidly into others, to say nothing of economic achievements in the line of cooperative purchasing by stewards, etc. No one man claims credit for all this. Briggs, and those who stand for him, craftily leave out all that Massachusetts stands for and pick for recrimination the very arrangements which the institutional authorities are specifically trying (and succeeding) to improve.

Really, Briggs speaks without information and in glittering generalities of which he should be ashamed, so little actual knowledge has he of our conditions.

How anyone could think of reporting to the governor or anyone else on insanity conditions in Massachusetts without investigation at first hand I cannot conceive.

Believe me, Briggs sinks into insignificance beside the men he publicly decries, he remains as illogical now as when he advocated glycothymoline for insanity, he has spoken without investigation and in defiance of public statements by men who have investigated, and he has diligently gone forth to secure aid in his campaign from men at a distance who regard him as the spokesman of a great reform party and who have written more or less thoroughly digested remarks concerning Briggs' contentions which they have later retracted. Your own initial statement to Briggs received currency at hearings. Did your later letter receive similar currency?

I have talked a little with Copp and Howard about the report which you suggested you might write. They welcome any report from you knowing that you would not speak unless you had carefully gone over conditions as they at present exist. They would be grateful for concrete or theoretical suggestions but agree with me that the coupling of your name with Briggs' is a matter to deplore.

As it stands, no report would be worse perhaps than any report, as Briggs seems to have gotten it about that Meyer is back of his criticisms, which really seem as if they applied to conditions 10 or 12 years since or even to still older conditions rather than those of the present day.

I know you will smile at my long-winded discursions concerning Briggs and will feel tempted to say that Massachusetts, not Briggs, is at stake. But I say, Briggs or no Briggs, the progress made in the last ten years in the condition of insanity in Massachusetts is at stake, and that the governor is likely to be filled with statements made without adequate investigation of present conditions.

I am sailing on the "Humidian" June 23 from Boston for Glasgow, being pretty well tired of the machinations of Briggs and other grave events of the season.

I wish you every joy of the season and hope I have not bored you by my defense of Massachusetts. If my infection had left my mind fully elastic, I could have written all this in far fewer paragraphs.

Adolf Meyer to Dr. Albert C. Getchel, June 13, 1912 (AMP, Series I).
Some time ago I was asked confidentially to make some suggestions as to the choice of capable and independent-minded persons for the Board of Trustees of the Worcester Hospital. I at once thought of you, and of President Sanford; but would like to get your personal reaction on some of the vital points.

I feel strongly that Massachusetts is at the juncture of either getting into the system of excessively large institutions with a hopeless setback of practical psychiatry and excessive institutionalizing of what should pervade the community; or then it will have a chance to rise to a more plastic system with smaller districts of work and correspondingly smaller institution units. As you know the State Board wants to make the unit 2000 or more, and intends to put Dr. Scribner in charge of all the Worcester institutions, and then make the men who really have to do the active and aggressive work subordinate to Dr. Scribner. The vicious feature of the Massachusetts system is that Boston has never had an adequate number of hospitals and provisions nearer than Boston so that from time to time a stream of cases would be let loose on Worcester or Taunton or Danvers, whereas Cambridge and Somerville contributed their cases almost altogether to Worcester. Now it is obvious that the Worcester Hospital is too far from the places from which the patients come to allow the hospital to investigate the conditions that produce the disease and to influence the environment in any sort of preventive activity on the ground of the information and the study of the case. Wholesale psychiatry can no doubt do a great deal, but I doubt whether it can do much for progress.

As you may remember the reason of my leaving Worcester was far less the attraction of higher salary and larger field than the inability to bring about an organization which really would be active and efficient and that largely owing to the inaccessibility of the Board of Trustees, and the general atmosphere of self-satisfaction, and the superstition that there was nothing better in the world anyhow. This may express the situation too bluntly, but indicates correctly what I had to contend with. Dr. Quinby was in favor of adding buildings where I think it would have been better to transform the existing building and to keep it small; it would then have been possible to limit the district of work to what would have been within reasonable reach of the hospital, and to do some extra-mural as well as institutional work. As you know, the present Board of Trustees has accepted the suggestion of the State Board to centralize, and it seems to me that inasmuch as I believe that within this year two appointments have to be made, it would be very essential to find open-minded and studious persons who would be willing to study the local facts, and also tendencies of work elsewhere; and to create, as far as possible, a spirit of progressiveness and not merely a spirit of administration. I do not know of a man whose judgment I would trust better than yours, and I should therefore welcome greatly suggestions and proposals from you.

It is, I believe, highly important to disregard the fact that apparently political issues are involved; I do not believe that myself; I merely believe that back of the unrest there is a deeply rooted feeling that things are not as they ought to be; and my study of the situation last summer certainly convinced me of the fact that there was every reason why a change for the better should not be retarded, and should not be expected from those who had made such an ardent stand for a policy adopted years ago.

I was very sorry that I happened to be in Worcester during the absence of you and your family. I should have greatly enjoyed seeing you, and reviving memories which are still very dear and warm in my mind.

Please consider the above confidential. I assure you that a cordial response will be greatly appreciated by me. The whole problem of improvement in the care of mental diseases is so close to my heart that I have to break down all the barriers of state limit.

When an Indiana physician became involved in leading a campaign in Indiana to improve conditions among the mentally ill, he solicited Meyer's advice. In the following exchange Meyer answered a series of specific questions about the structure and function of mental hospitals.

Dr. Charles P. Emerson to Adolf Meyer, December 29, 1913 (AMP, Series I).
Your recent note was so helpful to me and you were so willing that I am going to impose on you with another letter. Please feel perfectly free to refuse to answer this letter in case it imposes too much. We are beginning a campaign in Indiana for better care of the insane and it is necessary that I lead it because of my school position. It is so easy in any campaign to speak with more enthusiasm than accuracy and there will be plenty of physicians who will be all too eager to criticise any statement possible. They will study my statements with that end in view.

Would it be too much trouble for you to run over the following general statements and let me know whether you consider them as facts or reasonable working hypotheses or just dreams. Some of these I know you will agree to. Concerning others I am a little in doubt.

1st. Should every general hospital have a special building for the acute insane?

2nd. It is a crime to put the acutely insane patient in jail with criminals for from ten days (the minimum time here for the proper insanity commission to pass on the case) to three months as in some cases.

3rd. We certainly could cure some of the acutely insane and return them to their homes without commitment if we could treat them early enough.

4th. The longer they wait in the jail the longer the probable time it will take them later to improve.

5th. Some patients treated early would be curable and, if treated late, become incurable.

6th. It is just as necessary that a man with mental disease receive treatment for his mental condition as that a man with heart disease receive treatment for the heart condition.

7th. Indiana should be severely condemned in that our State institutions which receive the acute as well as the chronic cases have only one physician to every 150 to 400 patients and scarcely a trained nurse or a nurse in training in any State institution (except those in administrative positions).

8th. It is worthy of the severest condemnation that institutions with 1800 inmates should not have a hydrotherapeutic plant, a gymnasium, an occupational department, etc.

9th. It shows that there is something inherently wrong in our system in that one half the patients admitted last year to one of the institutions had already been insane for from one to twenty years. It is during those one to twenty years that they should have received their treatment and they might have done so had there not been such a prejudice against the State asylums.

10th. An institution without a general medical or nursing staff is an asylum even though the Indiana law decrees that it shall be called a hospital.

11th. About 70% of all admissions to the State asylums are theoretically cases which could improve sufficiently to return home if not recover (note the record for Pavilion F, Albany). Since only about 30% in some of our State institutions do recover sufficiently to return home our State institutions are preventing the improvement or recovery of many patients.

12th. To give proper care to sick medical patients requires one doctor to every twenty-five patients, one nurse to every four patients (the number of patients divided by all the nurses who at any time during the day or night work in one ward), and an expenditure of $2.10 per bed per day. The proper care of the acute insane would require at least one doctor to every twenty patients, one nurse to every two patients and at least $2.50 per bed per day. Since Indiana allows about 50¢ per patient per day, it is impossible that her patients can be receiving proper care.

13th. Hydrotherapeutics, occupation, gymnasium work and psychotherapy are indispensable in the proper care of acute insane. A better medical staff and better nursing corps would in the end save much money in Indiana.

14th. Some patients with typhoid fever scarcely know they are sick, others die. The disease is the same. Among the mental diseases we have the same differences in grade. Insanity is a term which does not specify the disease but the need of State control of the patient's person.

15th. It is thoroughly practical by treating the patients early while the symptoms are slight to reduce the population of our asylums.

These are in general the propositions that I expect to make this coming winter in talking to politicians and before a hostile audience of politicians and doctors. Do you think that these statements are too strong for me to make? I would certainly appreciate any assistance you may give me.

Should you just merely add "yes" or "no" after these statements and then return the letter, it might save you considerable time.

Adolf Meyer to Charles P. Emerson, January 2, 1914 (AMP, Series I).
Your letter is a most encouraging New Year's gift; it certainly is a most excellent opening of 1914. I am going to jot down some thoughts in connection with your questions, and shall send them on without very much care in the editing:

1. I feel that every general hospital should have if not a special building at least special provisions for the care of cases with difficulty of behavior and adjustment. In the first place come the deliria which fare very poorly in most general hospitals, and usually get restraint and drugging instead of a decent show and hydrotherapy. To extend this perfectly obvious need to the request of a special building for the acute insane, would depend on whether there are any physicians able to run such a place. As a matter of fact it does not take so much special equipment if one has the right kind of human equipment in the form of nurses and physicians. The best thing, therefore, would be to recommend that *some* provisions should exist everywhere, and that in a few centers these provisions should be developed according to the available talent. A few remarks on this issue are given in an article on the Phipps Clinic in the journal, the *Hospital*.

2. Your second point about jails is of course one touching a perfectly barbaric state of affairs, which cannot be ventilated too freely.

3. The question of commitment. That is a point on which there is much room for improvement. The fact that the hospitals of the State exclude patients who are not committed in some form, makes them so forbidding;

and the fact that most of the cases there *are* committed gives the whole institution a semi-legal stamp. The idea that there should be special insanity commissions is a residue of an antiquated period. There should be open door in the best sense of the word, and conditions inside which would attract patients with a spirit of hopefulness and helpfulness, so that a large number could come *under medical persuasion*. At the present time I have not a single case at the Clinic under commitment but use it when needed. I realise the difficulty, but I rather think it is best that physicians should have to exert some efforts and exercise their imagination and use their resources to the utmost, than that one should choose the easy road of clamming a man in line by a more then medical step. As soon as the institution is one *sought* by a sufficiently large number of people nobody will chafe seriously against having been taken there temporarily where there *was* reason for *doubt*. The second step where one's own medical persuasion becomes insufficient, should be that of consultation with two experienced and impartial physicians in the form of essentially a consultation to decide whether the patient shall or shall not be held for treatment even against his will under Health Board regulations. I would call this a reenforcement of persuasion, and it should have absolutely no legal features. As one of the considerations or options in this persuasion one should have the right to suggest to the patient—if there is any doubt whatever—that he could appeal to a medico-legal inquiry, and this should be made as expeditious and simple and direct as possible, deciding whether or not the patient's direction of his case shall be handed to a responsible representative or committee of the person.

This modifies the whole question of commitment so as to leave the medical issues in medical hands, and to let non-medical considerations come in when the patient wants to push the issue to the point of having a change in his legal status brought about in the form of appointment of a committee of the person. To this should be added as protection of the public against medical carelessness, some provisions fixing the responsibility of the physician in such cases.

This, you see, keeps out non-medical powers, and keeps the whole case free from one's having to raise the question of insanity, i.e. it keeps it merely on the basis of his presenting such a condition as requiring treatment under principles identical with the principles of quarantine, and based altogether on the legal powers of the Health Department.

4. I heartily subscribe.

5. The jail, like any kind of brutal force, *deception* and *underhand work*,

constitute a tremendous complication in the chance [*sic*] of mental cases; they are all equally condemnable. Concerning

6. I am sufficiently optimistic and aggressive to be convinced that there is a certain percentage of cases in which the treatment is making a vital difference; and while we have many failures I have to maintain this optimistic attitude.

7. Hence my approval of this.

8. Here comes up a question touched upon in a number of the subsequent points. Our hospitals for the insane are both State institutions. There is no doubt that a large percentage of the patients in our State institutions are essentially boarders, who nevertheless need medical supervision; but unfortunately they create a standard for the whole on account of the ease with which they are worked and because they, according to the law, give exactly the same revenue as the acute cases. As a matter of fact the *appearance* of economy of the hospitals for the insane as compared to general hospitals comes largely from the fact that there are so many mere boarders, many of them earning their way completely.

Now it is impossible to make hard and fast lines between the boarder and the patient in whom *time* and a chance for recovery are the most important factors. 25% of those who recover, recover after a stay of over one year; therefore we must see that the so-called asylum division, or colony, or whatever we want to call it, must maintain standards which form a basis for recovery to all those who *can* recover. My suggestion would be to change the internal organization of the medical work so as to encourage the *concentration of the actual treatment cases,* and to have the groups for time treatment and the boarders sufficiently distinct not to allow them to become the ruling factor in the organization of the work as a whole. I have for some time asked also, from the fiscal point of view, that institutions should be requested to estimate what the various groups of patients cost them. But this is an issue which I only mention because what we really want to do is to keep the asylum or colony care on the best possible level, that is, about that which prevails as the best standards in the better wards of our hospitals. On the other hand, the maximum improvement should come through an *organization de novo of treatment wards* organized more or less in the spirit of our Clinic, with one physician for 20 patients, as you outline, or whatever may be needed. Concerning

9. I would, with regard to the hydrotherapeutic plant, emphasize the necessity of one's needing not only a general hydrotherapeutic plant, but also provisions for permanent baths *on the wards*. The next point

10. depends very largely on the commitment frills, and on what hospitals of this kind are expected by the public to do for the public; that is to say, to points already discussed above.

11. Very true.

12. I should especially emphasize that it is not merely absolute recoveries that count, but *sufficient improvements* and recoveries to make life at home and in the community possible. Point

13. is answered above. It is essentially a question of organization of treatment services as distinct from the time treatment and the mere custodial services. With regard to

14. I should emphasize the fact that insanity is a term gradually to be eliminated by the question: *is the person able to cooperate or no longer able to cooperate in their own interests?*; and that obviously is practically the issue. Point

15. is no doubt true. The only thing is that so far the actual care given by our States is so limited that for a time there will be rather an increase of patients who need hospital care; but that is another question.

Allow me once more to thank you for your interest. It is very much in line with the tremendously earnest effort that Dr. Kempf tried to make last year; but it takes a great deal of judicious management and education. It will also take a great number of young men capable to replace the old obstacles—Hence my advice to Dr. Kempf last year, that it would be infinitely better to lay a good foundation by training than to devote too much attention to reform propaganda at the present time.

Throughout the nineteenth century the care of the insane had been divided between the state and local communities. Psychiatrists generally opposed local and county care and argued that the mentally ill were always better off in medically legitimated mental hospitals. Hence they opposed an experimental system adopted by Wisconsin in 1881 that mandated care for the chronic insane in local institutions. When Dr. C. Floyd Haviland (1875–1930) undertook an investigation of the care of the insane in Pennsylvania in 1915 and came out against the county care system, he came under attack by the Pennsylvania Board of Public Charities. During the controversy Dr. Thomas W. Salmon (1876–1927), medical director of the National Committee for Mental Hygiene, wrote to Meyer, and the two men exchanged views on the wisdom and desirability of confining the insane in state hospitals versus local asylums.

Thomas W. Salmon to Adolf Meyer, February 8, 1917 (AMP, Series II).
As you know, a determined effort, which has slowly gained public support, is being made in Pennsylvania to adopt the policy of complete State care for the insane. Dr. Haviland's report on "The Treatment and Care of the Insane in Pennsylvania" (copy of which is sent under separate enclosure) gives a graphic picture of the conditions existing in those local institutions for the insane which have been permitted to remain in the State.

Influential newspapers and humane-minded men and women have expressed their strong conviction that Pennsylvania should adopt full State care without delay. In the face of this movement, the Board of Commissioners of Public Charities, in their preliminary report which has just been issued, makes the following statement:

STATE CARE OF THE INSANE.

The overcrowding of the insane in the various institutions is no new subject. It is well known alike to you and your Board of Charities. It has been a matter of the utmost concern to us. Alienists are not yet agreed as to the causes, or even the best method of treatment of insanity. Different theories are being tried out and it will require years to ascertain what are the best methods of treatment and the most desirable forms of housing and care. Why then should we now fasten upon the State a system of entire State care which has not been proven to be the best, only to find, perchance, in the near future, that it must all be done over. In any event, we are persuaded that the immense amount of money required to provide State buildings in which to house all the insane, as has been advocated in some quarters, constitutes an insuperable objection to the proposal that the Commonwealth should now provide hospitals for all of this class of dependents. The records now show more recoveries and less complaints from the small institutions than from the large.

This statement is calculated to delude the members of the Legislature of Pennsylvania into believing that State care of the insane is an untried experiment or a procedure of doubtful value and is, of course, utterly unwarranted by the facts. State care has spread throughout the United States so that only seven other States now tolerate the maintenance by counties or cities of institutions for the insane. Dr. John A. Lichty, a member of the Committee on the Insane of this same Board, and Mr. Robert D. Dripps, Executive Secretary of the Public Charities Association of Pennsylvania, have stated the case for State care in Pennsylvania as strongly as it has been stated anywhere.

I know that you have devoted a considerable part of your lifetime to upholding the doctrine of State care of the insane poor and I want to ask whether you are not willing to write to Governor M. G. Brumbaugh, at Harrisburg, Penn., making clear the essential falsity of the statement of the Pennsylvania Board of Commissioners of Public Charities that State Care "has not been proven to be the best." I feel that the opinions of men like you would go far to convince the Governor and the Legislature that they are being misled, and will hasten the day when the insane poor of one of the greatest and richest States in the Union will share the benefits which are enjoyed by those in your own State.

Adolf Meyer to Thomas W. Salmon, February 10, 1917 (AMP, Series II).
I am greatly interested in this problem of State care. The great difficulty is to my mind the fact that there should be a clear understanding of the ratio or share of responsibility of the State and of the locality. To my mind, the State ought to take a share only to an extent sufficient to put into central control a sufficient amount of authority. That this is possible only where the purse string is involved is, I think, fairly certain, but it should not reach the point where the State disburses everything and local interests are no longer stirred. If, therefore, a proposition can be worked out which does justice to this problem, I shall certainly be most eager to endorse it. I am awaiting with interest Dr. Haviland's report.

We were very much shocked at the very sad blow to the Mabon household and to the New York State system. To my great regret I am unable to get away to be present at the funeral, as I had already arranged an important conference elsewhere.

Thomas W. Salmon to Adolf Meyer, February 17, 1917 (AMP, Series II).
I think that your letter of February 10th raises a very important point as to the share of dealing with mental diseases which is to be assumed by the State and by the smaller localities. I suppose that the part which will, by common consent, be assigned to the State will be that of dealing with well recognized cases requiring permanent or more or less continued care, while that in the community would be prompt and effective treatment of

recent and borderline cases and the provision of facilities for diagnosis under the most informal conditions.

The present issue in Pennsylvania is really only the continued or permanent care of the committed insane. Dr. Haviland's report and Dr. Sandy's recent confirmation of it show how far below the ordinary standards of humanity county care has been permitted to sink.

I am enclosing a copy of a bill which Senator Sage has introduced in New York. It seems to me that it opens a splendid opportunity of dealing with New York's problem in a more constructive manner. It is by no means certain that we should go on providing for additional institutions of exactly the same type as those we now have up to the promised limit of $20,000,000. I have strongly urged Senator Sage, if his bill becomes a law, to have a careful study made of the adoption of a colony system, the establishment of boarding out, the position of the State with regard to local psychopathic hospitals and more particularly the possibility of providing facilities for early diagnosis and prevention.

In this connection, I think you will be interested in a bill which has been introduced in the Massachusetts Legislature.

You will notice that Senator Sage's bill provides for an appropriation of $30,000 for expenses. Would it not be an excellent thing if $10,000 of this amount could be appropriated for Dr. Russell's services for one year and have him devote his time to the study of the problem and also act as advisor to the proposed commission?

When mental hospitals first came into existence in the early nineteenth century, they were relatively small. In 1851 the Association of Medical Superintendents of American Institutions for the Insane passed a resolution recommending a maximum of 250 patients for any single institution. For a variety of reasons, hospitals gradually grew in size. Some psychiatrists, including Adolf Meyer, opposed large central hospitals; others believed that large hospitals had certain inherent advantages. In the following letter to the chairman of the Michigan Hospital Commission, William A. White spelled out the case for large hospitals.

William A. White to R. G. Ferguson, February 21, 1927 (WAWP).
I have your letter of the 18th instant in re the size of Hospitals. My own opinion in regard to this matter is a very definite one. I am strongly in favor of the large hospital. If you will go over the history of hospitals for

the insane in this country, you will find that at various times in the course of events a maximum size has been indicated. At one time it was 500, then it was advanced to 1,000, and then to 1,500. To a certain extent I have felt that this steady advance was the result of making a virtue out of necessity, but the original idea was that a hospital should not be larger than would permit the superintendent to know each patient. I think such standards have survived their usefulness, and now whether a large hospital can give as good care to an individual patient as a small hospital depends entirely upon its organization and administration. For my part, I do not see that there is any limit to the size of a hospital which can furnish good care, except those limits that may be imposed by arbitrary local conditions such as geography or the growth about the institution of a city. In an institution, for example, of 5,000 patients the hospital would be divided up, let us say, into five portions of a thousand patients each and at the head of each one of these divisions there would be a man of the caliber and ability of a superintendent of a hospital of a thousand patients. It is rarely a question of efficiency of organization.

As to the question of cost I feel that the large hospital is more economical. Just where to draw the line I am not sure, because I think there is no fixed point, the line having to be drawn at different places at different times. One of the controlling elements in cost would be the ability to purchase in quantities which offered the greatest advantage. For example, such commodities as sugar, flour, cement can be purchased to best advantage in carload lots and a hospital to get the advantage of such purchases ought to be large enough to use such quantities.

The controlling factors in my mind, however, are the medical ones. As mental medicine has advanced in recent years it has called into its service an ever increasing number of specialists. There is now in our large mental hospitals not only the entire equipment of a general hospital, but such groups as the occupational therapists, the psychiatric social workers, etc. It is obvious to my mind, therefore, that the size of a hospital for mental cases ought to be large enough to distribute the top cost to best advantage, and as it seems to me that the top cost is constantly increasing, the size of the hospital will also have to correspondingly increase in order to accomplish this end.

Then there is another element bearing upon the medical care of patients which I think important. The larger the hospital the larger naturally the medical staff, and the larger the medical staff the more specialization there may be among its members. With a hospital of five thousand patients with

40 or 50 physicians, it means that if this medical group is properly organized, that a sick patient will have the advantages not of one or two physicians' opinions, but of the opinions emanating from a large group vari-
ously specialized. This is an advantage, I think, which makes the large
hospital capable of distinctly superior work to the smaller one, particularly
in these days when the field of medicine has become so extensive that no
half-dozen men can compass it.

   In the same way that the large hospital permits a large staff, the individuals of which have various interests, so a large hospital presents better
opportunities for proper classification of patients. They can be split up into a
wider variety of groups to their advantage. My own feeling, therefore, is
that a four or five thousand bed hospital at the present time presents the
possibilities, if properly organized, of maximum advantage to the patient,
and I should not be surprised, in fact I should expect to see this size increased rather than diminished as time goes on. I am fully aware that there
are many who do not agree with me in this position, but my experience
has led me to think in this way and I trust, as I have set it forth it may be of
use to you.

---

*The threat of violence in mental hospitals was perennial. Some patients proved
disruptive and threatened both themselves and others with physical harm. Some
attendants used extreme force, sometimes without adequate justification. The
human frailties of patients and attendants created a precarious balance that was
easily upset. In the following exchange with the first assistant secretary of the
U.S. Department of the Interior, William A. White defended his action in dis-
charging two attendants and upheld the propriety of accepting the validity of
patient testimony.*

   E. C. Pinney to William A. White, June 25, 1928 (WAWP).
During your absence another case of the dismissal of attendants for alleged
abuse of patients occurred, viz, [JHR] and one [B], whose first name I do
not recall. They are alleged to have had an altercation with a negro patient
in Howard Hall.

   [R's] story is that the negro snatched away his keys and that he had to
use force in order to recover the keys and prevent the patient from opening
the door and possibly releasing himself and other patients from the room;
that any injury the patient may have received was by falling over a bench.

However, Dr. Noyes reported to me that the matter had been gone into by the Board of Review, which was convinced that [R] and [B] had used unnecessary force.

You know my personal view with respect to the testimony of patients, not corroborated by those of sound mind. I am not disposed, however, to raise any question about the reinstatement of these men, but I do wish a little more diplomacy could be shown in these cases. It would make very much less trouble for the Department and would accomplish your purpose, if in cases where there is any doubt, attendants were permitted to resign instead of inflicting upon them the penalty of dismissal. In this particular case, these men insist that they used no more force than was absolutely necessary to control this violent patient, who, I am now informed, has been placed in a room by himself because of his violent disposition.

The two attendants do not desire to be reinstated, but they would like to have their resignations accepted, rather than bear for the rest of their careers the stigma of dismissal.

If you can find time, I wish you would review the record and advise me whether, under the circumstances, you would be willing to accept their resignations.

William A. White to E. C. Pinney, June 30, 1928 (WAWP).
I have your letter of the 25th instant *in re* the dismissal of Attendants [R] and [B] for the abuse of Patient [TC]. You raise certain issues in this letter and make certain suggestions, upon which I will comment as follows.

In the first place, you call attention to your view regarding testimony of patients of unsound mind. I appreciate your point of view perfectly but I can not assimilate it with my experience. If it were necessary, in order to dismiss a brutal attendant for the abuse of patients, to have evidence of witnesses of sound mind, a situation would be created which would make it physically impossible in the majority of cases to effect such a dismissal and would place a not inconsiderable number of patients in the Hospital who are helpless because of their mental disability at the mercy of such employees. It is the duty of every attendant to protect the patients in the Hospital whether they be under his immediate charge or not, and in the particular instance under discussion there were two attendants present and still the patient was not protected. How many employees would it be necessary to keep on a ward in order to be assured that one of them would stand up for the rights of the patient? Aside from such a situation as this, the attendant who desired to discipline a patient could do so with perfect freedom by a method which, I regret to say, has only too frequently been disclosed by investigations, and that is by taking him into the clothes room which adjoins each ward, locking the door and proceeding to inflict such punishment as he saw fit without any witnesses present whatever. It is difficult to see, if it were necessary for us to rely solely upon the testimony of witnesses of sound mind how such an abuse could ever be corrected.

Further than this, the matter of abuse of patients is one that is always in the forefront of the public consciousness whenever an institution of this character is under consideration. The history of this idea it is perhaps unnecessary to go into at this time, but in innumerable instances of investigations of hospitals for the care of mental disease this question has been called a vital issue. It behooves a hospital, therefore, to have a policy which is unequivocal, straightforward and clearly defined, so that when such matters come up there will never be any doubt in the mind of the public as to the way in which such matters are dealt with by those in positions of responsibility. I am very glad to say that Saint Elizabeths Hospital has always had such a record, and I believe it should be maintained.

Still further regarding this question, it is not only necessary that the institution should be known as standing under all circumstances for the welfare, safety and kind and considerate treatment of all its patients in the eyes of the public, but it is equally essential, in order that the institution should do its best work, that the patients themselves should feel the confidence in its management that such a policy as I have outlined alone will give them. It would indeed be an unfortunate thing if the patient population felt themselves at the mercy of attendants who might be brutal and inconsiderate, and knew that no plea that they might make would or could have consideration.

And finally with regard to this question, may I call attention to my experience to this effect: that repeatedly I have known of patients in institutions being called to the witness chair in Courts and having their testimony heard and considered, and that has happened frequently in the Courts of the District of Columbia. Upon the occasion some months back when Mr. Savage sued me in the Municipal Court, several of the witnesses were patients from Howard Hall. The Court and the jury were of course advised of this fact. The evidence of the patients was heard and considered and the jury no doubt gave it such weight as they thought it deserved. In at least one criminal case in which an attendant in the institution was the accused party, the conviction of that attendant was brought about solely through the evidence of patients. If I mistake not, the custom is that the legal status and the mental condition of the patient are called to the attention of the jury and the jury then considers his evidence for what they believe it to be worth. In regard to an investigation by the Board of Review at this Hospital, it seems to me that we not only are not estopped from taking the evidence of patients, but that it is our duty to get all the evidence that is available of whatever kind or character it may be when it appears that a patient has been mistreated, and then, having gathered that evidence, we are bound to act to the best of our judgment upon it. I can personally see no other course.

May I add in closing my comments on this general issue that many patients are perfectly well able to give testimony, in fact quite as able to give testimony as persons of sound mind; and I may say that many of them are better able to give testimony than are many people who have not been adjudicated. The idea that because a person's testimony is clear and coherent and to the point that therefore he is not suffering from mental disease, as is suggested in the Congressman's letter *in re* the patient in this case, is only based upon complete misinformation or rather lack of information regarding the mental state of those who are mentally ill. In fact the law in a rough way recognizes this when it recognizes that a person may be mentally ill in a medical sense and yet may perhaps possess testamentary capacity, that he may be mentally ill in a medical sense and yet may be criminally responsible, &c.

With respect to the matter of the resignations *versus* dismissals in instances of the abuse of patients. In a number of instances in the past I have, as a matter of fact, accepted an employee's resignation when he requested it. I must confess, however, that I do not see how it is possible to approach a problem of this sort with a request for a resignation. The only way under the law and the regulations in which this office can separate an employee from the service is by preferring charges and giving him an opportunity to answer. A request for a resignation would have no force of authority whatsoever; but if after the action of the Review Board and the approval of the Superintendent the employee requests that his resignation be accepted instead of his being dismissed, I think it is within the discretion of the Superintendent to decide and, as I have said, I have accepted resignations in the past. I think, however, that such resignations should only be accepted where no serious injury has been done to the patient, where it is merely desirable to dismiss the employees because they have actually struck a patient and in accordance with the policy of the institution such an act has to be dealt with, for the reasons above given, by dismissal. The patient may not have been in any way injured, and under those circumstances there is no desire on the part of this office, naturally, to interfere with the future employment in the Government of such an individual. In the present instance, however, I question the advisability of accepting the resignations of these two men. The injuries which were inflicted upon the patient were of such a serious nature as might easily have resulted in his death, in which case these two employees would have been guilty of homicide. It is through no good management or good judgment on their part that this patient did not die; and it does not seem to me, therefore, that it would be the part of a consistent policy to be willing to accept the resignations of men who had so outraged their position and authority and their relations with their charges as to conduct themselves in a way which was to all intents and purposes that of a murderer. This may be rather strong language and perhaps it is not wholly justifiable, because I have no reason to believe that either of these men intended any such result; but nevertheless had the patient died, under the law they would have been guilty of murder.

And finally, in response to your request to review the evidence in this case, I will say that I have talked the matter over with Dr. Noyes, who was not a member of the Board of Review, with Doctors Woolley, O'Malley and Silk, who were the members of the Board of Review, and with Dr. Lind, who has charge of the Howard Hall Service, and I have also read the record, and it seems to me quite clear that the action of the Board was fully justified by the circumstances. It must be borne in mind that in the evidence which we obtained, we were taking the evidence from a group of patients, aside from the attendants involved, with whom as physicians we have been in association for a considerable period of time, and that therefore these various personalities are known to us much better than the witness is known to the jury in a Court. The conduct of these attendants throughout the whole affair and their conflicting statements were such as to raise at once a doubt as to their honesty of purpose and their freedom from blame; and the testimony of patients, based upon a knowledge of their character, tendencies and possibilities, was confirmatory of this suspicion and directly indicated the nature and quality of the offense. I do not think under all the circumstances of the case that there is any reasonable doubt; and I understand that one of the attendants, at least as far as we are concerned, has accepted the verdict of the Board without comment or objection.

May I add to an already too long letter the general opinion of the members of the Staff who are dealing with these matters as members of the

Board of Review, which is to the effect that this method of dealing with the situation, namely, by a Board of Review, is much more protective of the employee and his rights than the strict following of the method which was formerly pursued under the Civil Service rules of simply notifying the employee of the charges, receiving his written answer to those charges and acting upon them.

The poverty of the American South played a decisive role in the history of public welfare in that region. In the following letter Dr. J. K. Hall, the distinguished southern psychiatrist and member of the General Hospital Board of Virginia, compared New York and Virginia mental hospitals and found the latter wanting.

J.K. Hall to Dr. H. B. Brackin, December 19, 1929 (JKHP).
On the 3rd and 4th of December I attended in New York the exercises in dedication of the New Psychiatric Institute in the new Medical Center. I suppose the building must have cost a million or two dollars and it seems to me to represent the last word in hospital construction. I went up to the dedication, both because I wanted to see the building and because the Director of the Institute, Dr. George H. Kirby, was an old college mate of mine at the University of North Carolina years ago. I regard that event as the most significant and impressive thing that has taken place in mental medicine in this country and perhaps in the world. The Medical Department of Columbia University, you know, is quartered there at the Medical Center on West 168th Street. There are the Presbyterian Hospital, the great Vanderbilt Clinic, the new Neurological Institute and the Psychiatric Institute. In the latter are 200 beds for mental patients, there is apparatus for research into the physical being, there is provision for a large outpatient service, and facilities for teaching both the medical students of Columbia University and postgraduate students. In other words, an effort is being made there to deal with maladjustment of all sorts in human beings as medical problems, and I suppose that the best medical and nursing skill that this country can afford will be brought to the service of the 200 patients in that institution.

I am daily and hourly all but overwhelmed by our need of more medical and nursing skill in our work with mental patients here in the South. I happen to be a member of the General Hospital Board in this state that has the oversight of all the five state hospitals. In these institutions there are about

7,500 patients and including the 5 superintendents there are certainly not 25 doctors on the staffs of these 5 institutions and certainly not a dozen trained nurses in the 5 hospitals. I believe that one or two of the hospitals have in them no nurses that have had any formal training at all. This is a terrible situation. The state hospitals, however, are not the only hospitals for the treatment of mental diseases that are in that predicament. We are constantly troubled here in this small institution by the lack of skill that we are able to bring to the bedside of the mentally sick patient. We do have 5 doctors on our staff but we are relatively ignorant and the nurses are, I am afraid, almost as ignorant as we are. When we opened this Sanatorium in the fall of 1911 we also opened and chartered a training school for nurses. I hardly know how we did it with the few patients that we had, with only two of us doctors here for several years, with meager equipment and poor quarters for nurses. At that time, however, the training school for nurses was not having to compete with the business world in reference to young ladies and we got along surprisingly well for several years and turned out, I think, some excellent graduate nurses. Later, however, we found it impossible to compete in our training facilities with the general hospitals and we had to give up the training school, but since then we have been giving a brief course for the purpose of training attendants. The young ladies who go through this training here are, after satisfactory examination, licensed by the Board of Examiners of Nurses as trained attendants and they are competent, I think, to go out and render fairly good nursing service. This work has not included the men attendants. Right now, however, I am in correspondence with a graduate man nurse in the hope that I may find it possible to induce him to come here and help me in organizing a class of training for some of the men attendants, most of whom come from North Carolina, and I know they can be enormously improved in their work by some training. Most of them, unfortunately, are limited in their education and I am probably going to have difficulty in making it possible for them to become licensed attendants, but I know that their knowledge can be extended, their skill can be increased, and they can be put in condition to render better service to the patients with more satisfaction to themselves.

Because I am not entirely familiar with the details of our school for training attendants I am asking Miss Louise Moss, the Superintendent of the School, to write to you in detail.

I am very much interested in what you are planning to do and I know that it can be carried through. Dr. Albert Anderson has a Training School for Nurses in the State Hospital at Raleigh and I think it is going along very well. Please call upon me for anything that I can do to help you in your high endeavor. I am exceedingly interested in what you are undertaking.

Conditions within state hospitals varied enormously. In some institutions psychiatrists found an environment that promoted trusting and effective therapeutic relationships with patients; in others the reverse was true, for the internal environment contradicted both medical and humanitarian goals. In the following letters Dr. Luisa Kerschbaumer described her experiences at St. Peter State Hospital (Minnesota) in highly negative terms. Trained in Vienna under Dr. Julius Wagner-Jauregg (who received the Nobel Prize in medicine for the development of malaria fever therapy for paresis), Kerschbaumer came to the United States in the mid-1920s and in 1927 became the first senior physician at St. Peter. Her European origins had not provided the ideal background for a position in such an institution. The fact that she was a woman also closed off any hopes of advancement with a public institution; virtually every superintendent of a state hospital was male.

Luisa Kerschbaumer to Smith Ely Jelliffe, March 2, 1939 (SEJP).
Thank you so much for your last nice letter.

Whatever you do for our poor sick hospital—in regard to Dr. H.—the Lord may reward you. Believe me, the fact that I stand this all is not anymore a matter of holding a job (or rather pay check), but I can't believe it that such can go on and on, it seems for ever!

A few days ago I discovered a fractured ulna on one of my patients. I had more than a "hunch" that the head nurse had done it but I had to keep my mouth shut. *I could not investigate—it would mean another brutal scene for me by the supt.* Then late one evening came an ethical nurse (an outside R.N.) to my apt.—the one for whom I fought with the chef cook to get her something to eat when she was in bed with fractured ribs and she was to be kicked out because she sees too much—well, this honest creature could not sleep anymore, she had to tell me to relieve her mind: that Mrs. S. the head nurse had broken my patient's arm. I returned sincerity with sincerity and told her frankly that I cannot do anything about it and that she will understand. She lost about 25 lbs in 3 months for grief. She cannot look on at the meanness our patients are treated with and that good people in this "hospital" are entirely helpless. —All I could do was to put a plaster cast on and feel sorry! So many fractured ribs or "possible fractured" ribs on patients' chest rays are reported from the x-ray readings from the U.! but who cares?! At present I have only 5 fracture cases, 4 legs and that arm, 2 casts under treatment. Of course there are "statements" made out—to smooth it over.

Incidentally, Miss McKey (an outside R.N.) caught in the White Elephant Bldg. one of our own breed nurses (from our Training School where we had them let [*sic*] pass!) how she just choked a patient. Of course, she was stunned and told her something whereupon the guilty nurse jumped and sassed at Miss McKey. Then Miss McKey went to the allmighty 6th grader, supt. of nurses and wanted that the guilty nurse should apologize or be fired. She refused to and, of course, she cannot get fired! This incident reached me from several parties, although everybody is warned to "never talk"! No word at staff meetings. In St. Peter we ethical doctors get to hear what is going on in this "hospital." We completely boycott the administrators. We never talk to them unless they ask a question then we answer briefly. It is an awful atmosphere. Some people ask me how I can ever manage to stand this all, I must have "iron nerves." A number of employees and even doctors are driven into neurosis and alcoholism—and this should be a "hospital" to "cure" such! Poor Miss McKey she looks like a different person, like much suffering. She told me she knows Dr. H. (she was in N.Y.) and I would be delighted to meet him (I made a poker face). They say she intends to find another job. She too drives away to mail her letters because our mail is "assorted" even by the chef cook! All the members of the clique are loitering around the mail box. Another nurse from the East remarks: "How long is this going to last?? It should be one clean sweep—" Work? "Work as little as possible, don't talk to nobody, gulp down your eats and crawl back in your apartment" is the prescription by Dr. W. (whose son had to climb those poles for the campaign) and he lived up to it for over 10 years! Many employees too never dare to say one word except: "I don't know" or "lovely" or "a nice day to-day" when it hails hazel nuts! You have to admit that such a life is worse than slavery. It is not only for the sake of the poor inmates but also for the sake of those employees that this tyranny should fall! "That bughouse trash" we are called in St. Peter or "she (or he) cannot amount to much otherwise they would not work in such a place" is another standard saying. Of course it is true for many but not for all. Responsibilities and economics play havoc with some people.

Of late we were offered a chiropractor to give treatments in this hospital!

And if we had a midwife to take care of some female employees—we would be complete.

I was told that Fergus Falls State Hospital has an osteopath as superintendent!

Dr. McK.—who is drowning his grief in something stronger than water—just returned from another trip from the Cities (his hobby is politics) and he is more puffing and spitting than ever. He broke the news that high salaried medical posts were bought during the last administration but also posts in better places were. I would not be surprised. When a supt. assnt. must be taught how to take spinals and what is schizophrenia, when he does not even know what delusions and hallucinations are—(I, myself, taught him the principles) and soon he was supt.! He told me himself that the "job" was "offered" to him because I told him frankly what I think of him.

I am just not a quitter but more like the grizzly that turns against his aggressor, otherwise I would have left long time ago. And then I think I can do some real good if I stay and help with the house cleaning. It is the tyranny, the abominable system that I hate more than the individuals involved.

My boss shows rarely up and then his face is swollen, very red and sometimes his lips are scarlet but it's not lipstick, then again he looks so drawn and of grayish skin color. He is still fighting to become the head of the General Hospital, Minneapolis. City stuff there is just as bad as here, I was told. There must be a curse on tax money that tax supported "hospitals" have such a wry face!

The patient whose life I had saved and whereupon I was almost fired and the guilty nurse was promoted—that patient improved and could go home. Her husband acted as if he were so glad to have her back and yet he always found an excuse not to take her. Then her niece forced him (against my advice) to take her home, and she told me that patient's sister and patient's husband are siding with each other and he put her here to get rid of her. "But," I said, "he could get rid of her only temporarily but not for ever by sending her here." She then made an awful remark. A few months later patient's sister came to my office and started to make me a scene that I had talked to the patient's niece! I merely left my office and her raving in it. Then she complained to the supt. about me but he said not one word to me. Then it was decided to return the patient not here anymore but to try her at Moose Lake State Hospital, Minnesota. —I could not tell the relatives that I had saved that patient's life (she would have been dead for sure when her political supt. assnt. had returned from his trip). My life saving probably would not have been appreciated by one party, anyhow—

So we are drifting around like on a sinking ship. I must admit that "Sammie" has a "tough" job "remodeling" certain hospitals! Thanks the Lord for my humor and my art work following that urge for creation.

When you have some books on hand, please send! . . .

P.S. Special regards from my adrenals that are not used to so much consideration!

Luisa Kerschbaumer to Smith Ely Jelliffe, September 16, 1940 (SEJP).
Oh, Dr. Jelliffe, if just Heaven or what not would help me out of this awful place! Of course, I realize fully my mistake. I should have left soon like other doctors who did "catch on" almost immediately but it must have been that I was so starved and frozen from the famine and lack of funds for fuel that I was glad first to get a meal and a little warmth, and I have the responsibility for my mother too, and then it took me longer than a born American Dr. to "catch on" and then I am so idealistic, too much so. I never had practical thoughts for my own advantage. And then I kept hoping like several others that such awful conditions would end soon but it seems they last for ever and ever!

You have no idea how it feels to be put under the dictatorship of an ugly, masculine, unbalanced six grader and when everybody knows how she got her poste!

Relatives of my patients complain about me that I do not put my almost dead patients to bed, but I cannot do it because the six grader Miss cancels my orders.

If I would only know a way out of this rotten asylum. Outside doctors just laugh about this hospital and even the affiliate nurses ridicule it.

You have no idea! Only one working here can grasp the racket.

Perhaps the *woman* physician is in my way or the Vienna University on account of the war now? Or don't they believe that I have that many qualifications as listed? I never thought of making more money of it. I am content with so little but I cannot stand this tyranny of crooks and brutes.

If I only knew what to do? I filled those blanks out for the Army service too.

Only Dr. Wolner (the grouch) and I are the only sober ones amongst the

8 doctors and the only ones to be found. All others are "out" or "sick" or drunk for weeks already in one stretch.

And I have no idea when the housecleaning will be?!

The financing of public mental hospitals differed from state to state. In the nineteenth century many states required payment from families of patients with some financial resources. In such cases the question of differential care within the hospital arose. As early as 1854 Samuel Gridley Howe, the famous mid-nineteenth-century reformer, warned of the dangers of a dual hospital system, one catering to poor and indigent patients and the other to more affluent groups. Nevertheless, differences persisted, both between private and public hospitals and within public institutions. In the following letter Dr. William D. Partlow (who became superintendent of the Alabama Insane Hospital in 1919) sketched out the way in which his state charged for hospital care and what effect it had on patients.

William D. Partlow to Dr. French H. Craddock,
December 12, 1940 (WDPP).

Answering your letter of December 10th,—the law regulating the commitment of paying and indigent patients to the State institutions presupposes that they will receive the same consideration in every respect, however, we do make the special consideration of giving paying patients separate dining rooms and separate dining room fare. They all receive the same attention, classification on the wards, nursing and medical attention, there being no difference except the paying patients have separate dining rooms and dining room fare.

The law regulating the commitment of patients to the hospital, Section 1446, of the Code of Alabama of 1925, provides that at the time the Judge of Probate is making commitment, he shall also investigate the financial ability of the relatives or the individual to pay and if found able to pay, shall make a small bond of $300.00 and pay in advance the amount decided upon and set by the Board of Trustees of the Hospitals. That amount at present is $30.00 per month, payable monthly or quarterly in advance.

The institution asks no question as to whether the person be paying or indigent. The Probate Judge determines the status.

To summarize, the Probate Judge committing a case determines whether they be paying or indigent. If paying, the person or some designated near relative usually makes payment of at least $30.00 in advance and the Probate Judge causes this small $300.00 bond to be made, each month the person pays this $30.00, he being given notice from the Steward of the Hospital. We draw nothing from the State Treasury for the support of paying patients.

All are treated alike, paying or indigent, in every respect except separate dining room fare which has a little advantage over the State patients.

I was very sorry not to be able to attend the Fox Hunt. I do like to attend these meetings, but have missed them all this year,—both State and National.

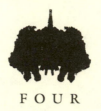

F O U R

Psychiatric Therapies

From their very founding in the early nineteenth century, mental hospitals provided patients with a variety of therapies. Generally speaking, nineteenth-century therapeutics tended to be eclectic and nonspecific. Given the absence of any kind of empirical data that might relate etiology, symptoms, and physiology, psychiatrists followed older and quite traditional medical practices. Like their colleagues in medicine, psychiatrists accepted the view that all parts of the body are interdependent and that health and disease grow out of the interaction of individuals with their environment. The goal of treatment, therefore, was to restore the normal balance, which would in turn contribute to the alleviation or cure of mental disease. Therapy included a balanced diet that would rebuild the digestive tract and nervous system, a healthful environment, exercise, fresh air, sunlight, as well as tonics and cathartics.

The holistic view characteristic of nineteenth-century psychiatry was based on the view that care and treatment were indissolubly linked. Indeed, even the concept of "management"—a word that appeared with a high degree of regularity in the psychiatric literature of that era—was imbued with medical overtones. By manipulating the patient's environment, the psychiatrist could overcome those past associations that had led to the disease and create an atmosphere in which the normal restorative elements could reassert themselves. For this reason, hospitals made provision for the employment of their patients, for religious observances, and for appropriate amusements, all of which were regarded as crucial elements in the therapeutic regimen.

Like their colleagues in general practice, institutional psychiatrists were also attracted to purely medical interventions. In particular, they employed drugs that tended to calm noisy and troublesome patients. The behavior of such patients often hampered their own recovery and interfered with the recovery of others. Psychiatrists thus regularly prescribed various sedatives and hypnotics including hyoscyamine, opium, morphine, sulphonal, calomel, and digitalis.

Throughout the remainder of the nineteenth century and into the twentieth century as well, therapeutic intervention in mental hospitals remained the rule rather than the exception. New therapies were adopted and discarded with regularity. During the 1890s, for example, psychiatrists experimented with thyroid extract, electrical treatment, and even on occasion such drastic surgical procedures as bilateral ovariectomy. Nor was it uncommon for psychiatrists to provide detailed rationalizations for innovative nonspecific therapies. Dr. Donald Gregg, a member of the staff of the influential and much emulated Boston Psychopathic Hospital, offered in 1914 three justifications for medical intervention: first, such interventions serve to combat in a direct way the processes that caused a disease; second, they strengthen the patient's general resistance; and third, they reassure "the patient or his friends that something is being done for him in accordance with the idea that still lies deep-rooted in most human minds that for every disease there is some curative drug." In an analysis of six wards with an average of ninety-five patients each, Gregg noted that, in a single month, 877 orders for medical treatment had been given. The two most widely used medical therapies were hydrotherapy (30 percent) and eliminatives (38 percent). The remaining therapies were divided between stimulants (6 percent), packs (9 percent), and depressants (3.5 percent), miscellaneous approaches accounting for the remaining 3.5 percent. Gregg also noted the availability of other interventions in the psychiatric armamentarium, including lumbar puncture to drain off excessive amounts of cerebrospinal fluid.[1]

Between World Wars I and II the pace of therapeutic innovation markedly quickened. The receptivity toward new therapies was understandable. Concerned with their decline in status relative to other specialists, psychiatrists were eager to employ physical therapies that would emulate the presumed successes of other branches of medical science such as surgery. In addition to their hopes of reestablishing ties and integrating themselves with a biologically oriented medicine, they were concerned as well with the welfare of their patients and were thus receptive to any therapy that enabled people to leave a mental hospital and function in the community.

1. Donald Gregg, "A Comparison of the Drugs Used in General and Mental Hospitals," *Boston Medical and Surgical Journal,* 171 (1914): 476–77.

Above all, the idea of therapeutic nihilism was completely unacceptable. Aside from the fact that the absence of therapy might undermine the legitimacy of their specialty and of mental hospitals, psychiatrists could not countenance the thought of doing nothing for their patients and thus consigning them to institutional oblivion. Consequently, they were attracted by any approach that might prove beneficial and lead to either cure or improvement.

One of the first to espouse a novel approach was Dr. Henry Cotton, a former student of Adolf Meyer and superintendent of the state hospital in Trenton, New Jersey. Cotton had become an ardent convert to the view that infections play a major role in the etiology of the psychoses. Persuaded that many infections spread from the teeth to other regions of the body—especially the tonsils, stomach, and lower intestinal tract—he came to the conclusion that the extraction of diseased teeth or the removal of infected tissues constituted an appropriate form of therapy. At the Trenton hospital Cotton pursued aggressive surgical therapies, including such major procedures as colectomies. Although few psychiatrists carried the focal infection theory to such extremes, many accepted at least its partial validity.

Without doubt the most significant therapeutic innovation of the 1920s grew out of the work of Julius Wagner-Jauregg, an Austrian psychiatrist who eventually received the Nobel Prize in 1927 for his work. Early in his career Wagner-Jauregg noted that mental symptoms occasionally disappeared in patients ill with typhoid fever. His observation led him in the late 1880s to undertake a study of the effects of fever on psychoses. For several decades he experimented with various means of inducing fever in psychotic patients and ultimately became interested in inducing malaria to produce the desired effect. During World War I Wagner-Jauregg obtained blood from a soldier infected with malaria and inoculated a number of paretic patients. The results appeared highly promising.

Wagner-Jauregg's work received an enthusiastic reception in the United States and Europe. Fever therapy, along with the use of such arsphenamine substances as tryparsamide, became the dominant mode of therapy in cases of paresis (the tertiary stage of syphilis, which accounted for about one-fifth of all male first admissions to mental hospitals). Their popularity was understandable. Both therapies were capable of being administered to large numbers of patients in institutions with only a modest medical staff, and both seemed to be based on a rational and scientific foundation. In one case, a specific substance killed the spirochete; in the other, a general reaction of the immunological system produced similar results. Throughout the 1930s, interest in fever therapy persisted.

The most striking therapeutic innovation of the 1930s was the introduction of what became known as "shock" treatment. The technique was originally developed by Manfred Sakel, a Viennese physician, who had observed mental changes in diabetic drug addicts whom he had treated with insulin. Sakel then employed the procedure on psychotic patients, especially schizophrenics. The injection of a sufficiently large dose of insulin drastically lowered the sugar content of the blood and thus induced a hypoglycemic or "shock" state. About the same time that insulin shock therapy came into use, Ladislas von Meduna, a Hungarian physician, developed a kind of variation on the technique that utilized a drug to induce convulsions in schizophrenics. The origins of this approach lay in his observations that epileptics were rarely schizophrenic; that convulsive attacks in schizophrenia had beneficial therapeutic results; and that epilepsy combined with schizophrenia seemed to have a brighter outlook for recovery than epilepsy without schizophrenia. Eventually Meduna settled on metrazol, a powerful drug capable of causing convulsions.

Between 1937 and 1940 the use of insulin and shock therapy swept across the United States with startling rapidity. The popularity of such a therapy was understandable. First, it was somatic and did not rely on verbal communication or vague environmental modifications. Second, psychiatrists were predisposed toward any therapeutic approach that offered some hope for schizophrenics. Third, it could, with care and discrimination, be used for substantial numbers of institutionalized patients. Finally, it harmonized with the medical model of mental disease, thus reinforcing the medical legitimacy of psychiatry. Concerned with some of the side effects and dangers of insulin and metrazol treatment, psychiatrists were quick to adopt electroshock therapy when that technique was introduced toward the end of the 1930s.

Nowhere was the receptivity toward radical therapies better illustrated than in the introduction and acceptance of prefrontal lobotomy. Developed by Dr. Egas Moniz in Portugal in 1935, prefrontal lobotomy was employed in the United States by Walter Freeman and James W. Watts at the George Washington University Hospital in 1936, and its use spread gradually.

Such aggressive therapeutic interventions posed serious ethical and scientific questions. Most of the innovations were empirical in nature and often lacking any rational or theoretical foundation. Even more important, the alleged claims of success were not based on sophisticated evaluations that carefully compared outcomes in both treated and untreated cases and also took into consideration the effect of a spirit of hope that accompanied all new interventions. Finally, few psychiatrists were aware of the ethical issue of using untested procedures on patients who lacked power and basic legal rights. In an early critique of aggressive therapies, Oskar Diethelm of the New York Hospital deplored in 1939 the activist bent of his colleagues and called for the imposition of experimental controls. In arguing for restraint, Diethelm implicitly criticized his fellow psychiatrists. "It is important in medicine," he observed, "to recognize fully the responsibility with regard to those who follow voluntarily, that is physicians; to those who follow blindly, that is lay people; and to those who are forced to follow, that is patients." The pleasure of being a pathfinder, he warned, was "alluring but leads to all the dangers of adventure."[2] In their correspondence, many of the leading psychiatrists of the interwar era echoed Diethelm's reservations.

Although most psychiatrists welcomed the new somatic therapies, they were far less enthusiastic about Freud and psychoanalysis. Despite the broad public interest in Freudian ideas in the interwar years, psychoanalysis had virtually no impact on patients in traditional mental hospitals. A few leading figures, including William A. White and Smith Ely Jelliffe, were enthusiastic supporters, but even they recognized the limitations of psychoanalysis in large institutions. Apathy or hostility were the characteristic reactions of the bulk of American psychiatrists to Freud and his followers.

Trained as physicians, psychiatrists rarely countenanced the thought of doing nothing with their patients. Even when conceding that they lacked effective diagnostic tools or classification systems, they were reluctant to express negative views on the future of their patients. Their optimistic outlook was evident in the writings of William Alanson White, who sought to bridge the gap between psychiatry and psychoanalysis. In the following correspondence White expressed his commitment to therapeutic optimism.

2. Oskar Diethelm, "An Historical View of Somatic Treatment in Psychiatry," *American Journal of Psychiatry*, 95 (1939): 1165–79.

W. A. Robison to William A. White, February 24, 1917 (WAWP).

I have learned thro Dr. Smith Ely Jelliffe, New York, that you are employing Freudian psychology in psychiatry in your hospital, and I am very desirous of learning with what success you are meeting—especially in the dementia Praecox paranoid cases.

I have started a fight for its adoption in the hospitals of my state, which are at present under the sole domination of strictly orthodox practitioners of materia medica.

William A. White to W. A. Robison, March 6, 1917 (WAWP).

I have your letter of the 24th ult. in re the use of Freudian psychology in this hospital. In response to your request for information I may inform you that for some considerable time past we have been attempting to deal with mental diseases from the psychological viewpoint. If you are acquainted with the history of the care of the so-called insane in this country you will know the remarkable fact that it is only in the past few years that mental diseases have been treated as mental diseases. They have more usually been treated as evidences of physical disorder. We have been approaching the subject from a mental point of view for a long time, and in recent years have gone at it from a psychotherapeutic standpoint. We have followed Professor Freud's work and are using his psychoanalytic methods, without, however, dogmatizing about it or allying ourselves with any special cult.

Our results it is naturally pretty difficult to formulate. A number of cases of very severe types of psychosis have gotten well and gone back to a constructive and productive life, and it would seem that their getting well has been because they were helped along those ways. The critic, of course, would say they would have gotten well anyway, and it is pretty hard to reply to such a statement. What would have happened is always difficult to tell. Aside from the effect on the particular patient, however, the effect upon the general attitude of the hospital towards the patient is exceedingly helpful. Mental diseases have ceased to be stupid affairs to be called by a certain name and then forgotten. They are getting to be filled with interest, and the medical officers themselves profit by the work, I am sure, in very great degree. This profit, of course, also is reflected all along the line and raises the standard of understanding and appreciation of the mental reactions to a higher notch.

William A. White to Dr. E. Stanley Abbot, November 4, 1920 (WAWP).
I have your very good letter of the third instant with reference to reading a
paper at the Medico-Psychological Association. I hesitate in these busy
days to promise papers which require so much time and thought to prepare. I have done so in recent years and then never been able to get around
to their presentation. However, it is my present intention to be in Boston
at the next meeting and take an active part in the discussion. The Dementia
Praecox problem interests me very much and I should like to contribute to
the symposium. Naturally in my busy administrative job I hardly have time
for prolonged analyses of Praecox cases, and so could hardly present a case
as you suggest, but I have given considerable thought to the Praecox problem and there are certain aspects of it which I would be very glad to consider briefly, two in particular, one diagnostic, and the other therapeutic.
On the diagnostic side I feel that we have no reliable criteria of diagnosis,
but I have a suggestion to make as to the direction in which to look for
such criteria. On the therapeutic side I feel that the pessimism, voiced for
example by Freud, as to the impossibility of improving the Praecox by
treatment, is not warranted. I should be very glad to incorporate these
ideas in a short paper which we might call tentatively "Some Considerations Bearing on the Diagnosis and Treatment of Dementia Praecox." . . .

---

*Beginning about 1919 Dr. Henry Cotton (1869–1933) of the Trenton State
Hospital, who was a former student of Adolf Meyer at Worcester State Hospital
in Massachusetts, began to publicize his belief that chronic, masked, or focal infections played a very important role in the etiology of mental illness. He also
claimed striking therapeutic successes through the removal of allegedly diseased
teeth and other infected tissues located in the stomach or intestinal tract. The
private reaction of most of the leaders of the specialty was decidedly negative.
Questions about Cotton's radical therapies (which included routine colectomies)
led to an investigation by Dr. Phyllis Greenacre (Meyer's associate at Johns
Hopkins) in 1924 and 1925. Greenacre's report, which remained private, discredited Cotton, who nevertheless remained in office until 1930. At that time
S. Katzenelbogen, also of Johns Hopkins, prepared another devastating report.
The trustees of Trenton State Hospital, although permitting Cotton to remain
at the institution as director of research until his death in 1933, virtually halted
the use of surgical procedures as a therapy for mental disease. The following
letters and documents provide insights into the debate over this controversial*

therapy. Especially noteworthy was the absence of any effort to restrain Cotton's right to employ aggressive therapies or to debate the issue of patients' welfare and rights.

> William A. White to Dr. L. M. Jones (superintendent, Georgia State Sanitarium), September 26, 1919 (WAWP).

I have your letter of the 24th instant. You ask my opinion about what I think of the teeth as causes of mental illness. My opinion is that the emphasis that has been laid upon infected teeth is a most unfortunate one. I believe that anything that impairs the general health of the individual may be a factor in causing a mental break, when naturally the break will occur along the lines in the personality make-up which are weakest. This of course does not mean that everybody who is mentally ill ought to have their teeth all pulled. I can conceive that it would be quite difficult to establish any connection oftentimes between infected teeth and poor health, and I am sure that people may have apical abscesses without any special involvement of their general health. We have at the present time two resident dentists and one consulting dentist. We are contemplating increasing this force perhaps by another man. We have 3500 patients and naturally there is a good deal of dental work to be done. We have X-ray apparatus and X-ray the mouths where necessary.

We have a visiting eye, ear, nose and throat specialist who spends half a day each week at the hospital and makes such examinations and gives such treatment as is necessary.

> J. K. Hall to Dr. Albert Anderson, July 27, 1922 (JKHP).

I have before me in manuscript form two papers which are going to be published in [the] August issue of *Southern Medicine and Surgery*. One is by Dr. Charles A. L. Reed, Cincinnati, and the title of the paper is "Diagnostic Surveys by Diagnostic Commissions for Asylum Populations." Reed would take entirely out of the hands of asylum doctors all examinations and diagnostic work on the patient. He would do this, I believe, because he thinks that asylum physicians are not in harmony with his theory about the relationship existing between infection and insanity, and for the further reason that he does not regard the asylum doctor as having sense and skill enough to make a proper physical examination.

The other paper is by Dr. Henry A. Cotton, of Trenton, New Jersey, and the title is "Focal Infection the Cause of Much Mental Disturbance." I think this is the paper that he had at McNairy's meeting last April. I do not know what the degree of relationship is that exists between focal infection as a causative factory of insanity, but I do believe that Cotton and Reed are both infected with red ants—Reed the more so. Cotton's theory and work is doing some good, but, in my opinion, it is doing more harm, because he is having lots of people deprived of their teeth and a portion of their alimentary canal that is probably useful to them. And then the worst feature of his preachment is that he raises hopes in the minds of relatives of insane people that cannot be realized. Cotton is unjudicious in his attitude and unsound in his reasoning. Of course, he finds foci of infection in insane people, but this is not conclusive proof at all that the nest of infection is the cause of the insanity. If I were to examine all the people in the world who have blue eyes I would probably likewise find foci of infection, but nobody of sense would be willing to believe that the foci of infection were the cause of the blue color of the iris. The world has been overflowing for the last few years with lots of damn fool theories, and I think it important for the welfare of humanity that some of us doctors at least retain what little sense we have and try to keep our feet on the ground.

By the way, I have to tell you a little joke which I heard from Rev. M. L. Kesler, which I think is apropos to the matter about which I am writing. My friend Kesler, you know, is rather long of leg and somewhat ungainly in appearance, like the Great Emancipator, and he is like the Great Emancipator in the respect also that he has nothing at all in his head except good sense. Luther Kesler was telling me and one or two other doctors at McNairy's meeting, that Abraham Lincoln was once asked by a gentleman—and Lincoln probably realized that the question was being put in a critical and somewhat reflective and perhaps in a more or less personal way—how long a gentleman's legs should be. Lincoln was apparently lost in reverie for a few moments and then he replied that he supposed a gentleman's legs ought to be long enough always to keep his feet on the ground. There are a good many short legged men in the world and unfortunately some of them are in the medical profession, and a few of them are psychiatrists.

Now, as Mr. J. P. Caldwell once said to me when getting down to his knitting, most of Cotton's attitude and all of Reed's attitude toward the present practice of psychiatry constitutes a reflection on the manner in which patients in State Hospitals are treated. Reed is so bold as to declare that patients in these institutions are not treated at all, and for that reason he advocates the arousal of public opinion to such a pitch that the examination, diagnosis and treatment of insane patients shall be taken entirely out of the hands of the present State Hospital authorities. There is undoubtedly a good deal of criticism of State Hospitals among the people today. Some of this criticism is well founded; a good deal of it is not. It will be a tragic affair, however, for the citizenship of the state to lose confidence in those men who have charge of their insane relatives in State Hospitals, and this tendency to indulge in unjust criticism of these State Hospitals ought to be combated and corrected. I am going to reply in my editorial department to both of these papers and to the general tendency as outline[d] by these papers. I am therefore obliged to call upon you for some data. I ought to know, in the first place, the number of patients that you have in your hospital each day; I ought to know the number of admissions, men and women separately, for a year's period; I ought to know the number of deaths for a year, men and women separately; and I ought to know out of the number that were admitted to your hospital during the last calendar year, for instance, just how many of these admissions were discharged from the hospital as recovered, or at least as able to return home and begin work again. This inquiry about recovery has reference to recoveries out of those actually admitted during a given period, and then I should know how many doctors are connected with the hospital, including you, how many nurses and attendants help in caring for the patients, and I ought to know what it costs a year to keep a patient in the State Hospital, and what it costs a day to keep a patient in the State Hospital. I ought to know also what you are doing in a medical way and what you are trying to do for your patients physically and mentally and spiritually. If you are not doing as much as you would like to be doing for the patient, I ought to know why this is the case. Is your Medical Staff too small, and your nursing force inadequate? If so why? Does the state not give you money enough to run the institution as it ought to be run. In other words, in answer to Cotton and Reed, if the patients in the insane asylums in the United States are not adequately and properly and intelligently treated is it because of laziness and ignorance of the doctors who have charge of these patients or is it because the states do not appropriate enough money for the proper care of these patients? Please tell me how big your medical staff ought to be; how large your nursing force should be, and what equipment you should have that you have not got. I ought to know something also about the adnexa; the industrial features of your hospital; the work shop, the laundry, the farm, the live stock, etc, etc, etc. Time is getting short and if I am to controvert Brother Reed and Brother Cotton I ought to have the data as soon as possible. If you will furnish me with the proper information I shall try to give them both hell, because I do not propose to see the State Hospitals unjustly assaulted. I do not believe that Reed's and Cotton's theories are true and I do not propose for the people of North Carolina to come under the influence of untruths if I can prevent it.

William A. White to J. G. Whiteside (secretary to U.S. Senator T. H. Caraway), November 14, 1922 (WAWP).

I have your letter of the 13th instant. You ask me about the work of my very good friend, Dr. Cotton. Dr. Cotton is one of the most enthusiastic and energetic workers in the field of psychiatry in this country, but like all forceful men who have ideas of their own he necessarily finds himself out of agreement with a good many of the profession, including myself. He attempts to cure mental diseases on the theory of its at least very frequent origin from some source of infection, such as the teeth, the tonsils, and the intestinal tract. My own personal view is that while there is some warrant for such a belief, which I am perfectly willing to admit, that Dr. Cotton goes to extremes in his views. In other words, I, myself, am not a believer in his theories, except that I am willing to acknowledge that here and there a patient may become mentally involved from such causes. I do not believe, however, that any such number of cases of mental illness are traceable to such causes as Dr. Cotton does. I would therefore hesitate a long time before I would subject an individual to the serious disfigurement of having all of her teeth pulled or to the dangers of a surgical operation, involving a removal of a considerable portion of the intestinal tract. I should want to be thoroughly convinced of the connection between any signs of infection in these territories and the actual mental disease, and it is just this connection which I fail to see in most of Dr. Cotton's work.

William A. White to Dr. A. T. Hobbs, March 7, 1924 (WAWP).

I am informed by Dr. Haviland that you would like a statement of my feeling toward the work of Dr. H. A. Cotton on focal infections, in order that you may gather from it and other similar statements the attitude of American psychiatrists toward Dr. Cotton's work for presentation at the Annual Meeting of the British Medico-Psychological Association, next spring. I take it that what you wish from me is a general statement telling you how I feel about the whole matter rather than a discussion of the specific details involved. A very comprehensive and pains-taking effort in this latter direction was made, as you know, by Doctors Kopeloff and Cheyney, whose published results are available in the same number of the *American Journal of Psychiatry* in which Dr. Cotton's presentation of his own case is set forth, namely the number for October 1922.

As you may know, for a number of years, I have been writing and talking about the necessity for considering the organism as a whole and proceeding upon the hypothesis that no adequate understanding of mental disease will ever be had except as it proceeds upon this basic assumption: that there is no way of understanding the psyche and its various manifestations either in health and disease,—no way of appreciating its placement in a general biological scheme of things, except as we study its evolution from this standpoint, and when we do this we must necessarily come to a realization that the history of the psyche is as old as the history of the body and that the two are never separate, but merely different aspects of the living organism. It is only from this broad biological point of view that psychiatry can be assured of its proper place and its progress based upon firm grounds. Recognizing the inextricable interrelations of somatic and psychic phenomena as expressions of the living organism as a whole, it is manifestly as illogical and as dangerous for future progress to approach the problems of that organism exclusively from either the somatic or the psychic side. Mental medicine needs to know very much more about the organic constitution and physiological functions than it has in the past and internal medicine needs to know very much more about psychological states, antecedents and mechanisms than it has known in the past. This very briefly and inadequately is my point of view and it can be seen readily how, from this point of view, I cannot bring myself into sympathy with the work of Dr. Cotton, who excludes, to all intents and purposes, entirely, everything from consideration on the mental side except that he makes certain conventional diagnoses of his patients, classifying them as dementia praecox, manic-depressive psychoses, etc. From that point on the entire discussion leaves the mental condition of the patient out of consideration and the results are expressed in statistical summaries. To my mind there cannot possibly be any satisfactory communication established between these two aspects of his patients so long as this hiatus remains, and any argument to prove his position, based upon further figures of the same character, leaves me cold, especially in the face of Kopeloff and Cheyney, previously mentioned, which from the same starting point, namely the conventional diagnoses and proceeding with the same technique, arrive at results which prove precisely that nothing has happened as a result of removal of focal infections except what would normally be expected in such types of psychoses. The hiatus between the conventional diagnoses and the statistical summary is, I am quite willing to grant, one of exceeding difficulty to fill in, and yet the existence of a difficulty cannot justify the unequivocal acceptance of conclusions which avoid it. Dr. Lewis, at this Hospital, has conducted an extensive investigation of the organ constitution of dementia praecox patients dying here. As a result we have become convinced that at least the malignant types of praecox that die in public institutions show consistently marked organ inferiority. Mott called attention to this inferiority as expressed in the gonads. It has been found in our autopsies there also and in addition there has been found inferiority of the thyroid and of the adrenals and of the circulatory system as a whole expressed by small heart, small vessels, etc. These inferiorities we believe are without question constitutional and not traceable to later disease. Our theory of the nature of praecox, therefore, takes into consideration these findings and is based in part upon the belief that praecox is fundamentally defectively organized organically, and that in a general way at least the malignancy of the praecox reaction is based upon the degree of organ deficiency. From such a point of view it can be readily seen how the results that Dr. Cotton claims cannot be understood by us as resulting for the reasons which he sets forth. We cannot believe that the removal of focal infection, no matter how carefully or thoroughly it be done, can affect the constitutional organic make-up of the individual. It of course might remove sources of ill health and therefore place him in a better position to take advantage of his functional capacities to the full, but this would only mean an added margin, usually a very small one, of adjustment, and I confess it is quite difficult for me to see how some of the confessedly or at least apparently very inconsiderable infections which are dealt with by Dr. Cotton have any very material effect upon the gross output of the individual. I do not understand the figures which Dr. Cotton gives. I cannot fit his extraordinary percentages of recoveries with my concept of what is going on in these patients. I can only wonder at what the explanation may be and I can see no way of arriving at a satisfactory explanation without actual first hand contact with the material. For example, I can well imagine that the publicity which has been given to Dr. Cotton's work may easily have attracted a large number of patients of the very mild types of psychoses and psychoneuroses who would under ordinary circumstances have made at least reasonably good adjustments spontaneously. I merely suggest this as a possible explanation. I have not the remotest idea whether it does explain any of the results in part or whole, or whether it does not.

Without prolonging this letter inexcusably, I may add that I feel very deeply that the work of Dr. Cotton has been exceedingly unfortunate for the cause of psychiatry. As I said in my introduction, the exclusive centering of the attention upon either the body or the mind of a sick individual is in my opinion a serious scientific error, and whether or not Dr. Cotton himself personally believes that all the problems of psychiatry can be solved from a somatic approach the implications of his work as it appears in print clearly warrant that assumption. Not only that, but they warrant the assumption that it is not even necessary that a complete organic and functional survey of the individual be made but that only detailed investigation along certain highly specialized, specific lines is necessary, namely along the line of investigation that is calculated to uncover focal infections, particularly in the teeth, the tonsils and the gastro-intestinal tract and also the genito-urinary tract. The individual as a whole, in other words, has shrunk to these proportions. I cannot conceive from my own point of view how such results can be accepted by the scientifically trained mind, and on the other hand I am sure this is a fair statement of the implications of Dr. Cotton's writings. Psychiatry becomes but an adjunct or the handmaiden of the gastroenterologist, the genito-urinary surgeon and the dentist, and man's crowning glory, his mind, receives no further consideration than this. Dr. Cotton's work, as it has appeared to us in the literature, with all the implications as they seem to me, I consider most profoundly unfortunate for psychiatry.

Adolf Meyer to Dr. R. Gjessing (Norway), January 27, 1927 (AMP, Series I).
Your most interesting and, I think, eminently fair account of your Trenton experience came just before I was pinched by a kind of "flu." Hence my slowness in reply.

Our investigation of a series of Dr. Cotton's cases did not give us the impression as if his own figures could be anywhere near correct. In principle I feel there is something to be expected. But the actual survey makes one feel that much of the result is due to the atmosphere of action and helpfulness which pervade the place, and that the diagnosis and estimation of the condition in the discharged cases is strongly colored by a policy rather than a painstaking scrutiny of the cases. I still feel that it is most deplorable that there is not the most careful control of the work made possible. Such an experiment will hardly ever become possible again. It takes the energy and also the onesidedness of Dr. Cotton to carry it through to the full extent.

Our very conservative attitude at the Phipps Clinic probably errs in the other direction. I am simply determined not to act without evidence and definite indications. I am not an obstructionist. Your young colleague, Dr. Anthonisen, whom I shall expect by October 1st, will, I hope, find the opportunities for work to his taste—a critical determination to demonstrate one's reasons and facts for therapeutic ventures.

If our reports ever get released, I shall send you Dr. Greenacre's account. We do not want to publish it without Dr. Cotton's side. He is, I think, working on it.

S. Katzenelbogen, "The Trenton State Hospital," c. late 1930
(mss. in AMP, Series I).

The object of my visit to the New Jersey State Hospital was to see how Dr. Cotton applies the conception of focal infection in his work with patients. He claims that infection of teeth occurs in practically 100 per cent of his patients; infected tonsils in about 80 per cent; involvement of the gastro-intestinal tract with consecutive toxemia in about 88 per cent of cases with the so-called "functional mental disorders"; finally infection of the sinuses and the genito-urinary system are to be found very frequently.

Without considering the problem of correlation, i.e., whether infected foci are incidental, contributing or essential factors in mental disorders, one cannot help being startled by the strikingly high percentage of cases in which infection was found in one or another system, as indicated by Dr. Cotton's statistics.

I was willing, however, to grant that the discrepancies between his findings and the general impression of other clinicians dealing with general medicine and psychiatry may be due to the fact that hardly any one has been so persistent and thorough in searching for infections of different organs, as Dr. Cotton has proven to be. *My primary interest, therefore, was to learn the means and ways which in the hands of Dr. Cotton have proven to be so remarkably effective in detecting septic foci.* The disclosure of the latter is imperative, it has been contended, for the reason that the "defocalization," by ridding the organism of the continuously invading poisons, would represent the only logical and effective treatment. With regard to this contention the following should be emphasized: In view of the fact that the treatment of defocalization comprises procedures which unavoidably cause the patient, to say the least, great inconveniences, such as being deprived of the teeth, and moreover, this treatment includes surgical interventions (laparectomy among other operations), one should require first of all, definite evidence that the organs considered to be involved are the seat of septic foci. For, it is well understood that Dr. Cotton ascribes the therapeutic results not to the above mentioned procedures as such, *comprising traumatic shock and in most cases general anesthesia,* but to the removal of [the] septic area and the thereafter following detoxication. On the other hand, in dealing with such drastic and risky therapeutic procedures one would quite naturally expect a very cautious consideration of each individual case, as to the possible evolution of the illness, consideration which would lead to the very inconvenient in their consequences interventions (pulling out the teeth), and particularly to dangerous operations, only as a last resort. With these ideas in mind I followed the work of Dr. Cotton and his associates. My observations were made at the following sources:

1. Staff meetings
2. Rounds with Dr. Cotton and staff
3. Laboratories and special departments for diagnosis and treatment
4. Charles Hospital (Private Hospital in Trenton which is provided almost entirely with Dr. Cotton's private patients)
5. The routine handling of the patient.

I. *Observations made at the Staff Meetings*

Usually three or four cases are presented for discussion. The patients are brought in after the record is summarized by the ward physician. The medical director or any member of the staff is entitled to examine the patient. A discussion follows and the diagnosis agreed upon is given to the stenographer by the medical director. The meetings take place every day and usually last about one hour.

In the presentation of each case I was struck by, to my mind, the very unsatisfactory examination of the mental status. I had the feeling that the work was done by someone who had had a very insufficient training in psychiatry or no training at all. More noteworthy is the fact that neither the medical nor the clinical director had shown sufficient interest in the psychiatric problem. I should like to emphasize this point for the following reason: In these conditions one is justified in believing that the statistics referring to the recovery rates in certain psychotic types may contain inaccuracies as to the diagnostic grouping of the cases.

Still more questionable may be the evaluation of improvement in view of the fact that the psychiatric examination is obviously inadequate. I must add that I was told by the members of the staff who worked for years under Dr. Cotton that there has been absolutely no change in the formulation of the cases since his resignation. Besides, members of the staff including Dr. Cotton, do not conceal their contempt for psychiatry *in so far as it does not subordinate the psychic status to the physical condition*. Their slogan, of which they are proud, is: treat the physical condition and the patient will recover from the secondary mental disorders.

The physical examination is done by the ward physician. As the records show it can hardly be credited with being nearly as completely and thoroughly done as one would expect from physicians who boast themselves of doing "medical" and consequently good psychiatric work and not merely "psychiatric work." The clinical examination is supplemented by a special survey of the mouth and throat by the dentist and the nose-throat man. The routine laboratory examinations in each patient are: a) g.i., X-ray (barium enema); barium by mouth very often; b) X-ray of the teeth in each case; c) gastric secretion very often. *Blood count,* including differentiation; Wa; *Blood chemistry:* Ca, glucose, chloride, alcali reserve. *C.S.F.:* cells, Wa, globuline; *Urine;* ab., etc. and microscopic examination. Also an electrocardiogram is being taken almost in every patient. A specialist in electrocardiography comes twice a week to the hospital to read the electrocardiograms. All these examinations are carried out, as I said, routinely. No one on the staff seems, however, to be sufficiently trained in physiopathology to be able to attempt an interpretation of the laboratory data and their possible correlation to the physical and mental findings in a given case. Following strictly the routine established by Dr. Cotton, his associates do not seem to take an interest in any other inquiry outside of the routine, even when the inquiry would appear strongly indicated in a given case. Thus, in accordance with Dr. Cotton's observation, N.P.N. and urea in blood have been found to be normal in almost all of his cases in the Hospital; these analyses are therefore, no longer being carried out in a routine way. . . .

I was also impressed by the frequent findings of hypocalcemia and acidosis. It became clear to me when I learned that Dr. Cotton considers blood Ca 9 mgm. per cent, as hypocalcemia and alcali reserve 60 as acidosis. Although he recognizes that in accordance with the common opinion normal Ca lies within 9–11 mgm per cent and normal alcali reserve between 52–75, still he sticks to his own standards, evidently for no other reason than that they fit the theory better. If it seems logical that infection should induce certain blood alterations, and the latter cannot be elicited in the light of the generally accepted normal standards, then it is again logical to admit that there is something wrong with the normals. "Besides, everything is clear in the light of the conception of focal infection; the latter is responsible for mental and physical disorders." That is what constantly comes out in the discussion with Dr. Cotton and his associates. In a conversation with the acting medical director he made the following statement: "Thanks to the concept of focal infection medicine becomes simple and every blacksmith will be able to practice it." This "simplicity" comes out in the usual diagnostic formulation: The diagnosis "Septic psychosis" is invariably put to the front. The type of psychosis is given as sub-title. "Defocalization" is consequently on the top of the various therapeutic procedures.

II. *Rounds with Dr. Cotton and Staff.*

Going through the surgical division I felt like being in a general hospital. Patients who had their teeth, tonsils removed, or had other surgical interventions kept quiet. The operation plus the anesthesia and the consecutive sickness quiets them, I thought. One is also favorably impressed by the work of the nurses, evidently well trained. They have here a school for nurses with a two years' training in this hospital and one year in a general hospital. Besides, the work they do here is exactly the same as in medical and surgical wards. Also the attendants do their work intelligently; apparently they are recruited from a better educated class than those of the Springfield State hospital, for instance. The nurses present some notes on the behavior of the patients, usually once a month, which go into the record. They do mainly as the physicians themselves, "real medical work, not like in other psychiatric institutions," according to the clinical director.

In my rounds with the ward physicians in other divisions I got quite a different impression. First of all, I felt sad, seeing hundreds of people without teeth. Only very few have sets of false teeth. The hospital takes care as to the pulling out of the teeth, but does not provide false teeth. In answering my question whether food is specially prepared for these patients, Dr. Cotton told me that they "get along all right with the ordinary food, gaining weight." Otherwise these already "defocalized" patients looked to me not different from those in the Springfield Hospital. "These patients will get well, when the poisons have been eliminated; you cannot expect it immediately after the cleaning up of the infections foci," I was told. They also explained to me that the improvement of the physical condition is to be expected before the recovery or improvement of the mental condition! . . .

In the State Hospital since the resignation of Dr. Cotton cholectomies have so far not been done. Dr. Stone does not seem to be enthusiastic about it and moreover by not favoring these operations he is sure to please the two boards of directors—The State and local boards. He continues doing laparatomies for release of adhesion. He is also, generally speaking, guided by the indications above mentioned but he requires more definite radiological signs of abnormality—and, as I was told, laparatomies are being performed much less frequently under the new directorship.

Routine Treatment.

1. The routine "defocalization" consists in: a) Removal of tonsils in each case except old senile patients; b) The extraction of the teeth is being done in the great majority of cases. Not infrequently they are prevented from pulling out all the teeth by the patient or by the relatives. This happens now much more frequently than it used to be with Dr. Cotton as medical director, for he invariably succeeded in getting permission in those cases in which nobody else on the staff could. The relative decrease of the number of cases with complete extraction of teeth is also due to the fact that under Dr. Stone's directorship the dentist has the last word in deciding upon extraction. The dentist is not quite so radical as Dr. Cotton is, but I felt from my interviews with him and from following his work that he also is quite badly infected with the idea of focal infection and is extremely easy in deciding upon extraction. Dr. Cotton told me that he had a hard time to persuade the dentist to adopt his views on the indications of extractions, but he apparently succeeded finally. c) Sinuses are found to be infected in about 25% of these cases and consequently washed and drained. d) The electrical coadulation of the cervix is being done quite frequently. e) The release of abdominal adhesions and cholectomy also enter into "defocalization," in accordance with the concept that the intestines are infected by stasis, although it is being done in cases in which there are no marked functional disturbances of the g.i. tract or none at all. As I mentioned above indications for laparatomy are sought in the radiological picture. *But the main motive is, on one hand the non-recovery,* and on the other hand the "thorough knowledge of the pathology of the intestines" and therefore the certainty of finding abnormalities in the removed colons and adhesions on laparatomy. For my part, I would say, without malice, that in their sacred efforts to do something for the patients since "psychiatrists do nothing for them" they resort to laparatomies because there are no other available points of attack of "septic foci" after the teeth and tonsils are removed and the cervix

coagulated. The colon can be removed, at a high cost of human life, it is true, but still it can be done, why not try it since the conviction is absolute that the survived patients will get well.

The other routine therapeutic procedures are:

2. Colonic irrigations (sodium bicarbane 60 gr. in 8 gallons of water) during 15 minutes or more every other day.

3. Moss wave given every other day. These two last treatments are completed in between 2-3 months.

4. Calcium therapy which is assumed to localize the infection.

5. Fischer's solution (alcaline) on account of the "acidosis" (when the alcali reserve is at *60* and below) which is being found very frequently.

6. Typhoid vaccine in intravenous injections. They use it as a sedative in disturbed cases. The patients have fever, chills and they quiet down. Those who have insight and had once the injection are threatened with being given a second one if they do not behave. The menace works well in this direction for criminals who are sent to the hospital from prisons, either for examination or for treatment.

7. Malaria therapy is also being used quite liberally, mainly as a means to make disturbed patients, including manic ones, more manageable. . . .

COMMENTS.

From the presentation of cases in the staff meetings and my private discussions with the members of the staff, I got the impression that the purely psychiatric work is rather poorly done: This may be ascribed to the two following factors:

1. The most important, if not the only one, is that those who are responsible for the work in the Institution do not cultivate interest in psychiatric problems in the members of the staff. The concept of focal infection is self-sufficient. The accurate discrimination between different types of psychosis matters very little, for the reason that *any psychosis would be of septic origin* and the type of psychosis would be determined by the individual predisposition.

2. The members of the staff including the heads of the institution, guiding the work of the ward physicians, have apparently not had sufficient training in psychiatry or hardly any training at all. However, this seems to me to be only a minor factor, because I have reason to believe that those, who are curious about problems which do not fit into the theory that focal infection and physical disturbances in general would be the primary cause of mental disorders, must do away with their "phantasies and talking here-

sies" if they want to hold their position and make advancement. The reading of the records may give, perhaps, a less unfavorable impression as to the
study of the mental status, because they very often contain in addition to
the examinations done in the hospital, different reports on examinations
made by psychiatrists, previously to the admission. And if I am right in
contending that the psychiatric study of the cases is generally insufficient
and inadequate, then the following conclusion imposes oneself:

1. The statistics with regard to recovery, improvement and the distri-
bution of recoveries and improvements among different types of psychosis
must contain inaccuracies introduced involuntarily and with the absolute
bona fide.

2. The various departments (X-ray, dental, otolaryngological) are in
charge of men who, apparently, know their work. The laboratories are
fairly well equipped and very active. It is a general hospital which presents
the necessary facilities for medical diagnosis and care in various branches
of medicine *except psychiatry*. By that I mean that no specific psychiatric
work is being done.

3. Applying the formula that mental disorders are caused by physical
diseases and therefore should be treated by medical and surgical procedures,
they overdo very much with regard to treatment. The malaria therapy in
manic depressive psychosis, the indiscriminate use of typhoid vaccine for
intravenous injection in order to make the patient more manageable is
unfortunate.

The extraction of the teeth does great harm to those who cannot afford
to pay for a set of false teeth; and these patients are numerous. While in the
hospital they suffer from indigestions, I was told, not being able to masti-
cate the ordinary food which they get there. At home, recovered, these
poor people have the same troubles, not being in a position to choose
food which they would be able to eat without teeth. In addition, they are
ashamed of being without teeth, since in their communities it is known to
be a token of a previous sojourn in the State Hospital. They abstain from
mixing with other people, refuse to go out and to look for a job, according
to the information I got from the social workers. Thus, many of those recovered develop reactive depression.

The release of abdominal adhesions may be justified in cases of strictures
interfering seriously with function or causing pain. In resorting to such an

operation one should bear in mind that any surgical abdominal intervention may be followed by adhesions. As to the major operation of cholectomy, I know only that in general pathology it is being resorted to only in cases of carcinoma; partial resection may be envisaged in cases of extremely pronounced megacolon. Most of the treatments routinely used may thus be justly criticized. They present, however, one favorable common feature which may account to a certain extent for the claimed favorable therapeutic results. And this is what one may call aggressiveness. The patient who has some insight sees that the Doctor takes a great interest in him. Moreover he cannot help feeling that something very drastic is being done to him. The treatment induces pain, fever, chills. The patient feels quite badly during the treatment and when he comes back to the *status quo ante,* he feels comparatively improved. Also the relatives are hopeful. When improvement or recovery takes place, it is attributed to the specific treatment without considering other factors, among which time is [a] not less important healing factor. In cases of failure they find, at least consolation in the fact that the physicians did whatever it was possible to do for their patient. On the other hand, the illness induced by the drastic procedures may have some effect. One knows that diabetes may improve during a fever disease—pneumonia, for instance. (This kind of observation had led, among other factors, to the now specific proteino therapy or fever therapy.)

All the treatments are carried out on behalf of the almighty "focal infection." In many, if not in most cases it is however, hard to see evidences of the existence of septic foci in the incriminated organs. This statement meets with the objection that they know more on the pathology of the g.i. tract than the critics who have never made systematic studies and could not possibly acquire the experience allowing to detect infection and an abnormal physical condition in cases in which no marked alteration [*sic*] are to be seen, neither clinically nor by the X-ray examination. At any rate, it is only fair to give credit to Dr. Cotton for the organization of a quite unusual State hospital. It provides facilities for diagnosis and *treatment of diseases belonging to the domain of general pathology.* It is not a boarding house, but a modern hospital in which the patients are taken care of. This hospital also presents facilities for research work. It contains a wealth of material which properly used, without preconceived ideas, may be used for very enlightening contributions, particularly in the domain of the g.i. tract.

The introduction of fever therapy posed some severe problems. The malarial plasmodium in the 1920s could not be cultivated or preserved for any length of time outside the human body; thus a malarial person had to be brought together with a paretic patient. Within mental hospitals there was a risk that grew out of the use of paretic donors, since the treponema pallidum *(the organism that caused syphilis) might be introduced into the blood of patients without syphilis. At St. Elizabeths Hospital William A. White was cognizant of the dangers and refused to authorize the use of syphilitic donors, but he was one of the very few psychiatrists who evinced any sensitivity toward the risks involved in therapeutic experimentation. The following exchange occurred between White and a physician on the hospital's staff.*

Watson W. Eldridge to William A. White, June 21, 1930 (WAWP).
. . . 4. The last two malaria control cases which were inoculated about ten days ago have as yet shown no paroxysms and I begin to suspect that we are about to lose our malaria strain once more.

5. In this connection I would like again to raise the question of inoculating with malaria from paretic to paretic, as is done in all other places in this country where malaria is used, of which I have been able to get any information. This procedure would permit us to have malaria for use a great deal larger proportion of the time than the present system permits. . . .

William A. White to Watson W. Eldridge, June 24, 1930 (WAWP).
I have your weekly inspection report, dated the 21st instant. In paragraph 5 you again raise the question of inoculating with malaria from paretic to paretic, suggesting that we proceed in that way in harmony with the practice that is followed everywhere else in the country, so far as you know. In reply to the suggestion I must reiterate that I am unqualifiedly opposed to this practice. I am fully aware of the advantages you claim for it, but I am also impressed with the disadvantages of such a practice and they seem to me, as they always have, of such a nature that I cannot consent to incurring them, at least so long as malaria can be obtained from Wasserman-free donors. If the time ever comes when this is impossible then it may be necessary to take up your suggestion, in which instance I am sure that many modifications would have to be made in our methods of procedure.

Watson W. Eldridge to William A. White, June 27, 1930 (WAWP).
I have your letter of June 24th commenting on Paragraph 5, of my weekly inspection report dated the 21st instant.

In your letter of comment you state that you cannot consent to the method of malarial inoculation proposed by me "at least so long as malaria can be obtained from Wasserman-free donors."

I presume, of course, that you refer to donors who are definitely non-specific both in regard to history and physical or laboratory examinations. This at least is what I have always understood you mean. However, in view of the wording of your letter and the possible chance that you may possibly mean simply "Wasserman-free donors" I beg to call your attention to the fact that a large number of our paretics are Wasserman-free. I think that I am safe in saying that approximately fifty percent may be so classified and if they could be used as donors the difficulties of the problem would be very greatly relieved.

May I request that you consider the matter from this standpoint and let me hear further from you in regard to it?

William A. White to Watson W. Eldridge, June 28, 1930 (WAWP).
Yours of the 27th received. While I may have used the term "Wasserman-free" donors, I felt that you knew perfectly well what I meant, and your letter confirms this. My meaning was as you suggest therein, that I will only consent to the use of definitely non-syphilitic donors.

When White learned about the early prefrontal lobotomies, he expressed his views in no uncertain terms.

William A. White to Smith Ely Jelliffe, August 7, 1936 (SEJP).
One of my friends has handed me a book by Egas Monz, who is Professor of Neurology at Lisbon, entitled "Tentatives Operatoires dans le Traitment de Certaines Psychoses." Needless to say I have not read it, but I gather that the idea is about like this. Chronically psychotic patients, particularly involutional melancholias do not get well because they cannot resolve their doubts. They stick on the horns of a dilemma and they are not able to go either this way or that. The possibility of these doubts resides in the frontal lobes. Therefore by removing the frontal lobes the patient ceases to be cursed by doubt and is well. I do not know all the details, but I think they stick in something through an opening on each side called a leucotome which is for the purpose of scooping out the white matter as the name

indicates. Other methods have been used, as injecting absolute alcohol, but the point is to destroy the organ that is responsible for the conflict which cannot be resolved. I am asked to subject my patients to this operation as a legitimate experiment in therapy. I do not very often trouble you with the various propositions that are handed up to me, but here is one which I would like to have you tell me what you think of in as few words as possible. I could express the whole matter in one word, but I do not want you to do that because it would be unmailable. However, something that is worth while in this situation may have escaped me, but you naturally know my disinclination to consider the destruction of the organ in which the difficulty lies as legitimate therapy.

Sakel's introduction of insulin shock treatment posed certain dilemmas for psychiatrists. The procedure, for example, seemed at variance with basic biological principles. Sakel himself was cognizant of this anomaly but insisted that his therapy could not be evaluated by ordinary scientific standards. Nevertheless, the absence of a rational basis for the new therapy was not an argument against its use, particularly if the results were promising. Sakel provided a possible working hypothesis, though he conceded that he could be wrong. Insulin shock therapy also raised other ethical issues. Should psychiatrists be permitted to experiment with untested therapies on chronic patients? To many, the answer to this question was not clear-cut, for by the 1930s mental hospitals were filled with tens of thousands of chronic patients who appeared destined to spend the rest of their lives in institutions. If there existed even a remote possibility of helping them, should they be deprived of the opportunity? In the following correspondence a number of leading figures expressed their views.

Hans Maier (Zurich) to C. M. Hincks (general director, National Committee for Mental Hygiene), October 7, 1936 (translated from German, AFMHP).
I was delighted once again to receive from you a sign of life. I hope that you have somebody who can translate this letter into English.

As regards the insulin treatment of Sakel, I should like to write to you—naturally only in a personal way—the following.

Sakel employed insulin treatment originally in connection with morphine withdrawal cases, and we had some excellent experiences with that. Then he began in Vienna to treat schizophrenics with insulin shock. The manner and method of public advertising for this therapy was very disagreeable to me. It was immediately publicized that Sakel had found a cure for schizophrenia. (In any event it seems to me impossible that Sakel was personally responsible for this.) I therefore have been reluctant to test the results, especially since the method is not without dangers. At first, the lecturer, Dr. Max Muller of Berne, traveled to Vienna, and began a year ago in a very careful fashion to investigate the experiments. The technique is now so well developed that with careful procedures, the constant presence of a physician and well trained personnel, there no longer exists any great danger. The experiences in Switzerland indicate that in newer cases of schizophrenia of not longer than a year and a half in duration, in a certain percentage of cases—though we have not sufficient experience as yet to check up on the results with scientific accuracy—good remissions can be obtained.

We have now been using this treatment for six months and have seen approximately two dozen such cases. It is my impression that it is incorrect to talk of a cure for schizophrenia, but rather that the patients for whom this treatment is successful subsequently become psychologically well oriented. This, however, is as strange as those cases which remit spontaneously or which have been treated with narcosis. I regard insulin therapy, insofar as I am now capable of judging, when it is undertaken in a very careful manner, to be a certain enrichment of our means to obtain remissions in schizophrenia. It is therefore a parallel therapy to treatment with narcosis.

Physiologically, the method is really interesting, but not researched enough. The theoretical formulations of Sakel are not conclusive, but that, however, does not preclude practical use. In the meantime I do not believe that this sort of treatment presently has a really healing effect upon the schizophrenic process. Sometimes one also sees successes in older cases than those of merely a year and a half duration. However, this was also the case with narcosis, and indeed also occurs spontaneously. One should use this method of treatment in the future, but it is surely not a cure all for schizophrenia and in any case one should be warned against attaching all too great an optimism thereto.

I hope that this information can be of some help to you. . . .

[P.S.] Just as I had written this letter, by chance Sakel himself came to visit me and I discussed the matter with him. His views made a very good impression on me and conveys a more careful impression in his oral expressions regarding his conclusions than many of his students. Moreover, next week he departs for New York so that you perhaps may soon have an opportunity to talk with him there. His address there is in care of Dr. Schilder.

Winfred Overholser (commissioner, Massachusetts Department of Mental Diseases) to C. M. Hincks, October 27, 1936 (AFMHP).
I appreciate your thoughtfulness in sending me a copy of the letter from Dr. Hans Maier regarding the insulin shock treatment in cases of schizophrenia. Apparently this is another instance in which a form of treatment which has been effective in some cases, has been popularized and prematurely hailed as a panacea. . . .

William A. White to C. M. Hincks, October 27, 1936 (AFMHP).
I have your letter of the 26th, with enclosures. Thank you very much for them. I have a suspicion that some of these schizophrenic patients get well with insulin shock treatment and other similar methods that are exceedingly painful and disagreeable in order to get out of the sanitarium where they use such methods or at least to escape their repetition. What do you think of that? . . .

Abraham Brill to William A. White, October 31, 1936 (WAWP).
. . . As to the meeting that I was sorry you could not attend: I had all the active psychiatrists of New York there. To mention a few: Parsons, Gregory, Casamajor, Hinsie, Hamilton, Lambert, etc. Sakel was asked many questions and it seems that they were all very impressed. Parsons made arrangements to have Sakel initiate the work in the Harlem Valley Hospital. This hospital was selected because of its proximity to Glueck's place, where Sakel has obligated himself to work for some time.

Bellevue has already started to treat four cases. The Psychiatric Institute is getting ready to start some cases, and I hope that you will soon put it into operation.

Glueck gave a sort of outline of the theories in his two papers. Sakel, himself, was very enlightening; he gives the impression of being a serious-minded person who knows what he is talking about. Now, we have all of us lived thru similar seductive cures for schizophrenia. I know that is in your mind, and I believe all of us have thought of it, but after all, schizophrenia is so hopeless that anything that holds out any hope should be tried. My only interest in this matter was to bring it before people who know the problem and will not try to make capital out of it for commercial and other reasons. . . .

Adolf Meyer to William A. White, December 17, 1936 (AMP, Series I).
The hypoglycaemic treatment has been taken up by us and I shall have the daughter of Professor Wilmanns, formerly in Heidelberg, to undertake this treatment, if possible at the Springfield Hospital and first in our own Clinic. There is no doubt about the value of the attitude of seeking help on the part of the patient that gets stimulated and the results reported by my Swiss friends are of a character that make it really an obligation to try it out. When Dr. Ruth Wilmanns comes, probably in January, I shall see that she also will get in contact with you so that you can hear from her what she has been able to observe. It is quite obvious that such a technique is not the only item in the treatment.

Dr. Sakel came to see us a couple of weeks ago. He made quite a good impression. He detached himself from exclusive association with Dr. Glueck. He did not make any extraordinary claims but together with the statements of Dr. O. L. Forel and of Muller published in the Schweizerische Medizinische Wochenschrift for October, 1936, I feel not only justified but under obligation to give the matter a trial.

Dr. Ewen Cameron who was with me three years and after his work in Canada and the publication of his quantitative psychiatry is now running a number of cases at Worcester State Hospital, told me that it is important not to combine the method too quickly with aggressive psychotherapy. You probably also have seen Joseph Wortis's article in Jelliffe's Journal. I consider him a dependable person. I am quite sure that I act in harmony with my best judgment if I say that in the proper hands it is justifiable to have the matter get a conscientious trial in a public institution. . . .

Before 1920 psychoanalysis did not appreciably influence American institutional psychiatry. Those who entered the specialty by working in a mental hospital had traditional medical training and hence were rarely exposed to psychoanalytic concepts. Moreover, there was a great deal of opposition toward Freudian ideas among physicians with a neurological orientation. In the decade before and after

Freud's only visit to the United States at the famous conference at Clark University in 1909, psychoanalytic ideas began to find a small but friendly audience. Meyer's initial reaction was not hostile; he saw a parallel between Freud's emphasis on the importance of childhood experiences and his own emphasis on the uniqueness of individuals, their life experiences, and their habit disorganization. William A. White was the most prominent convert to Freud, and helped to bridge the gap between psychoanalysis and psychiatry. Nevertheless, the relevance of psychoanalytic techniques to mental hospital patients—most of whom were psychotic or suffered from somatic disorders with accompanying behavioral symptoms—remained questionable. In 1937 Abraham Myerson (1881–1948), who was associated with the Boston Psychopathic Hospital and did some notable work on the inheritance of mental disorders, polled some of the leading psychiatrists on their attitudes toward Freud.[3] The responses of J. K. Hall and Adolf Meyer reveal the range of views.

Abraham Myerson to Adolf Meyer, November 23, 1937 (AMP, Series I).
I am making a survey of the reactions of the leaders in psychiatry to psychoanalysis and I am anxious to have your classification of yourself in this respect. For my own convenience I have divided the reactions into four groups:
1. Those individuals who completely accept psychoanalysis.
2. Those who feel very favorably inclined towards it but do not wholly accept it and are, to a certain extent, skeptical.
3. Those who, in the main, tend to reject its tenets but feel that Freud has contributed indirectly to the human understanding.
4. Those who feel that his work has, on the whole, hindered the progress of the understanding of the mental diseases and the neuroses and reject him entirely.
Thank you very much for your cooperation in this matter.

Adolf Meyer to Abraham Myerson, November 26, 1937 (AMP, Series I).
I am afraid I cannot classify myself as you would like me to do. I can classify some others that way, but have to think otherwise for myself and many others.

3. Myerson reported his poll results in his article "The Attitude of Neurologists, Psychiatrists and Psychologists towards Psychoanalysis," *American Journal of Psychiatry*, 96 (1939): 623–41.

Most psychiatrists are more or less proficient and interested and active in various lines and not sold out.

Most of those who are not analysts know little of analysis, by which term I should want to imply the one or the other of the camps of analysis.

There are those who can say they are well, moderately or poorly informed, and practicing one or another method and certain concepts. I should say I am moderately to well informed, but do not practice any of the methods beyond what falls in line with what is acceptable in objective psychobiology.

I am in the main critically inclined but inquiring and keep in fairly close contact with those who practice psychoanalysis and are familiar with the developments. I may say I am unable to be a blind follower, and criticize freely some analysts and their work, and some of the methods. I might say I criticize the followers frequently, and when they are attacked by outsiders I usually find flaws in the attacker.

(3) Facts and tenets are so interwoven that I am perhaps considered inconsistent in my attitude. I occasionally send patients to "analysts" and often advise caution when asked about analysis.

(4) The fourth category leaves me with serious doubts as to the wisdom of the way the statement is formulated. All depends on the person and individual and group judgment. It has "happened," and has stirred up more than anything else an interest in human ways of seeing man and his problems. It certainly has led to interesting progress and courage of convictions and it is up to the critics to do as well or better before they take the attitude described. It has at least been articulate and keen, but not sufficiently self-continent and also not neighborly.

In all this, we might of course take a very different attitude: The propaganda has been based on the promise of the only cure, and a sure cure; it had the element of plausibility and of a vigorous protest against the rigid dogma that one should not bother with anything short of the all-or-none, and that science should make no concessions; that absolute "hard boiled" determinism could be the only acceptable condition within which science could be science. Moreover the conception was of a kind that was strictly logical and could not possibly be disproven because any falling short of the complete proof was simply an incomplete analysis something due to resistances. One is taken back to Zeno's problem and some other false applications of logic, which one should avoid like poison. On the other hand, the doctrine of free association and the repression of the "intolerable," and the escape under disguise and the "murder will out" kind of pattern gives such a "naturalistic" tang to style so very much like the adolescent freshness and smartness that the old fogies and old maids were in for their well-deserved castigation and witch's dance. Could not every unprejudiced person see sufficient evidence of analogy on all sides? Yet what of analogy? Looseness of any such magnitude tempted the Ku Klux vigilantes who "obviously" are unfair and must be reached by counter measures, etc. Most of these reactions would seem to be "beside the point," but very favorable to a display in line with modern "adolescenthood," the remedy of which would probably be time rather than indulgence in argument or force—or an appreciation of the rule of the tertium quid; not all opposites divide the whole world into two completely inclusive as well as exclusive camps. Half-truth and three-quarter truth does not satisfy the seeker of truth. It seems best to avoid adding fuel to a fire which probably will have its charm for a time and will make room for more compatible and less wild forms of oxidation.

In the meantime, there are some of us who are not afraid to give in on a "go ahead and do your worst" kind of attitude; who quietly go ahead making the extremes unnecessary and laying bare the fallacies, and creating an increasingly large number of well informed active liberals neither in the vanguard or in the rearguard, nor mere standpatters. I feel in the main it is possible to keep aloof from sham-perfectionism and also from partisanship. I feel but rarely the urge to go far ahead of the attitude of inquiry to a need of finality which will take care of its own lack of necessity. There is such a thing as critical pragmatism. I also like decisiveness where one can cut across without killing part of what should survive to yield a convincing experiment. In all this statement I seem to be more tolerant than I actually am. I should rather rest the case with my deeds than with my words alone. When "*all* is said and done," there will be but little left of the conflicting elements. Hence, this is a personal statement, to be taken as whole, and one to be taken as personal communication, as I still hope to give a comprehensive review of the situation when I'll be through with another more central formulation.

Abraham Myerson to Adolf Meyer, November 30, 1937 (AMP, Series I).
Thank you very much for your long and interesting account of your reactions to the Freudian point of view or, more broadly, psychoanalysis. I assure you that your desire to keep this personal will be respected.

Meanwhile, let me say this about my own position which perhaps is misunderstood at the present time by a good many people who know me. First, I am a great admirer of Freud. I measure greatness not by the truth or non-truth of the individual's contribution, since that is not a matter that can be easily determined if it is at all determinable. I measure greatness by the influence a man has upon the thought and deeds of his time, and measured by this standard Freud is a great man and, I believe, an honest man, perhaps one of the most honest minds that has ever been on this planet. I also believe that psychoanalysis has indirectly done a great deal of good, in that it has, first of all, made us examine the human being more closely and has compelled us to seek to strip off the mask which separates the real motivation from the assumed or asserted motivation. Moreover, it has acted as a goad in that men opposed to it or reacting against it have been impelled to do better work in their own field, let us say of physiology or biology, in order to contribute something solid to the study of the human mind.

On the other hand, I believe that the method is utterly unscientific and furthermore open to all kinds of criticisms on the basis of candid evaluation of results. Apparently the Freudians know nothing at all about control experiments. They assume the validity of their postulates and seek to prove them, which is a most vicious way of operating, if at the same time one fiercely resents as they do any attack or any criticism of the postulates. For example, I believe that the method of free association is absolutely invalid; that you can take ten words from a time-table and by free association get the same complexes from anybody that you can from the material of a dream, since there are no closed places in the flow of the mind's operations. Furthermore, there is no such thing as a free association, since all associations are conditioned by the personality of the analyst and by the reaction of the patient to that analyst, as well as the reaction of the analyst to the patient. The whole theory of sex has been built up on the most slender possible basis, etc., etc. One could go on ad lib and ad nauseam, finding holes and flaws in the doctrines. Perhaps the word doctrine accounts for a good deal of my criticism. There is no place for doctrine in medicine or in science. There is no place for the Holier-Than-Thou attitude, and there is no place for an all-embracing philosophy which independently of experimentation and fact encompasses the mental universe.

When one sums up the assets and liabilities of the movement, it is probable that on the whole there has been some good accomplished. On the other hand, it has definitely hindered some of the younger psychiatrists from studying man objectively and with the instruments of present-day science.

I believe with Lecky that errors in many fields of science or thought are not so often disproved as they become obsolete. I am quite sure the day is coming with the advance in scientific instrumentation that the personalization of complexes, of the conscious and the unconscious, and the whole range and series of ghosts and phantoms which live in man's conscious and unconscious will be destroyed by objectively measurable chemical, biological, physical, truly psychological criteria and findings.

J. K. Hall to Abraham Myerson, June 1, 1938 (JKHP).
Not daily, but oftener than weekly, I have read your communication of January 25 addressed to me as an inquiry of my opinion of the value of psychoanalysis. I have allowed your letter to lie unresponded to because I have thought myself incompetent to formulate a statement about Freud's psychiatric philosophy. Had you sought the expression of my estimation of Aristotle's philosophy, of Plato's, of Herbert Spencer's, or even of Emerson's, I think I should have remained impolitely but helplessly mute. I should have said to you perhaps merely that you had asked too much of me. I think I recall with some degree of accuracy from my college days Emerson's statement that out of Plato even today amongst men of thought comes everything worthwhile. I still think that a large statement, but I am incompetent to refute it.

It is unfortunate that the procedure has been designated psychoanalysis; as unfortunate as the reference to a particular neurotic state as hysteria. The word is ponderously polysyllabic and objectionably pedantic. Much of modern psychiatric literature is cursed by linguistic repulsiveness. The attempt should always be made, it seems to me, to make the incomprehensible less so by simplicity of language. The very word psychoanalysis has fetched into our language, often with obvious effort, other terms of foggy meaning. Yet it is possible to speak of the profound things of life in simple words. That statement is confirmed by the Twenty-Third Psalm, by the so-called Sermon on the Mount, by much of the book of Job, by Patrick Henry's "give me liberty" oration, by Lincoln's Gettysburg address, by General Lee's farewell to his army, and by the innate eloquence of many an unlettered Negro whom I have heard preach. I doubt not at all that we psychiatric folks have inhibited the flow of psychiatric knowledge amongst the members of the medical profession by using a language the quality of which was objectionable to them. And I have no doubt that the use of a ponderous term, or of a neologism, has not infrequently induced some of us to believe we know what we do not know. But one should no more blame Freud for the perversion of language used by some of his disciples than one should blame Thomas Jefferson for the Fatherhood of The New Deal.

My thought is that the contribution of Sigmund Freud to the understanding of man's immaterial attributes is as great as Charles Darwin's work in the domain of the material. Each demonstrated the mighty influence of hidden forces—in man hidden so deep within him that he did not even suspect their existence. Darwin has enabled us to understand, for example, the reason for the rare gill-slit in the new-born child; Freud has made it equally as possible for us to grasp the reason that made unavoidable the kinship betwixt the Colonel's Lady and Judy O'Grady. In spite of Freud's stout insistence upon individualism the basic feature of his philosophy is human democracy; the emphatic statement that we mortals are much more alike than unlike. And insistence upon such democracy of thought and of feeling is responsible, I doubt not, for much of the hostility directed against psychoanalysis. For if we are not all snobs we should like to be.

My notion is that Freud's gift to the world is his discovery of the unconscious and its mighty influence in motivating human conduct. Freud has structuralized and individualized the unconscious. That achievement is comparable, I should say, to Harvey's discovery of the motion of the blood and to Virchow's demonstration of cellular disease.

The conception of the unconscious not only offers an explanation of much human behaviour that would remain not understood, but through the diagnostic effort that psychoanalysis begets and through the therapy that it makes possible it serves as a sort of mystic cord that binds patient and physician together in conjoint strength and sympathy.

One of my surgical friends is wont to say there is no minor surgery though there are many minor surgeons. If emotional or psychic or spiritual traumatization result from psychoanalytic practice it should be attributed perhaps to the inept analyst and not to psychoanalysis. Unless psychoanalysis be skillfully and judiciously used I think it should not be utilized at all. I believe in the helpfulness of psychoanalysis as I believe in the helpfulness of surgery. Freud's philosophy should be made use of, diagnostically and therapeutically, in those conditions in which it is indicated and only by those who are competent to use it.

Do I not cause you to think of the voice from the whirlwind: "Who is this that darkeneth counsel with words without knowledge?"

A major figure in American psychoanalysis between World War I and II, Smith Ely Jelliffe conducted a large correspondence and served as a clearing house for information and an encouragement to many. In the following exchange he expressed his views about psychoanalysis and his doubts about its applicability to institutional psychiatry.

James T. Fisher to Smith Ely Jelliffe, February 13, 1937 (SEJP).
It has been somewhere in the neighborhood of a year since I have had the honor of hearing from you, and I was reminded of your literary work last evening when I read your illuminating article on the subject of skin. It was most attractive and pleasing to read. It showed that you had some knowledge beside your particular hobby, psycho-analysis.

We are doing some scientific work in our clinic here with the Alpha-ray, securing most remarkable results in [a] haemoto-poetic way, even to the extent of inhibiting the growth of cancer, as well as doubling the red cells to the extent of a 100 per cent in a few weeks. I am wondering if you are acquainted with this particular type of physical and mental improvement.

I would like to hear from you relative to your conception of the big movement quite evident in the west, which you also have in the east, namely, state or social medicine. . . .

Smith Ely Jelliffe to Dr. James T. Fisher, February 18, 1937 (SEJP).
What makes you so stupid? Is it the California sun or the prunes that are so abundant? Psychoanalysis is only one kind of medical tool in one's work kit and it is no hobby of mine. *Medicine* is my hobby and you ought to know it by this time.

Yes I know something about Alpha Rays and I do not expect much from any of these purely physical agents to which the body has been exposed for a billion years and in spite of them has survived.

Personally there is too much politics in State Medicine for me to take much stock in it. As a rule politicians are nasty parasites living on the social body and they tend to break down most of what the hard working, keen thinking people in the world have built up.

For one real original person in the world doing something new there are a thousand parasites who louse like thrive on the results of his thinking. Medicine has grown to be a great body of value through the individual effort of such rare individuals. State Medicine and similar movements in my humble opinion tend in the opposite direction.

I have never known a real deserving person whom a real physician has ever denied their effort at trying to help. Here the definitions of "real deserving" and "real physician" are not easy to define.

Every time bureaucracy steps in they bring the manure in with them.

I send you a bibliography in which you may perceive I have been interested in many aspects of medicine. Why don't you loosen up and subscribe to the *Journal of Nervous and Mental Disease?*

Smith Ely Jelliffe to Luisa Kerschbaumer, April 18, 1940 (SEJP).
I fear you did not understand my last letter, i.e. re. the psychoanalysis.

Psychoanalysis in a mental hospital is practically useless. One has not the time, nor are the patients in the main of the type for whom it can be used. I simply meant try some mild obsessive case and practice. They are the best patients to work with to sharpen one's teeth on the technique.

If you have a patient with a "mild hysteria" they are the easiest to trace out the displacements. The sexual symbolism does not go so deep. It is more like an open book to read.

One can often take an hysterical's dream and see it translated almost verbatim in the symptoms.

Then move on to a mild compulsion neurosis. There are probably many on the wards, who, because of economic burdens and other things, add on enough symptoms to mask the original compulsion neurosis and make an apparent schizophrenic, which they are not.

It was a group of such that years ago Laforgue and de Saussure cleared up at St. Anne in Paris that convinced Prof. Claude of the value of psychoanalysis. They had nearly all been put down as "demence precoce."

Just think about it, at least. It will be as good as painting for sublimation, maybe.

When you finish the "Handbuch," no hurry, send it to my country address—Huletts Landing, Washington Co., New York. If by express send it to: Care George Peterson, Dresden Station, Washington Co., New York.

FIVE

Mental Hygiene

The ferment within American psychiatry at the turn of the century laid the foundations for what became known as the mental hygiene movement. The idea of preventing disease, of course, was not new. Nineteenth-century Americans had emphasized prophylactic approaches. Yet there were fundamental differences between twentieth century concepts of mental hygiene and earlier concepts of prevention. The latter was based on a fusion of religious and moral values and emphasized natural law, free will, and individual responsibility. Mental hygiene, in contrast, reflected a commitment to scientific modes of thought. Since disease was a product of environmental, hereditarian, and individual deficiencies, its eradication required both scientific knowledge and administrative action. Reflecting the modern belief that experts, as a group, had the knowledge to control their environment and thus to shape human behavior, mental hygienists launched a broad based crusade to create a better society.

Shortly after 1900 the appealing but vague commitment to mental hygiene assumed a variety of forms. One such form was embodied in the National Committee for Mental Hygiene. The NCMH was indissolubly linked with the life and career of Clifford W. Beers. Born in 1876, Beers graduated from Yale in 1897. When holding several jobs, he made an abortive suicide attempt. When his mental condition deteriorated, his family first sent him to a private mental hospital and then committed him to the Connecticut State Hospital for the Insane. After his release, he decided to write about his experiences in order to aid others struggling with the problem of mental illness. His goal was nothing less than the creation of a national movement on behalf of the mentally ill. After a subsequent stay at the Hartford Retreat, Beers wrote his classic *A Mind that Found Itself,* which was eventually published in 1908.

Beers recognized that the support of eminent psychiatrists was crucial to the success of his plan. He submitted various drafts of his manuscript to a number of leading figures, including Adolf Meyer, who by this time was a leading figure on the psychiatric scene. William James also became a source of encouragement as well as financial aid to Beers, who lacked a regular and stable income. Beers viewed *A Mind that Found Itself* as the prelude to the establishment of a national organization dedicated to the improvement of conditions in mental hospitals and supported by large grants from wealthy philanthropists.

In the two years preceding the creation of the NCMH in 1909, Beers turned to Meyer for advice. Meyer initially proposed the formation of a society for mental hygiene, a suggestion that met with Beers' approval and enthusiasm. The change in title ultimately proved of major significance, for a movement to promote health had replaced one concerned with improving institutional care and treatment of mentally ill patients. That prevention of mental illness proved an attractive idea to a variety of groups was understandable. To psychiatrists, hygienic concepts opened up new vistas and shifted attention away from their custodial role and inability to cure chronic institutionalized patients. Prevention also seemed to have the virtue of hastening the reintegration of psychiatry and medicine, since it invested psychiatry with the mantle of a biologically oriented specialty and put it in step with other medical prevention movements. To the emerging profession of social work seeking both identity and status, the movement offered the hope of collaboration with physicians on a more equal plane; the goal of mental hygiene was not limited to the treatment of individuals but involved as well the promotion of specific behavioral patterns within families and larger social groupings. The organizational mode was equally attractive in an era that placed great faith in formal structures that unified science and rational administration. Above all, the goal of prevention seemed certain to attract broad support from a public concerned with the seeming rise in the incidence of venereal diseases and alcoholism. Mental hygiene, in other words, was so broad and inclusive that it aroused little opposition.

During 1908 and 1909 Beers's relationship with Meyer began to deteriorate. Meyer first urged that Beers confine his activities to a single state. Beers acceded and in 1908 founded the Connecticut Society for Mental Hygiene, but basic conflicts between the two were perhaps unavoidable. Beers believed that lay people had to play the major role in founding and administering state societies; Meyer insisted that psychiatrists had to be the controlling force. When Beers began to move toward the creation of a national organization with its own funds, Meyer became even more alienated. Beers prevailed, and in early 1909 the NCMH came into existence. Its stated goals were extraordinarily broad: the NCMH would protect the nation's mental health; promote research on the etiology, treatment, and prevention of mental illness; enlist the aid of the federal government; and establish constituent state societies. By the end of 1910 an irrevocable break had occurred between these two strong-willed men, and Meyer severed his ties with the young organization.

The creation of the NCMH was but a beginning; still to be decided was its concrete mission. Above all, the committee had to find adequate and stable sources of funding. Ultimately financial assistance came from the Rockefeller Foundation and individual philanthropists, but in amounts that merely enabled the young organization to survive precariously. In 1912 Dr. Thomas W. Salmon joined the committee, and under his direction the organization began to conduct state surveys of conditions among the mentally ill. Salmon's vision, however, transcended the institutionalized mentally ill, and he began to redirect the organization's activities in other directions. Slowly but surely the committee's concerns broadened to include a variety of dependent and defective groups and a broad range of social problems. By the 1920s the original commitment to improving conditions among the institutionalized mentally ill had all but disappeared, thereby contributing still further to the growing chasm between psychiatrists and mental hospitals.

Though both its mission and its activities were vague and ill-defined, the NCMH projected a relatively hopeful outlook. Most of its members believed that mental disease could be prevented; they did not for the most part believe that mental illness was determined by inbred genetic or unchanging character qualities. Not all of those involved with mental hygiene, however, shared such benign and optimistic views. There was a side to mental hygiene that reflected fear rather than hope. By the turn of the century a number of people had come to the pessimistic conclusion that an alleged increase in degeneracy in general and mental illness in particular threatened the biological health of the American people. Given their belief that heredity rather than environment determined culture, they supported a variety of interventionist measures designed to preserve the alleged biological superiority of Americans: marriage regulation, immigration restriction, and involuntary sterilization of the mentally unfit.

Among psychiatrists the emphasis on mental hygiene aroused some controversy. Its amorphous nature led to considerable differences of opinion.

The private correspondence of psychiatrists and others illustrates the broad range of views concerning the definition and goals of mental hygiene, what constituted appropriate means, and even doubts about its intrinsic value.

When Clifford W. Beers (1876–1943) began writing his classic autobiography, he conceived of an organization dedicated to the improvement of conditions in mental hospitals. Such a goal, of course, did not preclude other subsidiary goals, including reform of state laws pertaining to the insane, but the emphasis was on the upgrading of institutions. In the following letter to William James (1842–1910), Beers sketched out his dreams and plans.

Clifford W. Beers to William James, April 16, 1907 (AFMHP).
In advising me not to be too sure about the market success of my book, or at least to prepare myself for possible disappointment in the matter of "sales," you prove yourself a friend—almost a relative. At one time or another those conversant with my project have offered like advice. And for this reason: My advisors seem to think that I will measure the success of my book by the number of copies sold; whereas, in truth, I shall consider a large sale itself only as an indication of success, and, under no circumstances, a small sale as proof of failure, inasmuch as my revelations must of necessity tend to correct the evils disclosed.

Of more importance to me than the wide circulation of my book is the formation of a society which shall carry out the plan for reform therein set forth. Should a "National Society For The Improvement of Conditions Among the Insane," be organized, as suggested in my book—or rather, manuscript—for the "Society" should at least be incorporated before my book is published, I shall consider my work a success, even though not more than a thousand copies of my book be sold. On the other hand, the sale of one hundred thousand copies, with no "Society" in existence to conserve the interest such a wide reading of my story would surely arouse would, to my mind, spell "Failure,"—this, too, despite the profit in money that would then accrue.

Those with whom I have discussed my project one and all admit that some kind of a "Society" should take hold and work for reform along the lines suggested in my book. Today there is no existing society which could carry out the proposed reforms nearly so well as a new organization instituted for that especial purpose. Hence, the question is: What sort of an organization is needed, and how may it be brought to a working perfection?

To this question I shall now address myself. Before approaching Mr. Carnegie (as I propose to do within a month) I must provide myself with authoritative opinions supporting my contention that there is both need and room for a "National Society For The Improvement Of Conditions Among The Insane." Your opinion; that of Dr. Page, as a Superintendent of a State Hospital for The Insane, the opinion of Dr. Blumer, as the Superintendent of an endowed Private Hospital for the Insane; together possibly with the opinions of members of the New York and Massachusetts State Lunacy Commissions, and a few of the managers of the State Charities Aid Association of New York (Mr. Joseph H. Choate, Mr. Francis Huntington, Miss Louisa Lee Schuyler, et al) should place me in a position to convince Mr. Carnegie that it is his duty, as it should and probably will be his pleasure, to finance the preliminary expenses of organization at least. And who can state with the force of proof that I may not even induce Mr. Carnegie to endow the projected "Society" as liberally as Mrs. Sage has endowed the Sage Foundation!

For the purposes of illustration I can do no better than to suggest that the "National Society" be so organized as to combine certain adaptable features of the Sage Foundation and the State Charities Aid Association of New York, which latter organization has done so much to raise the standard of hospital management in the state of its origin and activity.

Briefly, the Sage Foundation has an endowment of $10,000,000 and a yearly income of over $400,000. The object of the fund, says Mrs. Sage, is "the improvement of social and living conditions in the United States." Continuing Mrs. Sage says: "The means to that end will include research, publication, education, the establishment and maintenance of charitable and beneficial activities, agencies, and institutions already established. It will be within the scope of such a foundation to investigate and study the causes of adverse social conditions including ignorance, poverty, vice, to suggest how those conditions can be remedied or ameliorated, and to put in operation any appropriate means to that end . . . the foundation will be national in its scope and in its activities."

The Sage Foundation will be administered by a board of trustees consisting of Robert W. DeForest, Cleveland H. Dodge, Daniel C. Gilman, John M. Glenn, Miss Helen Gould, Mrs. William B. Rice, and Miss Louisa L. Schuyler. These trustees have in turn appointed an active Secretary who will set in motion the machinery of the society.

So much for the Sage Foundation. Now for a possible plan of organization for "The National Society For The Improvement Of Conditions Among The Insane."

In lieu of a better name let the one suggested stand. The object of the Society shall be the improvement of conditions not only among those *actually* insane, but among those thousands working among, or related by blood or any other tie to the two hundred thousand insane patients within or without our hospitals and asylums.

The means to that end will include research, publication, education (of the public, especially), the establishment of hospitals and sanatoriums of the most modern type which shall be so managed as to give the best results at a minimum cost; the organization of efficient agencies in each state in the Union where no such Association as the State Charities Aid of New York already exists, said agencies or "state societies" to co-operate with hospital officials and to perform such duties as are now performed by members of the aforementioned "State Charities Aid."

The proposed "National Society" should have a board of trustees consisting of men and women interested in the projected reforms and capable of directing the work in question. These in turn should select and appoint an active Secretary—a man possessed of a thorough knowledge of the inner workings of such a humanitarian enterprise as the one under discussion. It should devolve upon the Secretary to organize the permanent corps of workers needed by the "Society" in the performance of its task of reform and enlightenment.

The work of the "Society" should be national in scope. The projected organization should do for the Nation what the State Charities Aid Association of New York has done for New York—it should, indeed, do more, for it will work on broader lines.

The "National Society For The Improvement of Conditions Among The Insane" could accomplish results (I adopt phrases and adapt ideas suggested by the 1906 report of the State Charities Aid Association) "through the force of an educated, enlightened public opinion," and to this end could appoint or *cause* to be appointed volunteer, local Visiting Committees, and visitors, for State and private hospitals for the insane wherever located. These visitors need have no legal power,—in fact should have no legal power beyond that "of right of entrance," granted by statute. (Such a statute is in force in the State of New York). The visitors should work under control of the Board of Managers of the "National Society," reporting through the respective heads of each state branch of the society. The

State branches, while working independently, should report annually to the State Lunacy Commission of each State, or to such other Board or individual as may have charge of the care of the insane in a given State. That this system of visitation is both feasible and beneficial, the experience of the State Charities Aid proves. Their authorized visitors have been able to establish cordial relations with the State Lunacy Commission and also with the managements of the several hospitals for the insane. At the same time they have befriended the helpless and lonely patients.

The State Charities Aid has recently begun to assist certain patients discharged from hospitals for the insane. This so-called "after care of the insane" is of vital importance. For years it has been carried on in Europe, but, as yet, in this country little has been done along this line. A "National Society" could cause to be done in every state what is now being done in New York by the State Charities Aid Association. Each hospital for the insane in this country should have an "After Care Committee" as have four State Hospitals in New York, namely, Manhattan, Willard, Binghamton and Hudson River. "After Care" agents could be employed by the National Society (as is now done by the State Charities Aid) to help all local committees. The "After Care Committee" should work in close cooperation with the State Commission in Lunacy and Superintendents of the Hospitals. This work was undertaken last year for the first time by the State Charities Aid, which fact shows how woefully behind the times the United States is in this deserving work.

A "National Society" could frame and secure the passage of needed legislation in the several states,—each state branch of the society attending to the work in its respective sphere of activity. Insanity in Maine does not differ materially from insanity in California—if it differs at all, and model laws for one state should prove to be model ones for all others. Experts—in the employ of the "National Society"—could perfect and codify the laws relating to the insane and all institutions where insane persons are confined, then, barring slight changes made necessary by local conditions, these model statutes could, through State branches of the "National Society," be submitted to the several State Legislatures for enactment into law.

A liberally endowed "National Society," being independent of official appointment and of the public treasury would be in a peculiarly secure position in the matter of shaping legislation and securing the passage of "Humane" laws. Then, too, a "National Society" could, by eliminating pernicious political influences, protect and assist the doctors working among the insane.

Now for a few personal reasons for my insisting that a "National Society" be organized before my book is presented to the public. In publishing the story of my life—revelations which most people prefer to suppress—I feel that I am doing my share of the work outlined. Though the writing of my book, and the thought of publishing it (because of the end in view) has been and is a distinct pleasure, I cannot say that I shall continue to count my impending sacrifice of privacy a distinct pleasure unless I can assure myself that my plans for reform will be carried to a successful conclusion by the projected *permanent* organization.

Though several have said that there will be time enough to organize a "National Society" after my book has been published, I cannot agree that delay will prove advantageous. On the contrary delay will very likely complicate the situation. By organizing a "Society" before publication, such agitation as may result from my revelations will be under the control of men and women of the right sort. There are in this country today many worthy but unsuccessful reformers who have tried to organize some such "Society" as I have in mind. They have all failed because they had no such document as my book on which to base their project. Shocking accounts of abuse in Kentucky, for instance, have little or no effect on natives of other states; but a story of abuse which "rings true," as mine does, to the natives of every State in the Union, will without doubt arouse interest in each State and make it easy for a "National Society" to establish "State branches" along the lines of the State Charities Aid Association of New York. Inasmuch as those who have already read my Ms. (not fewer than fifty men and women) laid it down with the feeling that they should like to do something to assist the afflicted insane, would it not be sheer folly,—yes, cruelly thoughtless, to place my book on the market before a "National Society" should be established, ready to act as a powerhouse, wherein the good impulses of interested readers might be converted into pleasure and happiness for the inmates of our hospitals and asylums?

In my story I ask the reader to sign the following pledge: "I hereby testify that I am a believer in the Humane Principle of Non-Restraint in the treatment of the insane; I desire to be enrolled as one of its Advocates; and I promise to do what I reasonably can to advance its cause and help improve conditions among 'those afflicted thousand least able to speak for themselves.'"

With no "Society" in operation what incentive will there be for a reader to sign such a pledge? Yet, a majority of readers would sign and forward said pledge to a permanent organization which would make use of it in one way or another.

Another thing: I suggest a method whereby thousands of current magazines which are now thrown away might find their way into our State Hospitals. My suggestion has been pronounced "good" and feasible by every hospital official consulted. Yet that suggestion will prove of no value unless there shall be an organization which can act as the distributing agent to the extent of tabulating the "offers" and giving direction to the donors.

As to the amount of endowment necessary at the beginning I am in some doubt. At the start no large endowment will be needed unless the "National Society" shall exercise such functions as those now exercised by the General Education Board. Yet, I am of the opinion that it is desirable that the "National Society" should, within limits, act as a "professional almoner," distributing among the several States of the Union, completely equipped Psychopathic Hospitals (Psychiatrical Clinics), provided that the State in each instance shall provide a suitable site, and an endowment, or stipulated appropriation, for the continued maintenance of the hospital. Such a gift to the State is not unlike the gift of money to an institution of learning on the condition that a stipulated amount be raised by the beneficiary. The solution of the problem of insanity depends largely upon the establishment of Psychopathic Hospitals, especially those established in connection with the Medical Departments of our Universities. In my book I quote at length, the opinion of Dr. Stewart Paton on this subject. With modern institutions of this desirable type in operation, a basis for effectual reform in the treatment and care of insanity will be obtained. Then will come the establishing of cooperative sanatoriums, which will eventually do away with the run-for-gain type of sanatoriums. These cooperative institutions can be "promoted" as it were, by the "National Society," which, through its agents, can induce men of wealth to invest their money in such business-like, philanthropic enterprises.

Inasmuch as the idea embodied in the Psychopathic Hospital is new, there being no such hospital as that at Munich in *operation* in this country today, it seems likely that the prompt solution of the problem in hand depends upon philanthropists, and philanthropic organizations possessed of a many-million-dollar endowment. Whereas many Psychopathic Hospitals might be established within five years, or less, by a liberally endowed "National Society," or by public spirited men of wealth, such hospitals will not materialize for a generation in some States if the matter be left entirely to the States themselves.

The ramifications of an organization such as the projected "National Society For the Improvement of Conditions Among The Insane" are too numerous to discuss further at this time—luckily for the reader. However, this letter, together with your knowledge of my project as outlined in my manuscript should enable you to express an opinion regarding the feasibility of my plan for a "National Society."

I shall of course value criticism, for my aim is to arrive at the best solution of the particular problem before me.

In the hope of gaining the support of American psychiatrists, Beers circulated his unpublished manuscript to a number of leading figures in the specialty. One such was Dr. William McDonald, Jr., of the Butler Hospital for the Insane in Rhode Island (one of the older and more important private mental hospitals in the nation). In the following two letters, McDonald offered his reactions to Beers' manuscript. His responses illustrated the internal perceptions of institutional psychiatry, which differed sharply from those of other groups. McDonald's comments, which were by no means unfavorable, also suggested the presence of a growing split between, on the one hand, a medical specialty that claimed authority by virtue of the training and knowledge of its members and, on the other hand, lay people, government officials, and the public.

William McDonald, Jr., to Clifford W. Beers, June 7, 1907 (AFMHP).
I have read your manuscript with great care and attention. You have asked me to criticize frankly. I have done so as the following notes will show. It may seem to you that in places I have been severe. I have however not spared parts which seemed to me weak, believing that since your work on the whole is so creditable, it would be a shame to run the risk of spoiling it by retaining paragraphs which do not bear the stamp of truth and fairness. You will, of course, understand that I make all criticisms in a spirit of fellowship and with the desire to help rather than to hinder you in your work, and I realize that for you to attempt to correct all of the paragraphs which have seemed to me to be undesirable would mean the rewriting or omission of a considerable number of pages.

I think corrections which you have thus far made cover very well the points which I have previously raised.

The first criticism which I will make is in regard to the paragraph beginning p. 67, "It is an offense," etc. Once for all let me state that I believe you will strengthen your work enormously by being a little more fair and by looking at the matter a little more from the standpoint of those who have patients in charge. For a visitor to go to a patient's room without first making known his presence to those in charge is not an unpardonable offense merely because it does not give time to see that "everything is put in good order and the patient is in a presentable condition, and surrounded by conspicuous evidences of the tender care which his relatives imagine he receives at all times," or to give the doctor in charge time "to frame a specious address," etc. etc. But I am sure, if you will stop to consider a moment, you will realize what incalculable harm would be done if there were no such rule. There are always a large number of people filled with a morbid curiosity as to patients troubled with mental disturbance. Such people again and again visit our institutions merely to satisfy this morbid curiosity. If they could find their way directly to the patient, what protection would the patient have against these unfriendly, peering eyes? Again, it is a common trick of certain unscrupulous lawyers, of avaricious relatives and friends, or of mere acquaintances to seek private interviews with these sick persons in order to influence them to sign papers, to give over power of attorney, and often to sign checks for considerable amounts of money against the wishes of those who have the patient directly in charge and who have a right to exercise authority. Again, in these days of yellow journalism, reporters frequently seek to ascertain if such and such a patient is being cared for in the institution, or visit the hospital merely to obtain the opportunity to write up a thrilling, though not necessarily truthful, story concerning patients or the hospital. It is absolutely essential that all visitors should first report at the office or administration building. And patients should no more be subjected to the visits of the unannounced than you in your own house should be made to throw your doors wide open to any tramp who might see fit to disregard your natural desire for privacy. You are so nearly fair that you should not permit yourself to be tempted to make even the slightest exaggeration in order to present a good story. Give both sides of the argument and give the Devil his due.

We are making a strenuous endeavor to educate the public up to "the hospital idea." Though your book may do much good, it may also do harm in thwarting the best efforts of those who are endeavoring to combat the formerly prevalent opinion that mental disturbance is not an illness but a mysterious condition to which is attached a disgraceful stigma. . . .

On p. 88 you are inclined to criticize the physician for not verbally combating your delusions. Now a delusion *is* a delusion, and not merely a normal false belief, for the very reason that it is a false belief not founded upon experience, teaching or authority. . . . I think that you will find that every psychiatrist of large experience will tell you that he has never been able to argue a patient out of a delusion except where that patient has already begun to doubt for himself or has lost, at least to a degree, the morbid feelings and intellectual disorder in which the delusions have had their roots. At such a time the tactful physician may occasionally hasten the disappearance of the delusion by a few days or hours, but never by a number of months as you have stated.

Likewise in the following pages you make the common retrospective error of the recovered patient in giving too much credit for the abolition of your delusions, to the talkativeness of a single patient or to the effectiveness of this or that unessential incident of the days in which your mental state was changing and making itself ready for the uprooting of your false beliefs. . . . It was not your ingenious scheme which restored your reason, but conversely, your returning reason which made it possible for you to construct your ingenious scheme. Your senses no longer lied to you, and herein lay your salvation.

On p. 103 you speak of your "instantaneous return to reason." . . . Nevertheless, it is often only after hours, or days, or years of reasoning—none the less correct because slow in reaching the solution—that the truth is perceived. Your sudden "correction" occurred as the climax of weeks and months of *correcting* which was perhaps largely unconscious or indeed entirely unconscious. I know it will be hard for you to sacrifice this dramatic description of your seemingly sudden recovery, but mental illness, unlike physical illness, is usually corrected by a slow process, for it *is* illness and not a condition of *disequilibration* which can be righted by a turn of the balance wheel. Occasionally there are psychic injuries just as there are physical injuries, traumata, in which indeed the injurious agent may be removed with great suddenness, but these conditions are as a rule of short duration, and *your* mental trouble was not of this sort. . . .

On p. 119 at the top you speak of your thoughts as "stumbling over one another in their mad rush to present themselves to my enthroned reason." You of course realize that you were at that time merely experiencing the other swing of the pendulum and that, whereas your former depression had been accompanied as it usually is with retardation of thought and restriction of physical activity, so now elation was coupled with acceleration of thought and a pressure toward activity. But in both conditions there was abnormality of mental activity and judgment was deficient in both swings of the pendulum, so that it scarcely seems proper to speak of "reenthroned reason" since your reason was still defective, though the type of that defect had altered.

On the same page you say that "a genuinely interested physician would have been glad to have listened to your talk." This is quite true, but you should make it plain that you understand that it is impossible for the physician to listen as long as many manic patients would be willing to hold his ear. You have seen enough of such patients to know that when elated their talk is sometimes interminable, and, though the ideas expressed often seem of great value to the patient, the physician has to be on his way and must divide his time as his conscience dictates. . . .

I wish you might find it in your heart to tone down some of the harsh generalities which you have used in these pages; for example, your use of the word "hirelings" as applied to attendants. I fear that the public may gain from your book the idea that affairs in institutions for the care of the mentally ill are much worse off than the facts would warrant them in believing. You make general statements in speaking of attendants and physicians which might lead people to believe that your words apply to all institutions. In your endeavor to bring about reform, do not let it be thought that many of the reformations which you suggest should be enforced in the particular institution in which you were treated, have not already been carried out in the large majority of modern hospitals. I question if even now you would find at that institution many of the evils of which you are speaking. Give us credit for the progress of later years as shown in our rules of non-restraint, for the constant endeavor to use kindness, tact and skill and for the desire, by every means in our power, to bring about a cure.

On p. 140 you say "To place over me those I liked rather than attempt to make me adjust my unruly personality to those I hated would have caused attention and perhaps inconvenience; but would not the reward have been worth the pains. And if hospitals exist for the purpose of restoring patients to health, was I not by right entitled to these benefits?" But have you in your history allowed it to be sufficiently understood by the uninitiated that your own personality at this particular time was extremely unruly and that, while perhaps greater thoughtfulness might have been used in the selection of your physicians and attendants, it must not be forgotten that if every whim of every patient were to be indulged there would be such constant alteration in the arrangement and personnel of the staff that administration would be no longer possible? There are a number of such paragraphs in your work revealing lack of appreciation on your part—or at least sug-gest[ing] such a lack—of the enormous difficulties attending the care of the mentally ill and also there is a tendency, it seems to me, not to give credit for progress already made. To be frank, you are not always quite fair *in your text,* whereas from my personal knowledge of you, I believe you to be really fair-minded. . . . On p. 156 you describe minutely the camisole and on the following pages the tortures to which you were subjected by its use. If you mean to persuade the public that there is need of the arousal of a great wave of indignation which shall cause the camisole to be expelled from all institutions, your motive is a good one, but if you mean to let it be inferred that camisoles are commonly used, you will do a great injustice. I personally have not seen a camisole or a straight jacket in six years, except in a general hospital, and if you will inquire you will find that the use of such instruments of torture is to-day common in general hospitals which pride themselves on the employment of all modern and humane methods of treatment and you will find, on the other hand, that it has been abol-ished from an overwhelming majority of institutions for the care solely of the mentally ill. . . .

Again on p. 169, anent the padded cell. You speak of nine of our ten padded cells, as though such cells were common to all institutions. There is certainly no padded cell at Butler Hospital and, so far as I know, there never has been one. . . . They are commonly found in jails and prisons but not in hospitals. . . . You say that in each of the 226 public and 102 private hospitals for the insane in this country there are at least two violent wards; that is, that there are 756 violent wards in the country. Indeed you state that 15,000 patients are confined in such wards. You continue to say that these thousands live as it were near the very crater of a volcano of trouble, the remaining thousands live on uncertain slopes of this same volcano within a zone of constant danger.

I hardly know how to begin to criticize these statements. That they are exaggerated, I know. I am certain that they will add not a jot or a tittle to your book and believe, on the contrary, that if they were read at all widely infinite harm would result. Such an observant man as you have proven yourself to be by your keen descriptions of your past experience, must have noted in the daily papers of late the large number of wholesale family mur-ders committed. Only a short time ago a wellknown lady of Providence suddenly killed her husband and children; another threw herself and children from a steamboat plying between New York and Providence. I could mention a number of such murders if it were necessary to do so. The lady who destroyed her whole family was known to have been insane for some time but the husband had such a horror of hospitals (or, as these institutions are usually called by those who dread them, "asylums") that he had refused to have her committed. I have always been of the opinion that the vast majority of murders are committed by those who are really insane and who should have had proper treatment. I believe you have little conception of the way in which the relatives of the patient will exhaust every possible means of caring for such patients before seeking proper aid.

I wish you might have visited as many of the institutions of the world as it was my privilege to investigate three years ago. I have no recollection of having seen a single ward which would warrant the description which you have employed. And as for danger—while of course it cannot be eliminated entirely, it is not to be compared with the danger existing in many of the ordinary occupations and walks of life and it is surprising how few injuries result to patients, attendants or physicians where so many irresponsible patients are gathered together. Remember that it is the endeavor of modern superintendents to so conduct their institutions that there shall be no ward into which a visitor may not be freely conducted, providing he has the right to break in upon the privacy of the patients. Frequently the curious come to the hospital with a desire to see the "crazy people" and go away pondering deeply over the fact that they have found quiet where they expected to hear shrieks and a medley of insane jargon, and surprised when told that there are no maniacs, no padded cells, no straight jackets and no wards for wild patients. I have seen an attendant violently seized and almost kicked from the grounds for having been detected in using unnecessary force in leading a patient to his supper. The anger shown by the superintendent at that time was all the more memorable because of the infrequency of circumstances such as that which had called it forth. The description of your own behavior shows that all patients cannot be kept in a "polite ward." And so I must earnestly protest against the definition which you give for the wards in which "impolite patients" must often for a time be sequestered.

Your reference to the tearing of druggets, on p. 197, is extremely interesting, the more so as it adds to the collection which I already have of interpretations afterwards given by patients for the tearing of sheets, blankets, mattresses, etc. The real reason for this destructiveness with patients afflicted as you were, is the pressure toward activity. You say that your motive was not understood by those in charge, that they took your occupation as merely characteristic of wanton madness and that the habit of tearing druggets once acquired persisted as long as you were deprived of suitable clothes and held a prisoner in cold cells. I have seen a patient, whose conduct in the past reminds me very much of your own, tear sheets in strips exactly as you did and array herself in the most fanciful garments constructed from these strips. Her room was comfortably warm and she had sufficient clothing, though she persisted in removing her clothing entirely. She afterwards said that she tore these strips because she was not given thread and needle with which she could quietly occupy herself and that her desire to construct led her to manufacture from these strips garments suitable for the person of high degree whom she considered herself at that time to be. I do not mean to doubt your statements that you were cold and needed more clothing, but the tearing of the druggets had its origin in restlessness and intense desire for activity. These destructive traits are often purposeful and it is not surprising that you found a use for the strips. Your interpretation is, I fear, however largely retrospective and not the result of an exact analysis of your motives when you began the tearing.

On p. 223 is the statement, "Fortunately there are a few attendants possessed of manhood and a high sense of honor. These few—" etc. Such attendants are not few in number, and many of them are to be found in every institution working patiently, tactfully and with kindliness to alleviate suffering. I am sure you have no desire to do injustice to the class of attendants as a whole and that you will be willing to remove the damnation of your faint praise by being more liberal with well deserved commendation. . . . Page 264, "As was to be expected, this discharged and guilty attendant immediately secured a position in another hospital of the same character in a city not twenty miles distant." I wonder if you know that a black list is maintained in most hospitals and that as soon as an attendant is discharged his name is placed on the black list of one hospital and is sent immediately to other institutions so that they may be on their guard against hiring him. These black lists are kept up to date and an attendant once placed upon this list cannot gain a position in other institutions except under an assumed name and by testifying falsely as to his past. . . .

While these criticisms may seem to be very numerous and perhaps somewhat drastic, it may be said however that I have scrutinized carefully every word of the manuscript and have left nothing uncriticized which seemed to me to demand it. For the rest I have nothing but unstinted praise.

William McDonald, Jr., to Clifford W. Beers, September 6, 1907 (AFMHP).
. . . . On P. 398 and following pages, you recommend the establishment of hospitals for incurables. Personally, I question the wisdom of separating so-called incurable cases entirely from the curable. My reasons are as follows:

In the first place, who is to determine as to which cases are curable and which incurable? The longer I remain in the work the less certain do I become as to the incurability of any patient. After having seen a patient recover and go back to her work, who for 10 years had been the picture of a hopeless dement; after having seen another return to a normal state who for 12 years sat in one position with the head bent almost to the knees, the secretions running unnoted from mouth, nose and eyes, exhibiting the grossest beastliness in the taking of food; in short, presenting the picture of the severest type of mental deterioration: I say, after seeing such patient so far recover, I have become skeptical as to so-called stigmata of a hopeless condition.

Secondly, the very name "Hospital for Incurables" has always had a sinister and awful sound to me. I well remember in my boyhood having to pass by such a hospital every day on my way to school. Up over the front entrance was the sign in black and gold, "Hospital for Incurables." I never passed by this so-called "Hospital" without a feeling of awful pity for the patients who must read that sign while being carried beneath it into their living tomb.

In the special vocabulary of medicine there should never be found such words as "hopeless" and "incurable," any more than there is a place for "can't" in any dictionary. I also believe that the hospital idea should never be lost sight of, even in the institutions in which are congregated the less acute cases and those for which the outlook is less certainly favorable. . . .

In regard to the name for the society which you propose (P. 455), I would like to suggest that the word "insane" be omitted and some other suitable word substituted. The words "insane" and "insanity" have done much to retard psychiatric medicine and have impeded the development of proper legal protection and treatment of those afflicted with mental disturbance. . . .

On P. 461 your sentence, "And where no scandal exists that is all the more reason for agitation," strikes me as somewhat humourous. It reminds me strongly of your own mental attitude when you first began your tour of investigation and reform in the State Hospital. You stated to the Superintendent, I believe, or to one of his assistants that though you had never been in certain wards and had heard nothing concerning them, yet you knew that outrages were being committed there and that reforms should be instituted. Your sentiments likewise here are suggestive of a troublemaker rather than of the reformer. Scandal and agitation are not needed and as a rule result in little permanent benefit. The anger and resentment which is thus stirred up endures and in the end frustrates the so-called reform. What is needed is teaching, encouragement, suggestion, help rather than a criticism and condemnation. I am glad that you are trying to arouse public sentiment toward the betterment of conditions among our patients and it is to be hoped that your endeavors will result in the outstretching of many helpful hands to the men who are toiling and have for years toiled without encouragement and without proper salaries, without proper means and without anything to relieve the monotony of routine work of a most soul-grinding sort. I may as well say once [and] for all, in ending my criticism of your book, that I resent, as would thousands of my fellow workers, the insinuation which crops out here and there to the effect that the physicians have done little or nothing toward the improvement of conditions. Your own investigations must have been made with entirely blind eyes if they have not shown you the marvelous progress of recent years. This has been due not to public investigation, but to the steady working of a little army of professional men, handicapped by public ignorance and lethargy. You have little knowledge of the public and little knowledge of hospital physicians if you really believe the statement which you make upon the last page but one of your book. The form of the pledge which you propose to issue would be an insult to men who are not deserving of insults. If you knew as I know, the attitude of the public mind toward insanity you would not wish to see the experiment tried of "Packing all the drugs and all the doctors in the land over the seas and of installing in their places a body of amateurs with no equipment but consideration and sympathy." When you have seen a mother's love and tenderness bring about the absolute destruction of a daughter's mind as I have seen it do, you will be less sure that amateurs could replace men who have made the subject of mental disturbance a life study. You might as well send a group of loving, tender and sympathetic men and women into our operating rooms to relieve appendicitis, acute peritonitis, to remove tumors, to stop hemorrhages, to amputate mangled and useless limbs. The results would be as unfortunate for the patient in the one case as in the other. . . .

You have heretofore revealed an admirable degree of fair-mindedness for one who has suffered as you have. If you will take a cigar, sit down quietly in some cool spot, commune honestly with yourself, analyze the spirit of your words and seek to formulate a just opinion as to the work already accomplished, I am certain that you will regret having given tongue to those sentiments. I am so confident that this will be the case that I will not pursue the subject farther. Did I not possess this confidence I assure you that I could speak with a fervor that would leave little doubt as to my opinion of those final phrases.

I am sorry that such unfavorable comment must come at the end of my critical survey of a book which on the whole has aroused my admiration.

Meyer's initial reaction to Beers was favorable. Nevertheless, he saw Beers as a person who could aid in achieving the goals established by psychiatrists. In Meyer's eyes, the professional competency of the psychiatrist was the crucial element; he could not countenance the idea of lay people playing an independent role in policy determination. Meyer's insistence on psychiatric autonomy was a perennial issue, for it raised even broader questions about the proper relationship between professional groups and democratic government. In the following two letters Meyer spelled out his view of Beers's role in the mental hygiene movement.

Adolf Meyer to Dr. Henry S. Noble (superintendent, Connecticut State Hospital for the Insane), February 28, 1908 (AMP, Series II).
I assure you that the evening you gave us was a great pleasure and one of great gratification to us. I felt so absolutely sure of your attitude and of your great willingness to cooperate in any movement of value that I was rather more anxious to know whether there were any flaws in the statements of Mr. Beers, such as would have to be exposed in fairness to facts and such as might harm what I think represents his best intentions.

I am very glad to have your full statement of what I felt quite convinced of in the abstract, namely, that a great deal must have been done under your regime to meet situations such as, unfortunately, still exist in many places, and to my mind largely because the superintendents had become intimidated or tired concerning repeating to their boards of trustees and to the legislatures what after all looks like intolerable conditions. This I feel sure was the case at Worcester, and there I even hardly know whether the word intimidate can be used to exonerate the spirit of procrastination and the belief in sanction of conditions by their long duration. How these matters are to be met is rather difficult to see, but I feel inclined to think that a temperate and able committee with an efficient staff could serve as a valuable stimulator and do for the welfare of individual patients what the untiring missionary for hospitals and hospital sites, Dorothy [Dorothea] Dix, did in her day. Her ambition seems to have been governed by the thought of the "class of the insane," a sort of an inevitable percentage that has got to be provided for. The spirit of to-day is to get away from the class notion and to have provisions for groups of individuals, to start from their individual needs, to make a summing up of all these needs, and then to start out to get the means of meeting them,—this to my mind is the only way to break up the old habit of legislators, to merely think of a certain percentage of the annual budget having to go in the direction of a "class of the insane." A central committee ought to be able to do a great deal of good by pointing to the best standards, for alas I have hardly a doubt but that the Trustees of the Worcester hospital actually thought their hospital led the world. The organization of a movement within the State is another matter but to my mind of vital importance.

You are quite right that eternal vigilance is the only safe guard and its best assistant is a chance for physicians and attendants to get personally interested in the life and difficulties of the individual patients. There again we have to break up the idea that physicians and attendants are merely shepherds; the herd notion must be broken up; even in a hospital ward we should deal with an aggregate of individuals, and any physician or attendant who is not capable of seeing that to some extent, should be eliminated as a dangerous factor. That a great deal has been done by interested physicians in making a true history of the patient's condition and life, that I feel sure of; and any history which does not bring immediate returns to the advantage of the patient and the physician is a poor document. Some years ago Dr. Paton made a plea for better histories for the sake of accumulating facts for investigation. That would be a poor and abstract motive; on the other hand, we can say that the history to serve as a document of research must have shown its usefulness at the moment when it was made and the patient was at hand.

I strongly feel that we hospital physicians have a rare opportunity in Mr. Beers. It would be difficult to find a man with stronger convictions, and the point will be for those who have a wide experience to guide the energy that exists in him to make the most of the opportunities.

That you will get your modern hospital wards is a matter about which I have no doubt. I hope that they will have especially good provisions for cases of excitement, a matter which was wholly neglected in the special addition in the Worcester hospital much to my chagrin; and even on Ward's Island where the type of excited patients that we used to have in Worcester is practically unknown, there still is a tendency to aggregate unmanageable cases in a very inadequate part of the building.

Adolf Meyer to Julia C. Lathrop (Hull House, Chicago), October 22, 1908 (AMP, Series I).

We reached New York safely last Friday. Since then I have not found time to thank you for your hospitality and the opportunity to get a glimpse into things in Illinois, and possibly to do something to help a good cause. Mr. Graves has sent me a clipping of an editorial which might tend to show that the effort was not quite in vain; but I think much more interesting than that editorial is a letter I received from Doctor Greene, in reply to a note explaining to him why I could not come to Kankakee. He says— "I quite agree with all the methods proposed in your address at Rock Island, and if matters get in a settled state after the election until there is no likelihood of politics again upsetting the management, I hope to go to New York for a week or two, looking at conditions as they exist in that state, and the particular desire of having your advice on the best methods of procedure here."

I am not sanguine with regard to statements of this kind, but more than ever convinced of the fact that nothing at all can be done except along the lines of cooperation with the superintendents. I am on the point of breaking with Mr. Beers on this issue. He evidently is yielding to the advice of a lot of physicians who think that the movement should be a laymen's movement and that the officers of State hospitals should not become members. Under this policy I withdraw from the Committee, although Mr. Beers naively thinks that my difference of opinion would not interfere with my remaining a director, though somewhat inactive. I have not the slightest intention of figuring as an advertisement of a policy which I consider the most detrimental and the chronic sore of the problem of insanity in this country. The things have got to be done with and through the physicians of the hospitals, even if they get done slowly that way. I shall see Mr. Beers Friday evening.

Doctor Barrett told me of the impression Mr. Beers made on a visit to Danvers, Mass., where he saw him. It is perfectly obvious that his advisors favor a lay-movement because they do not wholly trust him and do not want to become implicated in a questionable move. The trouble with Mr. Beers has been that he is infinitely more concerned with securing funds than with doing other work. He is in the undesirable position of a philanthropist who wants to make a living out of his philanthropy. If he is assigned his place as a determined worker he is all right, but if, as Dr. Barrett said, he tries to impress on others that he is the "whole push" of the movement, that he appoints the officers of the association, etc., he is evidently making a mistake and justifies the lack of confidence and the disguised advice to make the thing a laymen's movement and a lobby for the legislature to secure appropriations and what not. I may be somewhat naive on that score, but I do not believe that appropriations can be maintained for any length of time on mere emotionalism. The sooner we spread among intelligent co-workers a correct knowledge of useful facts and an interest in helping us, the feeling of seriousness of the issue will come very naturally in our legislative bodies. There will be enough people who will ask before the election of a man whether or not he takes a sound stand or merely subordinates the problem to the political game.

I have written to Doctor Billings. I am sorry that I did not have a chance to have a good long talk with him, or still better, to have him present at the address and to hear him in discussion of the paper. I doubt very much whether he sees the things as he might if he were able to give the matter more time and to acquire a more intimate knowledge of the needs and possibilities. The conversation on his way to the hospital would have been absolutely insufficient to do anything.

Taking it all in all the visit to the West has opened my eyes to many difficulties and helped me considerably to formulate my ideas more definitely. I wish we could meet oftener and occasionally visit the hospital together.

I hope Miss Addams is fully restored; I was sorry not to see her, but very grateful to you for getting together some of my friends and persons interested in the common cause. . . .

P.S. I saw Mr. Beers last night (Oct. 23). The activity of the Connecticut society at the present time is essentially that of getting together life-members and a large membership. And all that practically on the ground that the reasons why the hospitals ask for various appropriations should be put before a larger number of people who shall be interested. Mr. Beers thus has enlisted quite a number of prominent taxpayers and hopes to do something efficient. The hospitals are standing aside, and in his opinion would not be fit to take any initiative under their present conditions and with their present personnel. He evidently has been talked into the believe [*sic*] that he should be Secretary of the National Committee. I told him that I thought only a man who had the absolute confidence of the hospitals on ground of well recognized knowledge of the ins and outs of the problem, should take that position so as to protect Mr. Beers against overtaxing and to give him the field in which he really can do most.

Our chief difference of opinion is this, that he is bearing in mind organization and chiefly organization, whereas I rather dread premature organization before a sufficient number of people know the best ways of cooperating with hospitals. I showed him a stenographic record of an after-care meeting at Willard to exemplify what material we have to collect before we can make a policy plain.

I do not quite know why I have the feeling that my Illinois address did not carry with some of the persons whom I had most expected to embrace the principles. It is evidently a matter not very easy to drive home, and still I feel that if we should organize a society now composed of persons not capable of an interest in that sort of a programme we would retard the perfectly feasible and eminently necessary step forward for quite a number of years to come. Mr. Beers realizes the point, and we shall write out the principles and send them to every one of the directors named so far with a desire to draw discussion so that the situation can be summed up and transmitted to the directors again before any organizing meeting takes place. Personally I am more than ever decided to cut loose from any movement which does not make cooperation with the hospitals and the ultimate raising of the hospitals to leadership of the movement the principal aim.

By 1910 the break between Beers and Meyer had become irrevocable and Meyer resigned from the National Committee. The following three letters illustrate the two polar positions. In the first, Dr. George Blumer (1872–1962), a member of the faculty, and shortly to become dean, of the Yale Medical School, supported Beers's position. The other letters by Meyer spell out in detail his analysis of the conflict with Beers.

George Blumer to Dr. Charles P. Emerson, c. April 1910 (AFMHP).
Mr. Beers has asked me to give you a line regarding my views on the Mental Hygiene Situation.

As I size it up Dr. Meyer, after helping to organize the movement, wants to back out unless he can have complete control. He now states that we are not ready to move yet &c &c, a policy of "masterly inactivity."

It seems to me that there is plenty to do, & that it will not help matters to wait, provided he can raise money to carry on the work.

This sums the matter up in a nutshell as I see it. The details Mr. Beers can supply.

Briefly

1. The work is needed.
2. A national Society is organized.
3. Are we to let it die because one member, possibly others agree with him, thinks we ought?

Adolf Meyer to Dr. Henry B. Favill (president, NCMH),
May 8, 1910 (AFMHP).

Careful consideration of the answer of Prof. Chittenden to my appeal for a specific discussion leaves after all no opening to me except that of asking whether you would not let me resign from the National Committee. It is obvious that the answer is also Mr. Beers's view and that Mr. Beers has lost confidence in me or rather that he has chosen to look to a different policy. My letter made my attitude plain enough. Prof. Chittenden's letter passes over all the points I raised, simply takes for granted that what should be discussed fairly and squarely would be settled in the end, and sees the main issue in the raising of money. I send you my letter and Prof. Chittenden's reply. I provoked the parting of the ways and stand by what I wrote. It is a matter of great regret to me if I cause complications for you. The attempt to combine my sincere devotion to the cause of organized work in mental hygiene and the equally sincere interest in Mr. Beers led me to concessions which are exploited too far to be compatible any longer with my judgment. We plainly need foci of strong local work. In the light of what Dr. Russell and others have to say, I know that we can do more by concentration on well defined fields than by helping to create a very uncertain central bureau inefficiently attached to any of the agencies on which we must depend for the actual work. For work along the lines laid down in the letter to Prof. Chittenden we would need no costly apparatus and could preserve a safe and efficient program and direct the money where it is bound to be most telling, viz—in the organization of clinics in the centers which are riper for that and in concentrating the available funds to make the work efficient and fit to spread. If the National Committee cannot accept this policy, I would rather help along the interests of mental hygiene from an independent position.

Adolf Meyer to Clifford W. Beers, August 14, 1910 (AFMHP).
The reason for my long silence is the fact that I found it too difficult to discuss at a distance the issues of your letter to me and to Mrs. Meyer without causing misunderstandings and touching unnecessarily upon matters which may no longer be actual. I have written to Dr. Russell that the matter was only submitted to Prof. Chittenden, that the fact that he did not even discuss it as an alternative forced me to the step I had said I would be forced to take, and that, once confronted with that situation, I saw myself forced to take the radical step of resigning from the Committee altogether. I cannot see how I could lend my name to a policy which I consider disastrous to you and to the whole constructive plan which I had shaped on ground of a long practical experience and not only as a "psychiatrist" as your present dominant advisors are pleased to put it. The solution which you were so ready to accept proved untenable and must be radical, unless I could be convinced that the Mental Hygiene movement was on safe and promising grounds. The whole matter rested with Prof. Chittenden and you, and as long as Dr. Favill has not acted yet, still does rest there.

The fundamental trouble, no doubt, lies in the fact that I had overrated your capacity and willingness to go through the school of experience in this most difficult problem of mankind, that our ideas of work for the actual cause split in the incident following my New Haven talk, and that my intention to help you in your personal affairs became very difficult through this realization and the growing distance, quite apart from the inevitable complication through my long absence in the West.

I was and am willing to go a long way to help you get another foundation; but I cannot let that conversation influence the cause of the Mental Hygiene movement as I support it not for myself and as I shall try to carry it out in a small way. I saw in it a safe place for you; but you chose a plan nearer your original aims and conceptions. My unwillingness to cross your path any more than was absolutely necessary led to a compromising attitude at the meeting in April. The advantage which was taken of this and as shown in the fact that there was not the same desire for common ground on the part of Prof. Chittenden then and after that, made my step inevitable.

I am afraid things have gone too far to be changed much. I am punished for my excessive confidence in the good will and capacity of cooperation of others. But I truly think you must not consider my withdrawal an obstacle or cause for worry *if* your plans and Prof. Chittenden's should be sound contrary to my view. I have never put myself in a conspicuous position personally and shall not be missed personally. Another matter is, of course, the soundness of the plan which is jeopardized, I think, by the elimination of my policy. But this is a different matter. I feel that your confidence in me and my personal judgment is too fundamentally altered to be reestablished. As far as I am concerned, I should not want you to try a mere attempt at accommodation. Nothing but conviction would appear to me safe enough as a foundation of the inevitably thorny path which, however, I am convinced, would bring you the worthiest rewards, modest, but substantial, and a stepping-stone for lasting improvement of things.

Dr. Russell will advise you well, but probably so gently, that you may not feel the contrasts fully enough at the time and then experience the results. Weigh his criticisms ten times as heavily as he puts them and you will get them at their real value. . . .

In 1912 Thomas W. Salmon (1876–1927) became associated with the NCMH. A physician with the U.S. Public Health Service, Salmon had conducted psychiatric examinations of immigrants at Ellis Island before their admission. Shocked by what he observed, he attempted to persuade the Public Health Service to improve physical conditions among insane immigrants denied entrance and awaiting deportation to their country of origin. He also published several articles critical of the policy of unrestricted immigration because it contributed to the rising number of patients in mental hospitals. When Salmon sent a piece on prevention of mental illness to Meyer, the latter offered some of his own views on the subject.

Adolf Meyer to Thomas W. Salmon, November 23, 1911 (AMP, Series I).
I have read your paper with great interest, and to save time I sum up its excellencies in the statement that it gives a very good programme of general lines of attack of prevention. The points in which it might be improved would seem to me to lie in the omission of any reiterations of the fact that there are *chances* for preventive work, so that you would get a little more space for concrete helps, or, at least, references to the same. For instance, in

discussing the psychoses connected with the acute infections we must admit that some individuals respond very easily with delirium, and that in
these it goes with cerebral oedema and fever reaction of the cells, and that
at least we can reduce the latter by proper hydrotherapeutic measures. Or
where you discuss alcoholism, I should point specifically to the necessity of
personal analysis of the nature and direction of the craving, and the means
of diverging it by suggestion, or by giving an outlet to better cravings. In
this connection it is absolutely essential to encourage the work of total ab-
stinence societies, the Father Matthew's movement, and finally to give first
class reference to the best methods of handling the alcoholic problem on
the part of the state and communities. (Gothenburg System etc)

Again, where you come to the question of mental hygiene I should make
a reference to the mental hygiene movement or to a description of it and
use all the space to making it clear how early children get into quandaries,
and how utterly naive people are in assuming that sex difficulties come only
where masturbation manifests itself; whereas, the foundation for most
aberrations and conditions of nervousness are laid before the age of four.
Hypocrisy or false shame, hammered into the children makes them often
enough incapable to take good advice when they hear it, and to develop a
normal conscience and responsibility of health. The next stage comes
where adolescent nervousness shows itself, and you simply *must* hammer it
in that at that period the errors of the early education must be corrected
when the first warnings appear, and that a wholesome, frank, constructive
guidance in life with regard to sexual and other ambitions must be made
possible, and that this is perfectly compatible with the highest ideals of
moral and religious training. My paper in *Psychological Clinic,* and Hoch's
papers on the Mental Causes may give you some concrete material.

You may, of course, feel that this goes beyond the limits of your space,
but my idea is to suppress what is a problem of future organisation and can
be referred to as a plan published elsewhere, and to use the space for as
many concrete helps and references of what has been tried, and is being
done *to-day*.

I feel with you that it is a remarkable progress that the bacteriologist
thinks of incorporating psychopathological issues. The time has evidently
come when people feel the need, and it is up to us to give them the right
material.

Although Salmon left his position at the NCMH in 1922 for a professorship at Columbia University's School of Medicine, the basic character of the NCMH did not change. By this time the committee's energies were focused on such subjects as delinquency and retardation, to cite only a few. The appointment of Dr. Frankwood E. Williams (1883–1936) as Salmon's replacement as medical director did nothing to restore the NCMH's original goal of improving conditions among the institutionalized mentally ill. The broadened scope of the mental hygiene movement was graphically illustrated in a proposal developed by Williams to study the "psychopathology of dependency," which was submitted to the Rockefeller foundation in 1925. The Foundation declined to consider the proposal.

Frankwood E. Williams to Edwin R. Embree (director, Rockefeller Foundation Division of Studies), May 1, 1925, with enclosed proposal (RFP).

I am authorized by the Executive Committee of The National Committee for Mental Hygiene to forward to you the enclosed proposal for an appropriation for a study of the psychopathology of dependency.

STATEMENT IN REFERENCE TO A PROPOSAL FOR A STUDY OF THE PSYCHOPATHOLOGY OF DEPENDENCY

More public and private funds are expended in the care and relief of that group in the community known as the "poor" or "dependent" than for any other single group—unless, perhaps, the group known as "delinquent." It is not possible to obtain accurate figures as to the number of dependent individuals there are in the United States, nor the amount of money that is annually expended in their care and maintenance. Certain figures are available, however, which indicate the extent to which public and private funds are absorbed by this group.

The National Information Bureau, on a basis of 129 cities with Community Chests, exclusive of New York, Boston and Chicago, estimated that there was expended in 1922 for *private* charity in this country $200,000,000.

The United States Department of Commerce reported that for 1919, $281,000,000 was expended from private and public funds for dependents.

The Department of Public Welfare of Massachusetts reports that for 1921–22 cities and towns of the State expended $6,642,000 for poor relief; the State expended $2,106,000 for the care of dependents exclusive of the care of the insane, etc.; while the Massachusetts private charitable organizations expended $32,000,000.

All of this money, of course, is not expended for "relief" in the ordinary sense, but it is expended to provide for the needs of individuals who cannot provide adequately for these needs themselves.

The Association for Improving the Condition of the Poor of New York City has a clientele of over 20,000 individuals (4,000 families) and expends annually a budget that exceeds $1,000,000. This is but one of several large charitable organizations in the City of New York and of many smaller ones. Similar organizations, of course, are at work in all parts of the United States.

It is assumed by those who support these organizations with their funds that dependency is due to economic stress, to accident, to the physical illness or death of bread-winners, and the like; that dependent individuals are those whom misfortune has overtaken; that they are essentially "normal" individuals who in their period of difficulty need assistance temporarily to help them back to economic independence and self-support. That there are such individuals among those who are dependent and that economic stress, illness and death do play an important part in causing individuals to become dependent, no one would seriously question. There are good reasons to believe, however, that these are not the only factors; in fact, to doubt whether in the great majority of cases, particularly of chronic dependency, that they are the fundamental factors.

The National Committee for Mental Hygiene in its community mental health surveys has, where possible, included as a part of its study an examination of a certain number of the clientele of the local charitable agencies. The number has usually been small as time and funds have not permitted more extensive examinations. The Committee has been led to believe, however, as the result of these studies that mental defect, mental ill health and instability play a much larger part in the causation of dependency than has been supposed; that in many instances the individual is dependent, not because he has not had proper opportunities or because misfortune has suddenly overcome him, but because he has been unable to accept those opportunities that have come to him or to meet the exigencies of living with any degree of adequacy, due to an inherent intellectual inadequacy in himself, to a mental or nervous disease that has taken away what adequacy he may once have had, or to a personality, psychopathological in type, that would make adequate adjustment to situations, without an understanding on the part of someone as to the special handicap, exceedingly difficult—in some cases impossible.

To determine whether this be a fact would be a matter of first-rate importance. Psychiatrists who have had experience in examining some of this human material are inclined to the view; social workers who have had many years of experience in working with dependents have for some time been suspecting it.

It became possible recently for The National Committee for Mental Hygiene to make a preliminary study of the subject, the object being to ascertain in a brief and intensive survey of representative material whether or not there was sufficient ground to warrant the undertaking of a more extensive study by which the point could be finally determined. This preliminary study was undertaken by invitation, at the Association of Improving the Condition of the Poor of New York City, an organization whose clientele is representative of the clientele of charitable organizations throughout the country. As the work of the Association is divided into divisions, an effort was made to study samples from each division, the only basis of selection being those whose presence could be obtained for examination; also, a "run-of-the-mine" sample of new clients applying to the Association who had not yet been assigned to a division.

The results of this study can be briefly summarized as follows:

Cases under the care of the Association five years or more (23 families studied):

Of the 34 adults examined, 31 presented a mental health problem of one kind or another—mental defect, mental or nervous disease, a psychopathological type of personality.

Of the 54 children examined, 21 presented mental health problems. Of these 21, it is important to note that only 2 were mentally defective; 19 were essentially promising children who already, however, are showing definite evidence of psychopathological personality traits and emotional maladjustment, conditions which at this stage are in many instances manageable, but which, if neglected, as they are at present, will undoubtedly result in handicapped, crippled adults who will be candidates of the next generation for charitable organizations.

It is to be noted, also, that of the 31 adults mentioned above, 14 were handicapped by more than one mental health problem; 5 with psychoneuroses, for example, were also mentally defective.

"Special Widow Group":

Of the 5 adults examined, 4 presented mental health problems.

Of the 19 children examined, 8 presented mental health problems.
Desertion Division (8 families studied):
Of the 12 adults examined, 11 presented problems of mental health.
Tuberculosis Division (10 families studied):
Of the 13 adults examined, 8 presented mental health problems.
Bureau of Relief (36 families studied):
Of 50 adults examined, 39 presented mental health problems.
Run-of-the-Mine—new cases applying (26 families studied):
Of the 36 adults examined, 25 presented mental health problems.
Of these, 8 presented more than one problem.
Of the 80 children examined, 29 presented mental health problems.
Thirty families were studied because the workers of the A.I.C.P.
themselves suspected that a mental condition was at the bottom of
the family trouble and dependency. This proved to be correct in the
case of 29 out of the 37 adults and of 2 of the 4 children.

The number of cases examined in this study is entirely too small to warrant generalization, but the Executive Committee of The National Committee for Mental Hygiene does believe that the examination of these cases
accomplishes the purpose for which the study was made in that it indicates
that a larger study from which generalizations can safely be made is not
only warranted but would seem to be necessary.

Should a comprehensive study reveal proportions anything like those
found in this preliminary study, a medical contribution to the field of dependency would be made of the very greatest importance. If the facts are as
indicated, many of the millions of dollars expended annually in the relief of
these individuals are being expended unwisely—through lack of knowledge. With the best of intentions, it would appear, money is annually being
shoveled into a hole. This money can be spent more effectively as many of
those individuals can be rehabilitated once their true condition is recognized for what it is and dealt with on that basis; particularly is this true of
the children in these families. A reorientation in the handling of dependents would seem indicated.

A study of the Psychopathology of Dependency would be as fundamental as the studios formerly made of the Psychopathology of Crime. The
first comprehensive study on this subject made by The National Committee for Mental Hygiene was completed less than eight years ago. The results at the time were questioned by some. Similar studies have since been

made by others in all parts of the country and the facts revealed in the original study confirmed. This has led in less than ten years to important changes in legislation, to the establishment of psychiatric clinics in connection with juvenile and adult courts, prisons and reformatories, to the establishment of child guidance clinics for the prevention of delinquency, to the appointment of psychiatrists as state criminologists in three states, to the establishment of a psychiatric clinic (with separate specially constructed building) at Sing Sing Prison to serve as the center of a reorganized correctional system for the State of New York, to the passage of legislation in Massachusetts, making mandatory the psychiatric examination of all prisoners committed to county jails for more than thirty days, of felons accused for the second time and of those charged with capital offense; and for the carrying out of these laws the establishment of a Division for the Examination of Prisoners in the Department of Nervous and Mental Diseases of the State.

A study of the Psychopathology of Dependency should bring as radical and productive changes in the field of dependency, and probably in even less time, as those in charge of social agencies are more ready to reorganize their work in response to new information than are courts and prisons.

A study at this time of the Psychopathology of Dependency would have two main purposes: (1) to determine by the examination of a sufficiently large series of unselected cases the part played by nervous and mental conditions in the production of dependency; (2) to work out a method and plan of organization by which social agencies dealing with dependents can reorganize their work so as to utilize knowledge of the mental handicaps of a client as a basis in planning their work of rehabilitation. It is believed that a study sufficiently comprehensive to establish these two points will require from three to five years. Material for such a study is available through the cooperation of the Association for Improving the Condition of the Poor of New York City. A capable staff of psychiatrists, psychologists and psychiatric social workers is likewise available at this time as the staff that has been making the preliminary studies is still intact.

The Executive Committee of The National Committee for Mental Hygiene would, therefore, propose an annual appropriation of $30,000 for a period of three years with the understanding that, if at the end of three years it appear wise to the Executive Committee of The National Committee for Mental Hygiene and the Board of The Rockefeller Foundation, the study be continued for two more years, with the further understanding that for the fourth year the appropriation be diminished 10% and for the fifth year 20%. The items of the budget proposed are as follows:

Director	$ 7,500
Assistant Psychiatrist	4,500
Psychologist	2,800
Vocational Assistant	2,000
Chief Psychiatric Social Worker	2,800
Psychiatric Social Worker	2,200
Psychiatric Social Worker	2,000
Clinic Secretary	1,800
3 Stenographers (@ $1,200)	3,600
Supplies	800
	$30,000

Edwin R. Embree to Frankwood E. Williams, May 28, 1925 (RFP).
At the meeting of the Rockefeller Foundation held yesterday, the opinion was expressed that studies of the psychopathology of dependency, while of unquestioned importance in themselves, should more properly be supported by an organization having a general interest in social matters and social welfare. The program which the Foundation is working out through the Division of Studies is so definitely biological in character that it has been thought best to restrict the studies considered to those having a definitely biological bearing.

I am exceedingly sorry to have to send you this disappointing reply. Of my personal interest in your proposal I need not assure you. On the other hand, I concur in the opinion that the Foundation's work should be concentrated upon the important biological aspects of mental and bodily growth. It is this consideration of general policy that excludes the important studies which you have suggested.

By the turn of the century, eugenicists were seeking to harness the authority of the state to a deterministic interpretation of heredity. They urged the passage of a variety of laws to restrict immigration from eastern and southern Europe (which was overwhelmingly Catholic and Jewish) on the grounds that groups from these regions were biologically inferior; to regulate marriage and prevent the propagation of defective people; and to segregate the feebleminded in institutions. They also supported laws providing for the sterilization of defective people. The development of salpingectomy (cutting and tying the fallopian tubes) and vasectomy (cutting and tying the vas deferens through a slit in the scrotum) in the 1890s offered relatively safe and simple surgical procedures. Success came in 1907 when Indiana passed the first law providing for the mandatory sterilization of confirmed criminals, idiots, imbeciles, and rapists when recommended by a board of experts. In the succeeding decade ten other states enacted comparable legislation, and by 1940 a total of thirty had such laws on the books. Most of this legislation applied to the mentally ill as well. Between 1907 and 1940 a total of 18,552 mentally ill people in state institutions were surgically sterilized. More than half of all sterilizations took place in California, which, together with Virginia and Kansas, accounted for three-fourths of the total. The majority of institutional psychiatrists either favored sterilization or at the very least remained silent on the subject of it. Opposition, on the other hand, was by no means absent. The following letters illustrate the diversity of views. William A. White, an acknowledged leader of the specialty, let no occasion pass without denouncing the practice; William D. Partlow, superintendent of the Alabama Insane Hospitals, was a strong proponent (although, interestingly enough, the 224 sterilizations in Alabama before 1940 did not include any patients in the mentally ill category).

Dr. Arthur P. Herring (secretary, Lunacy Commission of the State of Maryland) to William A. White, November 3, 1916 (WAWP).
The State Conference of Charities and Correction, including Maryland, Delaware and the District of Columbia, will meet in Baltimore on November 15, 16 and 17. At the general meeting, which will be held on Wednesday, the 15th, at 2 P.M., the subject of the mentally defective will be discussed. Dr. Vernon Briggs is coming down from Boston to tell us what is being done in Massachusetts for this class of patients and we would like very much if you would present in a general way the subject from the standpoint of prevention, especially as it relates to sterilization and segregation of the feeble-minded woman. . . .

William A. White to Arthur P. Herring, November 4, 1916 (WAWP).
I have your very good letter of the third instant. Thank you very much for your invitation to speak in Baltimore on the 15th instant. I am very much afraid, however, that you really do not want to hear from me after all, as I am very much opposed to the whole sterilization movement, and what I would say upon this subject might not fit into your general scheme of the meeting. I do not believe that there is the slightest particle of justi-

fication for the mutilating operations that are being advocated broadcast over the country at this time, and if I should happen to talk in Baltimore at your meeting I should unhesitatingly denounce the sterilization propaganda. If you want me to do that, why I may be able to accommodate you.

William A. White to Dr. (?) Fisher, c. November 1919 (WAWP).
I have your letter of the 4th instant. I will endeavor to write you further upon the subject that you are interested in. You are quite welcome to my opinion upon this matter, or anything else.

In the first place, the only theory of all the multitudinous theories to account for why we are what we are, the only one of these theories upon which we may base assumptions that warrant sterilization, is the Mendelian theory. Now if the Mendelian theory explained facts with anything remotely resembling the certainty of, for example, the atomic theory or the theory of gravity, or twenty other theories that I might mention, why then we might have something worth while to work upon, but when we consider that the Mendelian hypothesis is only one among a number of theories, that there is no unanimity among biologists as to its reliability, and that it has as yet been impossible to apply the hypothesis to man, except to the most limited extent, that even the very fundamental conceptions of the theory, the conceptions of dominance and recessiveness, and the yet more important conception of unit characters, are vague and indefinable and nobody knows what they mean, it seems to me preposterous that we should endeavor to formulate statutes upon it as a basis. I don't believe, and I don't believe anybody believes, who has studied law-making and how it comes about and what its effects are, that the making of a statute, the manufacturing of a law, the writing down of certain prohibitions by a legislative assembly can have any very material effect upon the race. The law and the lawyers, like religion and the clergy, represent the conservative forces of society. The faces of the lawyers and of the clergy are mostly turned backwards, and it requires a preponderance of righteousness to overcome them, and this is a very great advantage, because it makes it impossible to enflame a nation by some hair brained scheme because these conservative elements so preponderate that they cannot be overcome. I therefore don't believe that any statute is potent for good until it has come to express a great truth which has more or less already permeated the minds of the people who are to be subjected to its control. When a statute, then, in a sense becomes the reflection in law of the feelings of the people it will amount to something, and not much before. Now to enact into law a scheme for the sterilization of so-called defectives, based upon a theory which even scientific men are not at one about, against which there is a great deal of opposition and argument, and evidence of all sorts and character, which confessedly cannot be applied to man, except to an extremely limited extent, and the very concepts of which are vague to the extent of being indefinable; to base a statute upon any such foundation as that is inviting disaster. It is premature to the point of being abortive, and it puts off the day when legislation can be formulated that will be effective, because such legislation as can be formulated today must of necessity in its efforts be as disappointing as to make more effective legislation in the future be looked upon with grave suspicion.

My ideas about this whole matter are based a good deal upon practical experience. I see States formulating laws for the sterilization of defectives and organizing commissions to say who should be sterilized. I may be wrong, but I have yet to hear of the work of any one of these commissions. I don't see anything in the publications as to what they have done. I am not given to understand that they have been able to formulate any scheme of arriving at conclusions which invite scientific attention. On the contrary they appear to sit upon a case in a casual sort of way, determining that so and so is a defective, whatever that may mean, and that they ought not to procreate. Here in the Hospital we have had a field worker, educated at the Cold Springs Harbor Department of the Carnegie Foundation, and she has been working upon family histories and she has worked out many histories of families of patients in this Hospital, and she has spent weeks and weeks upon these records, and I challenge you or any other person to point to one of these carefully worked out families and give me in a single instance a prediction of what the heredity of any one of the numerous individuals therein contained will be shown by our charts that it actually is. Now if we cannot predict we have no right to interfere. It is simply and solely to my mind a case of "fools rushing in which angels fear to tread" and I have absolutely no sympathy with any such legislation for that reason. I have yet to see a chart upon which an absolute prediction could be made, except perhaps in the case of the union of two feeble-minded persons, and even there I would want to know something about the basis for the diagnosis of feeblemindedness.

I have seen numerous charts of other workers in this same field, men who advocated sterilization, and they have not been able to make any prediction, and why they advocate it I don't know. I am convinced that the more deeply one studies into the whole situation the more that he will feel, so to speak, that he is on holy ground and that he must keep his hands off. The everlasting tinkering with things is what I have no patience with. When we know something different for God's sake let us go forward with braveness in that knowledge, but until we know let us have some faith in the powers of nature that have brought us to our present kingdom. If what some of the alarmists say were true the race would be destroyed in the next three or four generations, but we know that there are no forces but that have been active for the last ten thousand years or more, and to assume suddenly that these things are going to arise up and destroy us is silly. Mott makes the very significant statement that in families in which there is insanity the insanity tends naturally of its own lack of impetus to die out in the third generation. Isn't it worth while considering such testimony as that? Must we brush all such things as that aside for the purpose of satisfying a sadistic orgy of cutting out testicles and ovaries, which in my mind still harks back to the horrors of twenty years ago when the surgeon cut out the ovaries with as much nonchalance as he would pear corns. The thousands and thousands of women who were sacrificed to that damnable period of surgery still horrifies me, and I am not willing to go into a new situation that involves unsexing and mutilating people until I have some pretty definite idea that I know what I am doing.

You have invited me to use strong language. I trust that I have satisfied your requirements. I feel that the whole matter is in doubt in your mind and for that reason I have yielded to the temptation to express myself in this way. If you can find a single commission anywhere in the United States engaged in doing this work that has done one quarter of the work upon family histories of the defectives that they have sterilized that my field worker has upon ours I would like to see that commission and know about their work. And unless they can do not one-fourth as much, but four times as much work, they haven't any business to come to a conclusion.

I invite your attention to my article on Heredity and Eugenics, I believe that's the title, in the forth-coming ponderous work on the *Treatment of Nervous and Mental Disease* in two large volumes, edited by Dr. Jelliffe of New York City and myself. I have a note from the printers this morning that they are sending me the galley proof, etc.

William D. Partlow to Dr. E. S. Gosney, March 26, 1934 (AVSP).
Acknowledging receipt of your courteous favor of March 22nd, I have received under separate cover from you your book, "Sterilization for Hu-

man Betterment," and other pamphlets to which you refer. I appreciate very much these publications.

Owing to the fact that we are and have been for several years sterilizing all inmates dismissed from our School for Feebleminded I am receiving a good many inquiries on the subject. We have up to the present time I believe sterilized 184.

Under separate cover I am mailing you copy of my last annual report covering our institutions.

For many years I have advocated the sterilization of certain types of constitutional hereditary deficients, including feebleminded, insane, repeating criminals, chronic drug and alcoholic addicts, epileptics, etc. I agree with you that an educational program is first necessary to produce and expose facts in order that others may make the same deductions and decisions that come to us who are in immediate contact with the problem.

By the late 1920s and 1930s expressions of doubt about the direction of the mental hygiene movement were not uncommon. Given the difficulty of specifying with any degree of precision the etiology of mental illness, how was it possible to talk about prevention? Indeed, figures such as Meyer and others thought that mental hygiene was often a synonym for propaganda. The following letters by Meyer and Maxwell Gitelson (1902–1965), a psychiatrist and psychoanalyst who served as president of the American Psychoanalytic Association in 1955–1956, reveal a pervasive sense of doubt about the very concept of mental hygiene.

Abraham Flexner (General Education Board) to Adolf Meyer, April 15, 1927 (AMP, Series III).

Doctor Vincent has referred to us his correspondence with you about mental hygiene, and we are trying to clear our minds as to the proper relationship between psychiatry, neurology, mental hygiene, and hygiene. Perhaps, in the first instance, the difficulty is one of definition. Would you be willing to help me clear my own mind by stating to me precisely the field, which, in your judgment, belongs to each of these subjects and then, in the second place, the points at which they touch or overlap?

Adolf Meyer to Abraham Flexner, April 20, 1927 (AMP, Series III).

Your inquiry of April 15 just reached me. It deals with a problem which would require a fuller discussion than a letter because it is not possible to cope with all the possible issues and questions that may well arise in the minds of inquirers of widely different experience and interests.

To my mind *psychiatry* should include all the disorders in which a knowledge of personality-functions and psychopathology is involved. That this *includes* a solid foundation in general medicine, neurology, and especially in the discrete and in the outspoken mental disorders is obvious. It is therefore not a mere issue of "psychoanalysis" or mere psychopathology and psychotherapy nor a question merely of "insanity," but it includes all mental diseases and the mentally conditioned neuroses and the conditions in which the personality or mental functions are secondarily involved (toxic and organic psychoses and many psychoneuroses).

Neurology should limit itself to those conditions which involve the problems of neurophysiology and neural anatomy and histology, and which do not clearly and necessarily include psychobiological problems (by which I mean the working and the effects of "memories" and emotions and personality and habit disorders). The idea that functional "nervousness" when it does not spell "insanity" should go to the "neurologist" has no scientific justification. There is no split between psychopathology and psychiatry from the point of view of research; the only separation is due to popular prejudice and to the fact that there are many physicians (and surgical specialists as well) who feel ready to treat "psychoneuroses" and "neuroses" without any psychiatric training. On the other hand, neurology and psychiatry have to deal with the same basic *organ,* the nervous system. Neurology studies all the detachable parts of the nervous system and nervous functions, whereas psychiatry studies the nervous system as far as it serves the integration of the personality. There will always be considerable overlapping. The aphasias and apraxias, for instance, are common fields; they should not be studied without the best that psychobiology can offer, and they must work with the best that can be offered by the anatomy and histology and experimental study of the cerebral cortex. But it is so specifically a human problem that it is not open to animal experimentation. Neurology also has to give consideration to what hysteria and hypnosis can produce, but hysteria and hypnosis belong intrinsically to psychobiology and psychopathology.

Mental hygiene is a difficult field, one dangerously over-advertised without adequate basic research.

The mental hygiene movement is a creation largely of our own American work. It required for its frank development a sense of possibilities to overcome the inertia and misconceptions in man's traditions concerning health and life. It began with the American form of child-study, and the interest in schools, and modern "after-care" and social work (see Schedule for the study of mental abnormalities in Children, *Handbook Illinois Society for Child-Study,* 1895; After-care and prophylaxis and the hospital physician, *Jour. Nerv. and Ment. Dis.,* 1907; Case work in social service, and medical and social cooperation in nervous and mental disease, National Conference of Charities, 1911; *Suggestions of Modern Science Concerning Education,* by Jennings, Watson, Meyer, and Thomas, 1926). It began to crystallize in a more sweeping form when an unusual human urge in Mr. Clifford W. Beers was swung from an attitude of vindication and desire for legislative investigation of all kinds of institutions for the insane into a thought of constructive work, as Mental Hygiene (*The Mind That Found Itself,* 5th ed., p.265). The result has been remarkable. The problem was easy to recognize. As a matter of fact, it had a somewhat one-sided development largely because of the fact that it has not been in the hands of the actual workers and investigators, but largely in the hands of organizers without research interest in the basic sciences involved. The work and domain of mental hygiene is best defined by the departments necessary to turn it from preaching and propaganda into teaching and research based on field and laboratory work. It has to cover the health and efficiency of all the mentally integrated functions, the behavior and conduct of the organism or personality as dependent on growth and experience. It includes not only what might lead to diseases or disorders of the personality but also the fluctuations and deviations of efficiency.

Hygiene might be called an effort of medicine to make itself unnecessary. It is a way of infiltrating the normal ways of life with the means of obviating damaging conditions and processes.

That in this task mental hygiene should have been omitted in our School of Hygiene in the face of my recommendations in 1919 is due to the teachings of the passing generation which left the human aspect of human science to a psychology of a dualistic parallelistic character which is being overcome but slowly since the nineties of the last century and really only since behaviorism and psychobiology exist on a natural-history basis including all the aspects and functions of man. Behaviorism was a side-product of academic psychology teaching. Psychobiology is a side-product of medical and psychiatric teaching aiming to make unnecessary too one-sided Freudian systematization, combining the best available laboratory research and the study of childhood and adult behavior problems. It so happened that psychology was still associated with a moribund type of philosophical teaching and a physiological tendency lacking a sense for the foot-measure of experience and clinging too much to the microscopic chronoscope. With it all went the fear of studying human and animal life on the same basis. Aspirations in the direction of fool-proof medicine and fool-proof hygiene leaving out the behavioristic aspects of man were based on a lack of understanding of the natural-history aspects and natural-history study of the human individual and groups, left too naively to defensive philosophy and theology and pedagogy and law (see in contrast my address at the Bloomingdale Centenary). The need of a change was realized and met by some of us overtaxed psychiatrists, and picked up by the social workers and lay-movements, and it is time that the deplorable consequences of the running ahead of propaganda be corrected.

Hygiene deserves special institutes, but I am inclined to think that in view of the great expense in money and actual basic labor the work in psychiatry and in mental hygiene had best be developed in closer conjunction than the work of general medicine and general and special hygiene is at the present time. A model neuro-psychiatric division of research and teaching should form a unit-group which to-day is too much disrupted owing to accidental interests, and because it has never been granted the possibilities of a frank development under broadly trained leadership, except perhaps in the Forschungsanstalt planned by Kraepelin, which lacks the combination of psychiatry and neurology and hygiene characteristic of the American development.

Mental hygiene should not be announced unless it can rest on a basis of research in

1. Psychobiology—with research in personality-study in the various periods of life from infancy to advanced age, and with special attention to the needs and emergencies out of which disorders of "health, happiness and efficiency" can develop. I considered Miles who worked at the Carnegie Institution Laboratory the *technically* best trained man for such a fundamental department.

2. The field of pre-school and school hygiene, from the angle of behavior adaptation and school problems—a department requiring field work and possibilities for specific research, not only testing but especially also study of individual and home and play problems.

3. Factory and industrial hygiene—partly in personnel selection and partly in hygiene of work and recreation, and study of labor problems.

4. Court work, especially in juvenile and domestic relations court—

field work and study of the methods applicable to specific problems and investigations.

5. Work with patients of all ages with some such principle as that of my article in the *Psychological Clinic,* 1908, II, 4: "What do histories of cases of insanity teach us concerning preventive mental hygiene during the years of school life?" or my article quoted in Stanley Hall's *Adolescence*.

These departments would give the foundation of such research and practical work as should be the basis of instruction. There would have to be in a curriculum such requirements of general medicine and of general hygiene as would yield persons of practical training, capable of research and teaching.

It is, I believe, of importance that one should realize *certain practical aspects* of the development and present status of this field in this country.

In the first place, with regard to *psychiatry*. Psychiatry is carrying a load of handicaps inherent in traditions and in the nature of its practical problems. As a matter of fact any one who treats mental diseases of the full-fledged character is apt to be put in a class by himself, to be shunned by families and patients because of the odium of "insanity." Hence the urge with some of us to include in our field all those branches of work which put the emphasis not on end-stages but on the developments and prevention, and therefore on mental hygiene, as indicated by most of the work of our American psychiatry. Hence also the great need of support of centers of work capable of covering this field so as to make them more independent of popular chance prejudice and the high cost of maintaining conditions that will hold the largely voluntary patients in the face of public prejudice and the cry of "the insane division of the Hopkins," not to mention other even more prejudicial terms. At present the clinical work has to carry the burden of furnishing hospital and university an annual return in hospital and medical fees amounting to more than $125,000—naturally a very heavy burden on the staff.

There is not to-day a well-rounded and well-founded organization for the study of psychiatry in this country. Nor has there ever been an opportunity to bring together a plan that would serve either a community or the purposes of research with maximal efficiency and economy: Work at the root, i.e., hygiene studies; studies of the outstanding diseases with all the laboratory resources and autopsy-controls; organization of graduate teaching. We have many excellent part-steps capable of a worth-while rounding off and capable of competing favorably with the European efforts.

The division of the fields of psychiatry, neurology, mental hygiene and hygiene is a necessarily pragmatic one. Some of us want to avoid controversy by speaking of neuropsychiatry as a group-unit, with the implication that whoever takes part of the field for his specialty should have reasonably thorough training in the whole field. The psychiatrist needs them all. The neurologist usually makes the bulk of his living on psychiatric or at least psychopathological cases who wish to be called "nervous." Since the neurosurgeon and the syphilis departments leave but few organic cases to the "organic neurologist," the neurologist's field has become very narrow (no matter how important academically and from the point of view of nerve and brain physiology of man it actually is), unless he be a surgeon and a psychopathologist or at least one who likes to treat functional "nervous" cases as well as organic ones, as is done in the orthopedic hospital in Philadelphia. That these cases are mainly psychopathologically determined does not seem to make any difference as long as anybody seems to be authorized to figure as psychopathologist who is willing to indulge in "talking-cure" or who has undergone a personal psychoanalysis with or without a personal disorder. It would seem justified to-day to require some supervised and controlled training in this responsible field at any rate for those who teach. Psychiatry requires its own psychobiological laboratory, its internal medicine department prepared for research in the direction of metabolism, endocrinology, the role of infections, and especially also pharmacological studies; and it requires special facilities to coordinate the complex material derived from the clinical work—a task deplorably underrated in most of our organization, and difficult to maintain without support for clinical research in addition to the subsidiary laboratories. The neurophysiological and neurohistological division has problems in many ways akin to those of the neurology department, but in such specialized fields that a special laboratory must be continued.

Neurology has its prototype to-day in the spirit and practice of research and teaching represented by Stanley Cobb. It is obviously and clearly a field best covered by a department with fairly independent equipment in laboratories and clinical facilities, but in closest conjunction with the similar equipment and facilities of the psychiatric department.

Mental hygiene has had an uneven evolution. It received its fullest development through the War, but was unfortunately over-advertised before it could lay its best foundations. The National Committee is at present in the hands of a group strongly inclined to exploit child guidance, and the adolescent and college problems, often on but little psychiatric and mainly psychoanalytic training, with a strong bias to draw in lay persons. It is the only field which has received considerable support, largely through the Commonwealth Fund with its annual budget of over $400,000, spent on work unfortunately divorced from substantial and fundamental work in psychiatry generally and in psychopathology and the basic sciences. The Institute to be started in New York is a continuation of the same Child Guidance program. Dr. Adler's group and program in Chicago is also essentially juvenile research. Yale gives a promise of collaboration of the necessary groups if the psychiatric department can be developed properly. At Johns Hopkins, mental hygiene is taught incidentally to psychiatric work with wholly inadequate support (a subsidy of $500.—a year); yet in the main it is on a sound basis as far as it goes, as part of the psychiatric outpatient department.

I should greatly appreciate an opportunity to discuss more fully the questions that may arise in the minds of those concerned with this whole field. Indeed I wish it were possible to get an opportunity to get relief from routine for a sufficient period to bring into accessible form what may be needed and helpful for orientation in this most urgent and most promising field of human endeavor.

Adolf Meyer to Dr. William Gerry Morgan, July 2, 1930 (AMP, Series I).
I have just read with much satisfaction your thoughtful presidential address. It is a strange situation. Obviously much more should be done among those who teach medicine to understand the actual needs of both the individual and the public in general. I have felt all along that what is needed is a formulation of pathology paying more attention to the actual human facts and needs and including in this a consideration of the personality, more in harmony with common sense than with psychoanalytic pseudophilosophy and dependence on Christian Science and kindred placebos.

What you say of mental hygiene is certainly true. It was Chittenden and George Blumer who took the control and guidance of Beers out of my hand about 1910, after I had given him the idea of mental hygiene; and after Salmon passed away it got into the hands of a group who might be better charged with "infantilism" than with paternalism—they got everybody upset over "the child." There is a lot of good work being done, no doubt. But it certainly is a pity that the medical profession does not rise more wisely in support of a reasonably conservative progressiveness including more stability in the adult. Nobody likes the debunking process; but it has to be done and probably best so through the establishment of substantial work which will place the responsibility on those who create more unrest than samples of work. I hope we shall before long have a mental hygiene division which shall be in a position to give an honest account of its actual work without having to swell the unfortunate noise and propaganda that has become necessary to maintain the salaries and professionalism of so many half-doctors and new "professions" under the name of mental hygiene, and under the praise of unattainable panaceas. This infantilistic paternalism is indeed a danger because it makes so many people cultivate the present-day excess of individualism "because the people want it"—or really because the people can be tempted to buy it as such—with a dissolution of any real cohesion among what you call "the backbone of our government." Our middle class seems utterly disconcerted. The fear of being called a Babbitt or a yokel for not being up to the latest wrinkle of psychoanalytic and sex-pathological propaganda, and the literary feeding with largely destructive material, and the ease with which we treat our efforts at government and at training social morality with ridicule without any steps toward construction—all these tendencies feed the drifting and the unwillingness to tackle the reshaping of certain dependable standards that would be better than our spineless laisser faire. Does our much quoted Bill of Rights really contain encouragement along the lines of "the right to be sick" and "the right to be drunk as a lord"—or can we avoid extremes of infantilism and extremes of paternalism by a bit more determination of coherent common sense in public life somewhere between government and lawlessness?

We have a nice task ahead in giving the alcohol problem a constructive instead of merely prohibitive or bootleg status. What can be done to reach those who create the alcohol problem? Those who really *do* call for remedy? How can we inculcate a conscience of health? We do not want paternalism nor do we want to make it look as if all we needed was to pick on the child or to emancipate it so that the parents are driven to give up the job. We need certain agreements on responsibilities in matters of health and behavior. We need appropriate education and standards and a formation of public opinion. Why only extremes? We cannot have more and more schools and hospitals and "clinics" and penitentiaries and reformatories, but somehow we need elements of constructive stability somewhere in our civic and social life and government and a government of freedom and solidarity. It will not come out of nothing. No civilization lives without effort. We may be tired of the Anti-Saloon League, supported by a good share of the well-meaning backbone of middle-class people. But where are the wiser guides? And what do we do to them and for them when we have them?

Somehow your address got me pondering quite a little. What a period of contradiction! Papers like yours make one think and, I hope, look for sound progress somewhere between paternalism and haphazard drifting. A better accounting of sufficiently well organized work, and teaching in keeping with what could convince the taxpayer, and less stimulation of false appetites. On the other hand, a restitution of public interest that may make it unnecessary to resort to excessive law-making and inefficient government.

Dr. Earle Saxe (director, the Southard School of the Menninger Clinic) to
Maxwell Gitelson, December 16, 1939 (MGP).

Because of your interest in children we thought you might like to read the enclosed article on "Solving the Problem Child" by Fred C. Kelly, which appeared in the November issue of the *Reader's Digest.*

The way in which this article came to be written is rather interesting. Mr. Kelly, whose articles have appeared in *Harpers,* the *Saturday Evening Post,* and elsewhere, came to Topeka two years ago to gather material for a story about the Kansas Legislative Council. In connection with the investigations of the Council were reports on conditions and procedures in the state hospitals for the mentally ill.

Becoming interested in the subject of mental illness, its origins and treatment, Mr. Kelly visited the Southard School. Watching the children at work and play and observing the methods used for their re-education, he said, "I had never before realized that it is the problem child who is doomed to mental illness in adult life. The solution of the problem should be treatment of the maladjusted personality in childhood before it becomes a burden to society."

Last summer he decided to write an article on this idea and returned to the Southard School for a second time.

We believe that he succeeded in catching the spirit of the work of our school. The chief importance of such articles in popular magazines, however, is that they tend to awaken people everywhere to the deplorable, if not criminal, neglect of unhappy, maladjusted children. At least this is our belief, and we hope that you agree with us. We should be very glad to have you write us your reactions to the article.

Maxwell Gitelson to Earle Saxe, December 19, 1939 (MGP).
Mr. Kelly wrote an intelligent article. However, my own question about such articles is the one which I entertain about the whole mental hygiene movement. Its capacity for creating a need has developed far in advance of its capacity for meeting the developed need. It seems to me that the social problem in psychiatry today is not to sensitize people further, but to give ourselves a little time to catch up with the already existing demands for help.

My own clinical experience has been replete with the present necessity to tone down expectations in terms of what we were actually in a position to offer, both in child psychiatry and adult psychiatry.

Earle Saxe to Maxwell Gitelson, January 20, 1940 (MGP).
I think you are quite right that the public demand for mental hygiene far exceeds present facilities for meeting the need. In fact we were somewhat hesitant about permitting the article to appear, and after it did and following the reaction that we had from the public, we sent out reprints to a number of leaders interested in child psychiatry in order to get their reaction.

I also agree with you that the mental hygiene conscious public expects more than we are able to give in the present state of child and adult psychiatry. It is unfortunate that many look upon it as a panacea for all ills. I believe this is more particularly true of the non-medical public.

In an attempt to meet this, we have organized a Mental Hygiene Institute, held each summer in June, for teachers and parents. In this way we hope we can contribute our small part to this major problem.

The Boundaries of Psychiatry

In its formative years in the early and mid-nineteenth century, psychiatry was an elite part of the medical profession. When the American Medical Association was founded in 1847, there was no disposition on the part of the Association of Medical Superintendents of American Institutions for the insane to affiliate with the new organization. Indeed, a motion to that effect was defeated in 1853, and efforts by the AMA to reopen the issue during the 1860s proved unavailing. Generally speaking, superintendents of mental hospitals thought their special concerns and higher status would suffer if they were subordinated to the varied concerns of the medical profession as a whole. Moreover, probably most were fearful of the divisive sectarian conflicts that plagued the medical profession in the mid-nineteenth century and thought it wise to keep a safe distance.

By 1900 this situation had changed dramatically. Traditional medical practice as well as concepts of disease had undergone a fundamental transformation. Increasingly medicine's roots were to be found in a biologically oriented science aided by a new kind of technology. The specific germ theory of disease, which seemed empirically verifiable, gave rise to a new classification system based on etiology rather than symptomatology, thus holding out the hope of developing curative interventions. Medical schools and hospitals were assuming their modern form. In twentieth-century America the high status of the medical profession quickly became the model par excellence for groups seeking comparable recognition and legitimacy.

Psychiatry, by contrast, seemed to be mired in an unchanging past. The specialty was still identified with traditional mental hospitals seemingly untouched by the scientific, technological, and economic changes transforming medicine. Psychiatric nosology remained descriptive; with the exception of paresis, the etiology of mental illness remained a mystery.

Laboratory research was primitive to nonexistent; the specialty had no roots in medical schools; and its relationship to scientific medicine was amorphous at best.

Concerned about their declining status among their medical brethren as well as the public at large, psychiatrists attempted to reorient their specialty. The basis of membership in the Association of Medical Superintendents of American Institutions for the Insane was broadened to include assistant physicians in the late 1880s, and in 1892 the name was changed to the American Medico-Psychological Association. Practitioners heralded the impending reintegration of psychiatry and medicine. "How marvellous have been the changes that have brought us to the conceptions we hold to-day of the scientific principles that underlie our medical art," Edward Cowles of the McLean Asylum noted in 1897. Cowles emphasized in particular two recent additions to psychiatric thought that held great promise for the future: the "toxic causation of disease" and the "new methods of investigating the anatomy and physiology of the nervous system." Taken together, both demonstrated that the treatment of mental disease was "being brought more closely than ever to common ground with general diseases." That same year, Bernard Sachs, the distinguished New York neurologist and former pupil of Theodore Meynert (author of an influential work that attempted to classify all mental disorders on the basis on anatomy), conceded that psychiatry had "lain dormant for many years." On the other hand, there was "no other branch of medical science" that presented "as many interesting problems." "The past of psychiatry," he noted, "has been full of discouragement; the present is involved in a maze of uncertainty, but the future is full of hope."[1]

The sought-after transformation of psychiatry was evident in a variety of developments. One involved the creation of new organizational forms, including the research institute and the psychopathic hospital; a second was the establishment of psychiatric wards and outpatient departments in general hospitals. The emphasis on mental hygiene was still another manifestation of the thrust to move the specialty beyond the walls of traditional mental hospitals.

In redefining the functions and responsibilities of their specialty, psychi-

1. Edward Cowles, "The Relation of Mental Diseases to General Medicine," *Boston Medical and Surgical Journal*, 137 (1897): 277–82; Bernard Sachs, "Advances in Neurology and Their Relation to Psychiatry," *American Journal of Insanity*, 54 (1897): 17.

atrists helped to create an environment conducive to the emergence of other mental health professions, including psychiatric social work and clinical psychology. Furthermore, their outward reach brought them into contact with a variety of social and behavioral scientists concerned with normal and abnormal behavior of both individuals and groups. Initially psychiatrists welcomed the involvement and assistance of these new occupational groups and disciplines. They looked forward to the creation of a broad coalition that, under psychiatric leadership, could assume responsibility for treatment and prevention.

The hopes of forging productive interprofessional relations, however, quickly created a series of unanticipated problems. For one thing, there were significant differences between the underlying assumptions and approaches of psychiatry and those of other disciplines. The roots of psychiatry, for example, were in a biologically based medicine, whereas the roots of psychology were in philosophy. The former had for the most part been less concerned with the kinds of problems that psychologists dealt with in the late nineteenth and early twentieth centuries, and the attempts to forge links between the two were beset by various difficulties.

Equally important, the effort of nonpsychiatric groups to forge professional identities led to conflicts over authority and jurisdiction. The young profession of psychiatric social work, to cite one illustration, rested on the belief that the social environment played a vital role in shaping individual behavior. Thus the psychiatric social worker, through social casework, provided indispensable assistance to the psychiatrist by gathering the background data on family and community environment without which an understanding of disease processes would be incomplete. The specialty, observed George M. Stevenson in his introduction to Lois M. French's classic analysis in 1940, found "its ultimate validation in the treatment and prevention of mental diseases, in the alleviation of lesser emotional ills and behavior disturbances, and in mental hygiene education, which aims to bring about a more effective and satisfying way of living." Such claims, of course, were remarkably similar to those of psychiatrists and created the potential for conflict. Even E. E. Southard—who pioneered in establishing a social service department at Boston Psychopathic Hospital and co-authored a classic text on psychiatric social work—expressed reservations about a specialty whose development he had fostered and supported. "I am afraid I must confess to one at least, namely, that psychiatric social work must be dominated far more than certain other branches of medico-social work, and again far more than certain other branches of social ser-

vice at large, by the physician and alienist. . . . [D]ecisions concerning
medico-social therapy . . . are decisions which are, in my opinion, medical
decisions . . . hardly to be entrusted to such social workers as the schools
have yet developed."[2]

Southard's comments reflected a series of concerns. Having urged the
creation of an inclusive mental health coalition, psychiatrists were now
compelled to define the boundaries between themselves and other emerging professional groups. If the lines of demarcation remained vague, there
was the distinct threat that psychiatric hegemony over the care and treatment of the mentally ill would come under serious challenge. Indeed, the
creation of professional organizations among psychiatric social workers,
clinical psychologists, and occupational therapists—as well as the existence
of academic associations in the social and behavioral sciences—sharpened
the possibilities of conflict. Moreover, vague boundaries also posed the risk
that psychoanalysis and other medical specialties might transgress upon
psychiatric authority. By the 1920s and 1930s, therefore, psychiatrists
were beginning to respond to perceived challenges. Their responses were
often ambiguous, for they recognized that others had legitimate concerns
in dealing with the mentally ill. The fact that psychiatrists were seeking to
integrate themselves into the framework of scientific medicine meant that
they would respond more softly to other medical specialties. The effort to
clarify boundaries and to specify lines of authority reveals much about
psychiatry's development during the first part of the twentieth century.

---

*When Adolf Meyer came to Johns Hopkins as director of the Henry Phipps Psy-
chiatric Clinic and professor of psychiatry, he was receptive to a course in psychology for medical students. In 1912 John B. Watson (1878–1958), then director of
the Psychological Laboratory at Hopkins, prepared a document sketching out the
content of such a course. Watson had received his Ph.D. in psychology from the
University of Chicago. His doctoral dissertation dealt with the psychological development of the white rat. Ultimately he came to the conclusion that animal
psychology could serve as a model for human psychology; he thus rejected the prevailing emphasis on introspective techniques. Watson became an exponent of*

2. Lois M. French, *Psychiatric Social Work* (New York, 1940), x; E. E. Southard in
L. Vernon Briggs, *History of the Psychopathic Hospital Boston, Massachusetts* (Boston,
1922), 173.

behavioristic psychology and the importance of the stimulus–response mechanism. Between 1912 and 1916 Meyer and Watson discussed the role of the psychologist in the medical curriculum and their philosophical and scientific differences; their correspondence illuminates some of the tensions between psychiatry and psychology.

Adolf Meyer to John B. Watson, January 11, 1912 (AMP, Series I).
Both in Washington and on re-reading your paper I felt rather strongly that after all we are still over-emphasizing conflicts between psychology and psychopathology. I fully believe in the give and take spirit, and I really believe that that is in the main the most general attitude among workers. The fact that I had a rebuff from Titchener is, of course, evidence to the contrary; at the same time, the meeting in Washington made me believe that that was due to misunderstanding and temperamental unwillingness to agree on common ground.

With regard to the psycho-analytical school, I feel that you overemphasize conflicts. Don't you think that to some extent this is due to the fact that you deal with conflicts between those who are working with facts and others who only know them through literature. I know of course what annoys you in the Freudian literature: it is the emphasis on fragments which are made to stand for the whole trouble, yet we see in the actual descriptions the main study of the facts in all their breadth, and it is only because the specific complexes or sexual trauma which you emphasize forms the most concrete material singled out for speaking purposes. Moreover, what happens in late adolescence is the breaking down in conflicts. To speak of the study as a cult sounds to me rather too much like what the straight-laced antagonistic German-Austrian neurologists are trying to make of it when they put a taboo on the whole line of investigation and refuse to review the material in their journals. Of the phrases that you attack those of "suppression," "psychic censors," and so on, are, after all, not as bewildering as they look, and with regard to latent and manifest content, and symbolism and substitution, the problem is not nearly as difficult as it would look from your criticism; and to call the whole "faculty psychology" is like calling Jennings' work "vitalism," or the discussions of foundations of functional psychology "meta-physics."

I know exactly what points make you sensitive, and I thoroughly approve of a very critical attitude, but I should like best of all to have the criticisms coupled with emphasis on the actual attempts at reducing the process of "substitution" "sublimation" etc. to understandable terms. I have all along made efforts in this line, but either insufficiency in my presentation or insufficient propinquity has made it so hard to follow up the matters and to bring them to a practical point of common understanding.

In all these discussions which attack the whole *school*, we furnish fuel to the spirit of conflict rather than of work. Titchener wrote to me that he could put the whole range of Freudian facts in terms of psychology, and I urged him to do it so that we would know what concrete facts we were talking about; but when it comes to it it is easier to back down, and to enumerate the number of faithful adherents and the number of years studying philosophy, and the fact that he had the refusal of a position at the very moment when I criticized him—as if all these things had anything to do with the facts.

What you say of the sub-conscious I quite agree with if at least we are willing to consider as a topic of psychology not only the actual manifestations but also the dispositions or potentialities for mental activity which should be kept apart from the disposition of activities of a merely physiological level. The behavior of these dispositions and the behavior of the actions in consciousness would require a terminology which certainly might be made an improvement on the first attempts tried by those who made the earliest studies in hypnotism and certain psychopathological facts.

With these frank statements I do not urge any change in the paper, but I should like myself a clearer mutual understanding of the difficulties. While I am not a Freudian in the sense of being surrendered body and soul, I think the majority are very much like myself, and it will be to the advantage of all concerned to make the most of what is acceptable.

One of the best things might be to go over some of the concrete material that you wish to criticize, and to restate it in better terms so that we might be sure that we are tilling the same ground.

With regard to the actual outline of the course, I feel that what you suggest should be part of the second year and not of the third year; the third year would then take up the elementary psychopathology, so that the fourth year could be devoted to the more complex conditions.

You remarked the other day that my notes for Washington were more intelligible than previous statements. I am, of course, not a judge as to whether you would consider it profitable, or possible, to bring some of those previous attempts to a level of intelligibility. The best thing there too would be discussion of the concrete difficulties, and your forcing me to bring matters into intelligible terms. I begin to appreciate more and more some of the institutions of good old Europe which bring men together on the pretense not of a five-course dinner, with all its formalities and complexities, but for a cup of coffee, or possibly more dangerous beverages, or in a jolly little excursion to a mountain top, or what not. Why on earth is it not possible to get some substitutes in those regions.

John B. Watson to Adolf Meyer, January 16, 1912 (AMP, Series I).
I am deeply grateful to you for the letter you wrote me in regard to my paper. Since it would consume a large amount of space if I attempted to discuss adequately the various points you mention can't we meet over in the laboratory some night and talk this matter out? I should like for Burrow, Taneyhill, and Huey to come over to[o]. On this side we would have Dunlap, Johnson, Wells, Bassett, and Lovejoy to act as moderator, but we would make him promise to keep out of the discussion until he receives our permission! I believe we can clear up our own ideas to some extent.

I don't think you fully understood me about what I said in regard to your Washington paper. I merely meant that your style was easier and your sentences more logically put together than in some of your earlier papers. I have never found what I think [is] your position—a difficult one to understand. If you will let me be frank I may say that the criticism I would make, is that you had written your Bulletin articles rather carelessly. You are perfectly logical in your position. You speak of mental conflicts warps, twists, etc., as actual mental affairs. This I can understand and believe in. The "subconscious" of Prince and of Freud, and the suppressed ideas of these and other psychoanalysts are not conscious experiences: They can become a part of conscious experience when the proper methods are used just as any other "past experience" of the psychologists may be recalled. Freud, Jones and others talk of them as actually existing conscious processes. My whole point is that these phenomena may be discussed wholly from an objective standpoint up to the point where *reinstatement* occurs. When reinstatement does occur the material is open to introspection. Why use the nonsensical terms of "conscious subconscious" or use the figure of Freud's "endopsychic censor" an illustration of which he gave at the Clark meeting.

You made the point, of course, that I am not dealing with abnormal cases directly. This is quite true but neither does the psychoanalyst confine himself to the clinical material. I have been hard at work upon normal subjects for sometime now. Upon dreams, Jung's method, etc. I have never made these studies for purposes of publication, but I have worked first hand with the method, so that your *criticism* is not quite true to the fact. I shall not attempt to discuss the matter any further in letter. I think you will find me open to conviction along any of the lines you suggest. I believe thoroughly in the method of psychoanalysis but outside of the work of Freud and to some extent that of Jung I feel that most of it is a matter of logical presupposition; such fellows as Jones make a closed system, they assume what they are looking for, and consequently there is no possibility of ever attacking them scientifically or convincing them that another viewpoint is possible.

Adolf Meyer to John B. Watson, May 29, 1916 (AMP, Series I).
My reaction to your paper "What is Mental Disease?" resolves itself into the simple summary, that you would like to see all the psychopathological facts treated under the paradigma of conditioned reflexes, with the elimination of *all* and every reference to psyche or mental, etc. You listened to a rather painful paper on neurasthenia by Riggs and to some remarks by Barker and myself, and felt troubled by the use of the word "mental" and drew some sweeping conclusions as to the reasons why Barker and I approved of Riggs—although as far as I remember my "approval" contained but scant praise of his performance and my views have little in common with Barker's.

The paper as it stands now shows that even at J.H.U. the incumbent of one chair can claim that he has for several years been "trying to understand" the position and attitude of his neighbor although the effort has led so far to little more than an effort through platonic intuition. You wrote me a few years ago that you understood what I published but objected to the carelessness of the contributions to the Bulletin. Now I would feel justified to claim after the perusal of this paper that the understanding must have been very one-sided and the effort to clear up uncertainties very small. It amounts to continuing to treat those who use the word mental or psychobiological as neophytes, and to refusing any statement which deals with any other concept except motor habit.

The reason why neurasthenia was said to be properly described as a psychobiological disorder is sadly misrepresented. The example of the neurasthenic dog is a piece of ridicule—probably not intended as such—bound to fall back upon the author as too ridiculous to carry its point or to be misquoted for ridicule of the psychologist who never would indulge in any such antics as you ascribe to him on receiving your dog. The references to Freud and to the specific "incest-motive," the floating affects, etc. deal with formulations which are not very happily applied. To discuss psychopathology as habit-disorders is a fairly old scheme by this time; to treat all the non-motor psychobiological links as speech disorders is however too generalizing a generalization to satisfy the physician studying the facts as they are.

The worst feature of the paper is its exclusive pioneer tone. Your application of the concept of conditioned reflexes is acceptable enough as far as it attempts to make fairly clear what the term may be made to mean; but to use it as you do as a formulation with the character of a dogma of exclusive salvation is a mere evasion of a psychophobic character, reminding me very much of the tone of the traditional "atheist" or the evolutionist a la Clevenger: it over-exploits a special term from a neutral territory to make any possible reference to the old gods unnecessary, but it is not capable of any tolerance such as would give a simple and natural formulation to the main points which force themselves upon the physician. The application of the very quotation taken from James and the scrutiny of the factors apart from "civilization" which cause the misshapen result in the neurasthenic would show the wisdom of retaining a frank open-mindedness for the world of imagination in a broader sense than you choose to refer to in your discussion of language.

If you strip your paper of the misrepresentation of our discussion of neurasthenia, and if you speak simply and plainly of the concept of conditioned reflex and its possible usefulness as a soother against psychophobia colics, and if you show the relation of your views to those of others who have done a fair amount of work in the field, you will obtain the thanks of the medical workers. As it is the paper is merely another of the half-cocked pioneer schemes, devoid of any serious attempt to do justice to others and attempting to handle a field concerning which you are obviously too uninformed.

I consider the attitude immature and suspect it of being *hopelessly* narrow, another one of those panaceas which make an impression on some students and create confusion in a good many more. Or may I hope that the attitude is not hopeless?

If the paper appears and brings out discussion, we shall see whether it tends to promote progress and clearness, or rather the fortification of the hopelessly dogmatic distorters of the biological and psychodynamic formulations. I am prepared to see it hailed by all those who want to give a dig to my effort to formulate a sensible objective psychobiology, but only used for the generalization of a scientific phrase.

The fundamental fact of the paper would be difficult to get at by the average medical reader. He would only in a vague manner get the impression that the evasion of common-sense psychology which he had been taught in an anatomo-functional jargon, was here translated into terms of motor habits, and he will probably be happy to acquire the new jargon of conditioned reflexes so as to evade the necessity of getting square with the psychobiology which some of us teach.

Behaviorism physiologizes the data of experience, while some of us consider it wise to speak in our first preliminary surveys in terms of common experience, actuated by the sense of economy concerning the advisability of translation of the immediate data into a special jargon. Psychobiology sees no harm in using the data as they present themselves, and the usual terminology; indeed I personally feel that most physicians and most students have not the necessary capacity to work with a new and expurgated code without cutting out many good traits of common sense and introducing their own uncontrollable pet notions under the haze of a new terminology. I feel that they show their mettle much more quickly when using the plain language which is put to the test of daily use, than when using a jargon back of which they can hide any amount of ignorance of the concepts and data of the work of other investigators.

Natural history and science and [logos] after all are the formulations of principles and the methods of their application. Wherever science takes the facts of controlled observation in as natural and direct and controllable a fashion as possible, it is safest. There are schools using the economy of principles to the utmost; others prefer to advocate economy of preliminary transmutation. Why not let them work side by side? I am delighted to give you full sway; but why should you assume the militant attitude of discrediting what evidently you are not concerned with?

I have not the conviction that you have given any consideration to our problem, and I feel that it is not wise or fair to throw a doctrine of purism and exclusive salvation on the physician while you still continue as editor of the *Psychological Review* and the *Psychological Bulletin*, hoisting all kinds of Psychology on the public. I naturally do not assume any attitude of censorship; but I feel that this publication would lead to discussions on my part which had better remain unpublished.

John B. Watson to Adolf Meyer, June 1, 1916 (AMP, Series I).
Thank you for your reactions to my paper. They were rather stronger than I had looked for. You have so long complained about Titchener and the others not giving a functional point of view, that I would suppose you would rather welcome such a point of view, which you might accept with-

out metaphysical objections. Every science has its metaphysical presuppositions; and there is no question but that in your last paper, as Lovejoy has pointed out, you have taken at least two irreconcilable positions. Of course you may not feel the force of this, because you say you are dealing with the common sense terminology which cannot do any harm. But the terminology you are using has no meaning for me; it has no meaning for Holt—you will notice that he has come completely over to my position and has just announced in the Bulletin a course in human behavior; nor do I believe that in three years time either your terminology nor psychological terminology in general will be as useful nor as helpful as you seem to think. This is why I am trying to take time by the forelock; I offered my paper in all humbleness saying in the beginning that I knew more about terminology than I did about any disease. You reply curtly that the only advice you have to offer is that I examine three or five cases of neurasthenia. While I do not wish to set myself up as knowing anything about the psychiatric end of neurasthenia, I may suggest that in the past three years I have done a large amount of work in psychopathology of everyday life. I have run across the same mechanisms that my inference leads me to think that you find in your admissions to the Clinic. While this does not meet your very proper suggestions that I examine a few cases of neurasthenia, I think it does give even me, laboratory theorizer as I am, the right to make the suggestions I have made in my paper. I shall publish the article in the *Journal of Philosophy, Psychology and Scientific Methods*, and shall be willing to leave the matter in the hands of our colleagues. . . .

P.S. I hope you understand that I am not trying to butt in on your preserves. I have a theory of psychology which I am trying to develop into a system. I tentatively try it out first in one field and then in another. This is my sole interest. As soon as I find that the system can be worked in psychopathology my interest in psychopathology will be connected with the men who are in it rather than with the subject itself.

Adolf Meyer to John B. Watson, June 2, 1916 (AMP, Series I).
I am glad to have your reply. I want to assure you that the main thing I have in mind is to avoid unnecessary confusion among those who have to do their daily work with mental cases. If we cultivate some regard for the principle "live and let live" there will be very much better results attained than by putting a whole class of workers under taboo. I am most certainly free from that failing. I should not have the slightest objection to any of

your formulations as long as you feel inclined to avoid a dogma of exclusive salvation. When you say that I replied curtly that the only advice I had to give was that you examine three or five cases of neurasthenia, you exclude from your attention the notes which I wrote on the paper. I suppose I should have said the only other advice and I also feel the only practical advice I have to offer is to examine a few cases.

I think I can formulate my position most satisfactorily in these words: I need the possibility of recording the observations as I make them as an intermediate step between the patient's complaints and the ultimate solution, which it might take weeks or months to reach. Of that work I want to see a record kept and that in terms which are as clearly objective as possible. With regard to all these points it will be easier to get on common ground in the observation of actual facts and for that I expect there will be opportunities next year.

As to Lovejoy's remark as to the two irreconcilable positions I am not convinced as yet. I think that there and in many other points there are ways of understanding each other better if one makes an effort to shake off for the time one's own exclusive dogmas. The difficulty I find with your forms of exclusiveness is that it forces certain facts and certain men into a position in which they might be more closely affiliated with Titchener than with you, and I am quite clear in my own mind that my position does not call for that.

In order to make things as plain as possible, I should like to say that I have no objection to formulating the facts in terms of conditioned reflexes. The only claim is that the wide range of possibility of such occurrences makes necessary further distinctions and that it would be wrong to throw into chaos the intermediate steps of information.

Adolf Meyer to John B. Watson, June 3, 1916 (AMP, Series I).
I am glad that you did not get my first reaction, if my pencil notes and my advice to examine three to five cases were a stronger reaction than you looked for and seemed curt. I did not send you what I wrote first and decided to limit myself to the notes written between the lines of the paper. The fact is that I am rather impatient of any dogma of exclusive salvation and of any peremptory declaration that but one method is "scientific." I am delighted to see a man work with all his might with a method that is suited to his temperament and unquestionably safe ground and a gain; but I equally strongly deplore his having to go out of his way claiming that any one who might care to work with a somewhat different pattern would

therefore be either a neophyte or a hopeless blunderer not worth an effort to be understood. You may say that you did not understand what we mean by mental; why then not ask some questions? Your references to what you think determines our reasoning certainly are a caricature. As to your own paper, I should be helped most if I saw you work out 3–5 cases of psycho-neuroses or psychoses, as I suggested in my note.

That our study of psychobiological reactions should be limited to the pattern of conditioned reflexes is to me a claim akin to that of any over-emphasis of any one-sided & [?] advance. It recalls the overemphasis of the neurone of the nineties. Fortunately the pattern of the conditioned reflexes is a working method and not merely a working *formulation* such as the neurone theory was [*sic*] or you might call my concept of integration. But even that perfectly sincere praise does not justify a dogma of exclusive sal-vation. You may point out the *advantages* of the study of man in terms of conditioned reflexes; you may even say that you might readily see the whole of psychopathology put into terms of conditioned reflexes; but do you not risk being presumptuous when you say that therefore every other way or principle is utterly superfluous or positively unintelligible?

Your "neurasthenic dog" is a permissible product of imagination. Your statement of what the physician would do with it is however, a farce, and that and the reason given for our acceptance of Riggs's main claim show exactly where and why you fail to understand the physician. I, for my part, am not going to misrepresent you if I can help it, and therefore I shall pa-tiently wait for the examination of a few cases so as not to do you injustice. You refer, however, merely to what I know were but very platonic efforts to understand psychopathologists.

Lovejoy may have shown that *he* might ascribe at least two irreconcilable positions to me. He quite appropriately put his statement in the form of questions. My terminology, you say, has no meaning to you. The reason is not difficult to find. You have never put any questions. These things do not come by intuition; nor will mere assertion lead to conviction. Neighborly work will no doubt do more; and that is why I offered you the hospitality of our Clinic.

Your temperament as shown in your work is not unlike Loeb's. You have to shut out everything that might confuse your outlook. It always is enter-taining but as far as convincing *him* useless to debate with Loeb. It is most satisfactory to take him for what he gives and not to ask for any assimila-tion of one's own viewpoint. So it may be with you.

With regard to terminology and to any one's having to take time by the forelock I am not so keen; but if you think you have been fair and humble in your paper, I simply have to say that I did not get that impression. As to the right to make the suggestions you have made in your paper—who would dispute that? And as to any preserves of mine, you will, I hope, have more opportunity in the future than you have used in the past to learn to know my liberality and hospitality. When, of course, it comes to the question whether my terminology would have to be surrendered because you do not understand it (which, by the way I cannot [take] quite seriously) and because the terminology of the conditioned reflex is good enough for you—well, there I shall use my judgment quietly and without any dogma of exclusive salvation. That is a point on which our bringing up differs. My forefathers have been free of the dogma of exclusive salvation since 1521; and I never had any need of eliminating a whole sphere of life interests as you did when you shed the Baptist shell. That is probably why I am much more tolerant in what I formulate as critical common sense; and I certainly do not see why we should spoil that which is most likely to help physicians in the task of formulating what lies between the complaint and needs of the patient and the final scientific solution.

You may have much more up your sleeve than your paper showed. You will find me receptive for all but one thing: intolerance and the dogma of exclusive salvation.

Titchener could not find a greater support theoretically than by your formulations. He will at once say: Do as you please; but you do not touch "*my* problems." And I am afraid many will feel with him; whereas with my point of view, I feel that I can rise above Titchener's viewpoint and take in all that is substantial in his and in yours. As to the absence of metaphysical objections, I grant that you keep from rousing them on your positive side. You make your task easy. But you certainly do not hesitate to sacrifice metaphysical advantages such as the integration concept furnishes together with plain tolerance for much that I should not like to miss from psychobiology.

Has Dunlap's collection of terminology come out yet? To write on the sense of the terminology would take a volume. Would he have the temperament needed for such a giant task of critical review? . . .

When the psychoanalytic movement emerged in mature form, the possibilities of conflict with traditional psychiatry increased sharply. Aside from intrinsic difficulties between the two, psychoanalysis developed some of the characteristics of a beleaguered religious sect persuaded that its members had a monopoly on truth. The result was not only conflict within psychoanalysis but conflict between psycho-analysis and psychiatry. The relationship between Meyer and Edward J. Kempf (1885–1971) is an example of how discussions over differences led to conflict. Although Meyer had been influenced by Freud before 1910, he grew steadily more hostile toward psychoanalysis in his later career. Kempf, on the other hand, moved from psychiatry toward psychoanalysis. As early as 1912 he was using Freudian methods at the Indianapolis State Hospital. After encountering diffi-culties with the hospital's superintendent (which led to his dismissal), he joined Meyer's staff at the Phipps Clinic at Hopkins and subsequently went to St. Eliza-beths Hospital in Washington, D.C. In 1918 Kempf and Meyer corresponded over the former's The Autonomic Functions and the Personality *(1918), which the latter had read in manuscript form. In this work, Kempf suggested that the psychoses were amenable to psychoanalytically oriented therapy. Their correspondence reveals the rifts that ensued.*

Edward J. Kempf to Adolf Meyer, December 21, 1918 (AMP, Series I).
I have always been convinced of the sincerity of your search for a con-ception of the personality that would put psychiatry in a truly scientific position, and for me you stand as a critical resistance which I must be able to meet successfully in order to present my theses in a convincing manner and eliminate its indefinite and unconvincing material. When on the Phipp's staff I felt deeply complimented by your impression that I might be able to contribute something of value to understanding the dynamic at-tributes of the personality and to this end I have worked consistently and patiently. This monograph is the best I have been able to do and I now hope that my critics and reviewers will point out the *specific* instances in which I make erroneous deductions or have failed to eliminate the possi-bility of quite different conclusions.

When I sent a copy of the monograph to you last year I hoped that you would mark the specific passages that were unconvincing and suggest wherein I might present my argument in more convincing style. When this was not done I was forced to go ahead and expose the whole thesis to gen-eral criticism which I hope will now be thorough.

Perhaps it would have been better to follow James' polemical methods of showing wherein my point of view and conclusions are better than the most important contemporary theories. This method, however, although useful in its way, threatened so seriously to confuse the reader with my im-pressions of the other man's impressions that I decided it would be better to present my thesis, with due acknowledgement, for what it was worth and the other man could take it or leave it. The principle is that, if it is useful or correct, it will take care of itself.

I do not believe, Dr. Meyer, that I am nearly so dogmatic as you often say I am. I have no use for dogmas that cover up the unknown or ignorance, such as that discouraging, vague, and undefinable dogma which is besetting psychiatry, namely, that an inherent defect, or constitutional inferiority is the foundation of the psychosis or psychopath's difficulties. I was raised under dogmas and no one hates them more than I do, but, on the other hand, I believe working hypotheses and theories, and fundamental principles have the *utmost* value. The student becomes forced into a mechanical position without them and his curiosity is ruined.

I cannot believe that you do not believe that nature has inherent fundamental mechanisms, principles, or laws, by which it consistently works and that probably most of them are knowable and that the *knowing of them*, in itself, will be of the *utmost* value.

This is the thing that charms me and appeals to me as the soundest common sense. I cannot believe that psychiatry can amount to anything (I am excluding organic neuropathology) until we become trained in seeing behavior, including consciousness and its contents, as symptomatic of the activities of the autonomic apparatus.

This belief naturally sees the various segments of the autonomic apparatus as the cause of typical segmental cravings; such as hunger for food, (a craving for acquisition of stimuli and their assimilation) and a compulsion to vomit (a craving for emission and avoiding of stimuli) as specific examples. The cravings originating in the pelvic segment are very similar in their acquisitive and avertive influences upon behavior. The book is surely not "a mass of pleadings which bring up strings of facts more or less related to the issue but rarely, if ever, convincing of the independent validity of a clearly pronounced and utilized claim," because, if I understand this correctly, I make especial emphasis of the independent physiological origin of the cravings for food, to vomit and to urinate, etc. I purposely left out the most potent influence of all, in modern civilization, the sexual cravings, because I thought it best to reserve this until my conception of the personality was being given at least some consideration.

I think that Cannon's and Carlson's work on hunger and Sherrington's data on the desire to urinate establish that autonomic motor and vascular changes and postural tensions, occur slightly preceding and concomitantly with our awareness of the craving, and similarly our thoughts of how to satisfy the craving are the symptoms in consciousness of the slightly preceding and concomitant efforts of the craving to find gratification, the thoughts being nothing less than sensory pictures of the seeking muscular movements.

The different cravings become *conditioned, through experience,* to use certain movements and environmental means to obtain gratification and similarly avoid others. The ungratified craving persists because the tension in the particular autonomic segment that initiates the craving has not been relaxed (gratified) by an appropriate stimulus which has to be acquired. This persistent postural tension gives rise to a persistent sensory stream which passes through consciousness as the persistent thought, etc.

Now *consciousness of self* or of a thought is *the organism acting as a unity,* more or less as the degree of consciousness is elaborated or constricted, to the sensation producing *activity,* of anyone or several of its parts.

You have often told me that my reasoning is *tautological.* This used to amaze and confuse me and for years I have actually been trying to discover wherein this is so. Do you mean that I am unduly repetitious, or repeat old stuff, or reason in circles? The first fault, of course, is a matter of experience and training, getting conditioned to become aware of the surfeit when it occurs; but the second fault I cannot admit, entirely, and so far as reasoning in circles, we must recognize that the mechanism of the individual and the environment is a circle, as well as the proprioceptive circuit, and the influence of the affective craving on the content of consciousness and the influence of thought upon the affective craving is functionally a circle.

I feel convinced, perhaps a little like Columbus when he concluded that the earth was round, that by studying the influence of autonomic postural tensions upon behavior and thought that we are going to discover a new world of human interest. Particularly if we discover the method of initiating and sustaining postural tensions that are conducive to a constructive growth of the personality.

I have been studying this for some time and, although what I see is hazy and distant, I am sure I see an influential something which I would like to work at when my book on psychopathology has gone to the publisher.

This work, I would like to say before closing, will be composed almost entirely of cases which are so worked out as to speak for themselves, I hope.

Next week I want to visit Baltimore and if you are not too busy I would like to talk over some of the sections of the monograph that seem to me convincing and, more so, those that are not satisfactory.

Adolf Meyer to Edward J. Kempf, December 24, 1918 (AMP, Series I).
You make a justified complaint when you ask why I did not raise my questions when you let me read the manuscript. There is one explanation in the fact that I wondered what you would do with the very fundamental criticisms of Dr. Cobb (which I think found their way into a parenthesis?). The other is an aversion to what might prove to be obstruction. But I should have asked somewhere for a simple building up of the definite sets of facts and manifestations of your conception, stripped of all other implications. Some well defined & circumscribed situations which would bring out the *whole sets* of facts which you want to use for your generalizations. You *might* have discussed definitely and distinctly the hunger postures and their role, and the vomiting and urination postures—as long as you meant to leave the sex-craving postures for your psychopathology. These specific entities I should like to see or read shown up so clearly that the reader would have no doubt as to the value of giving them primary attention and not only incidental attention such as I would be inclined to give them (provided that I should find it worth while for some definite reasons). Could you help me on the right track with a few page indications? Or am I "all off"? Point out reactions in which the consideration of the psychobiological determining factors in terms of various segments of the autonomic apparatus proves essential or at least helpful and a starting point for new attacks. I suspect that practically all your lines of attack can be formulated fully and more economically within the psychobiological level (including the cravings and emotions), and that the great interest in the autonomic share is a reaction to the early antimaterialistic soul-meanings still haunting your thoughts of the psychobiological level and evidence of non-assimilation of my integration concept.

The sample reactions I ask for probably are in the book; but they are drowned in material which gets away from the issue.

I feel that it is all right that the book is published—evidently with much more material than I saw in the manuscript, or am I wrong on this point? And did I then mainly look for the above points and then turn it over to Dr. Cobb on account of some doubts in the very foundations? I raise this perfectly frank question incidentally; the main query of this letter is for a few reactions or situations, if possible easily reproduced and open to study, which would bring out the facts used for your generalization and leading to a definite and clear temptation to see the facts in these terms hence forth.

Edward J. Kempf to Adolf Meyer, December 27, 1918 (AMP, Series I).
I feel that our communications about our respective views of the personality are going to be very beneficial, at least to me, in that it gives me a chance to compare what seem to me fundamental factors with your impressions of such things. It is evident that, like in all semi-controversies we will have to be goodnatured in order to endure the criticisms. That is to say, I do not want to finish up with the dissatisfying conviction, which is so common now among psychologists and psychopathologists, that the other fellow will not frankly expose his ideas to criticism but expresses them with such defensive reservations and alterations as to make them inaccessible.

The monograph, as you now have it, is not exactly the same as the manuscript I submitted to you. It would be difficult to point out the exact changes but they consist of considerable addition of explanatory material, quite a little simplifying of sentences and the addition of Doctor Cobb's references. No fundamental changes were made, but on the whole I found that the manuscript was too condensed in some of its most important sections, which is probably still the case, because I am realizing more fully that people like to *read* a book but not *study* it.

It has rather surprised me that you are inclined to persist in considering the points made by Doctor Cobb as "fundamental" to the theory because I am unable, even since you emphasized it, to see in it anything more important *than a side issue.* That is to say, it does not seem to me to have really any bearing on the theory, as such, whether the striped muscle has a dual nature or not. The important fact is that the autonomic apparatus regulates its own tonus and the striped muscles' tonus and largely its metabolism, and thereby fundamentally determines the nature of the kinaesthetic stream, and this, in turn, the content of consciousness.

I am sure you will grant me the same privilege, that I am glad to see you have taken, namely, of bringing up the personal side of my monograph. I am sure that nothing of any value can be accomplished in science or art by anyone, except as an accident, unless he is quite willing to permit his selections or expressions expose the secrets of his own personality. I may honestly say that I expected that your repressions would try to evade the issues this monograph was designed to meet, by passing it off as an attempt to solve a personal problem. This conclusion was logically forced upon me by your avoiding making a truly specific criticism of any points in the manuscript. In the first paragraph of my preface I therefore said frankly why I wrote the book. To encourage myself, because it takes courage to face this subtly suppressive method of avoiding issues, I reread Darwin's autobiography and wrote an analytical study of the affective sources of his theory. You can imagine my delight when, most unexpectedly, I found that Wallace, who independently formulated the same theory, but emphasized the struggle for life, whereas Darwin emphasized natural sexual selection, also revealed his personal difficulty in his theory.

Now tell me it I am not right; that it matters not how personal the source of the work, the important fact is, *does it tell the truth and reveal the processes of nature*.

I am confident that your respect for the sacred issues of the science of psychopathology and the need of the interest of the medical profession for its future will allow me to say that your integration concept, as you are teaching it, is not meeting our needs or the needs of the medical students. I am including the medical students, not so much from what they had to say four years ago, but from what they now tell me, namely, that they cannot understand your psychobiological concept or your beliefs as to what are the causes of the functional psychoses.

I believe, Dr. Meyer, if I may most respectfully say this, that this obscureness is due to your tendency to protect your own repressions. This tendency most assuredly will prevent one from becoming fully aware of many important features in the psychoses and in his own personality. This has been my own personal experience. I think one has no chance to think against his repressions unless he is willing to endure the discomforts of recognizing them.

My impression of the present state of your *resistance* to the *essential features* of my monograph, I cannot defend its flaws and whatever mistakes and valueless material may later be shown to exist in it, is that your sense of its proportions and value is unconsciously influenced by personal interests that you do not care to become frankly aware of.

Please believe me. This letter is written with the most sincere respect for your position and an earnest desire to get somewhere with our psychopathology. I am looking forward, with an open mind, to the criticisms of the more intelligent medical student, who, upon approaching psychiatry with an unprejudiced point of view, will study my theory of the physiological mechanisms of the personality.

I am now in the midst of correcting the final (?) manuscript of my psychopathology and am quite engrossed with fitting details to their best advantage, but I will go over the monograph as soon as possible and make up a list of page numbers upon which are to be found what I regard as the important facts and conclusions.

I am also sending you a reprint of my article on Darwin, which article I am, by the way, using with other case material in the chapter on the *anxiety neuroses*. In the coming January number of the *Psychoanalytic Review* I will have an article on "The Psychoanalytic Treatment of Dementia Praecox" with the report of a case. This case forms an important part of one of the chapters on the psychopathology of dementia praecox and brings out the mechanism of dissociation of the (sexual) affective cravings from the socialized ego. . . .

P.S.—I might say now in reference to the postural tensions of the bladder causing the desire or craving to urinate is discussed on page 25, and hunger, on pages 33, 34, 36, 44, 55 and 72.

The compulsion of the preparation for and the act of urinating is so universal as an experience following the onset of the craving that it does not seem necessary to go into its details. I think possibly, I am not sure, that an example of the difference in our points of view is to be had in the manner in which you phrased the question as to the "hunger postures" and "vomiting and urination postures." If you mean "hunger postures" in the sense of the postures of hunger in which hunger is used in the possessive, then I can answer that I do not believe such a thing exists. But if you mean in the sense of the gastric movements and postural tensions which cause awareness of the itching sensations of hunger and this, in turn, compels proficient movements to obtain relief for it then we should have no difficulty in understanding each other. My whole conception of all the affections and sentiments is built up on this *simple* physiological mechanism. It is of course necessary to show how the tensions may persist almost indefinitely and how they become conditioned to react when certain incidents occur. For an example of this, one needs but to analyze in himself the manifold sensations of tension that he feels when he is angry, and which, upon a little introspective consideration, will be found to constitute the feelings of angriness.

One can easily find examples in himself of how his autonomic reactions, which cause awareness of *anger,* are conditioned to become aroused when certain subjects are mentioned or certain people assume a particular attitude even years after the initial conditioning experience occurred.

Edward J. Kempf to Adolf Meyer, January 2, 1919 (AMP, Series I).
As you have requested, I have gone through my monograph and picked out some of the more essential facts and interpretations. Upon going over

the pages I must say, with your criticism in mind, about the manner in which essentials were submerged by details, that I was quite surprised to find that most of the essential conclusions are repeated in italics as the preceding discussions of them are finished. In many instances also Restatements are added in paragraph form.

In the introduction I took particular pains to point out what I thought were essentials and repeated them in the table of contents and listed them in the index in order to make them easy to find.

One cannot present a study of the autonomic functions and the personality in one-hundred and fifty pages without condensing the material so that almost every sentence is essential. This of course makes slow reading and does not permit the more important facts to stand out prominently. To meet this need I used most of the phenomena as section headings and listed them in the table of contents. . . .

If it should later become worth while to get out another edition I will certainly bear in mind your valuable criticisms about calling attention to the reader that so and so is regarded as a significant fact and when associated with certain other facts (specified) the following conclusion is indicated.

Adolf Meyer to Edward J. Kempf, January 8, 1919 (AMP, Series I).
Through a mishap your letter of December 27 didn't come to my hand until this morning. There is no reason for you to think that there is any sensitiveness on my part. I am perfectly willing to have you come out quite frankly with any specific explanation of my repression. I know too much in this direction to assume that I do not want to cultivate any; but I am perfectly willing to face what comes up. On the other hand, I do not think that circumspection and seeing more than one thing is necessarily due to repression. When you say that "your sense of its (your work's) proportions and value is unconsciously influenced by personal interests that you do not care to become frankly aware of," I feel that you owe me a frank statement. I realize that besides the possibility of repressions there is also a great probability of limitations, and one of my limitations is that of time and therefore a desire for an economy of presentation and expression, which I realize from my own experience is not always easy.

With regard to the ability of some of the students (and as far as that goes, the body of students) to have a full conception of my views, that might be expecting too much of them as well as of me. As far as I can see, the only alternative for them is whether one is Freudian or not, and whether they have any special concept back of that is very often a question. On the other hand, I know that a fair number of the students get a point of view of practical common-sense which allows them to use their judgment and experience in what they observe and to have their minds open to whatever is offered and reasonably shown to be of substantial help.

I hope to have some time to look more definitely into the places you point out. It is very probable that your psychopathology will have to bring the facts more quickly in the form in which I have to see things.

Your brushing aside of Dr. Cobb's objection is, I think, very fundamental. It is very much like one of the last public speeches of Van Gieson at the meeting of 1899, when he said that no matter whether the neurone retraction theory was proved wrong or not, he stood by the hypothesis. I suppose there is one of my repressions. I should like to know whether it would be in any way symptomatic.

With regard to your postscript and your reference to my phrasing of the hunger postures, I want to assure you that I cannot understand what you would mean by "hunger in the possessive." What you say of gastric movements, etc. is intelligible to me. The question is whether this self-evident type of mechanism can be demonstrated with sufficient clearness to make its mention and demonstration worth while in specific cases.

Edward J. Kempf to Adolf Meyer, January 12, 1919 (AMP, Series I).
Since you ask me to explain what I meant in my December 27th letter by the reference to "personal interests which you do not care to become frankly aware of," and which influence your sense of proportions of the essential points in the monograph, and, of course, also the work of others, I will give my impressions of your position and your attitude.

You occupy the foremost chair of psychopathology in America and one of the most important in the medical sciences. The serious obligations this position forces upon you, through the natural expectations of most men who are interested in solving the riddles of psychiatry, that you should guide, if not largely contribute to, the development of insight into human behavior, automatically places you in a defensive position if this is not done. It seems that this defense influences you to be unduly resistant to the contributions to psychiatry which may shift the general acknowledgement of progressive thinking to other striving centers because that would reflect upon your own unproductiveness.

The natural solution of this dilemma would be either to become aggressive and productive in a manner that would merit the acknowledgement of leadership or defensively avoid frank issues as much as possible. The non-committal attitude prevents clear self-expression so as to remain inaccessible to direct analysis. Such things of course are largely the cause of defensive evasiveness which may be a temporary advantage, in that it precludes the possibility of many errors; but, if it becomes a consistent characteristic, it eventually leads to the reputation of being afraid to come out into the open. As a former member of your staff, for the high reputation of which I have, naturally, ardent wishes, I may say that the general attitude of psychiatric criticism is no longer when is Meyer going to commit himself to definite issues and say what he believes and why, but the opinion is now, he cannot be induced to do this.

It certainly is any man's privilege to hold back until his hour to strike comes, but it seems that the obligations of your position require at least a certain amount of expression of opinion and exposure of views to a counter-review. The necessity that psychopathology shall progress requires this. For example, the predominant influence of the affections upon thought emphasizes the importance of working out the physiology of the affections and the mechanisms by which the affective cravings adjust to one another. Since this is a paramount issue why should it be obscured by defensive evasions? My monograph tries to get directly at this thing, and in sending it to you I hope for a pointed estimation of its essential claims, stated as nearly as possible in a manner that is open to discussion. That would show, quite clearly, where we stand in relation to one another and what I have to build up or throw away in order to get on a uniform basis with you. So far I am unable to understand how you think "the psychobiological level" works.

Now, other psychiatrist's, who have been in your school, say that you cannot be gotten to express yourself so as to be open to critical examination. If this is true it would be such a misfortune that I cannot believe it. Take, for example, the controversy of physiologists over the dual nature of the striped muscle cell. I regard this of secondary importance because, if the autonomic affective apparatus controls the tonus of the striped muscle cell and thus, largely, the kinaesthetic stream and the content of consciousness, what difference does it make to my theory whether the striped muscle cell's tonus is regulated through its being a dual cell or because some other physiological arrangement exists? That is to say, it does not seem of fundamental importance to the theory of evolution, as such, as to whether man ascended from a spider or a fish, but that he did ascend according to certain autonomic principles of adjustment is of the utmost importance because they can be applied to his present problems of adjustment.

Now, to use this point of controversy as an example, although I hope it will not prevent more important issues from being digested, it seems to me that it ought to follow, naturally, that you would state *why* you think Doctor Cobb's reference has fundamental importance and *what it seems to signify*. This sort of critical attitude would, of course, in proportion to its correctness, satisfy the general desire and need for frank, critical reviews. There are many things that are not worth considering and this may be the actual value of my work, upon this hangs my fate, and I must be willing to abide by it, but it is high time that psychopathologists learn to commit themselves to an evaluation of the influence of the affections in the psychoses, with care of right or wrong, but not fear of it, in order to get somewhere.

Before leaving an explanation of what I regard as your personal resistances, I would like to add that the prudish resistance of the ascetic element in Johns Hopkins Hospital no doubt reenforces your own aversions to fully evaluating the influence of the sexual affections upon normal and abnormal thought and behavior, but I think your general dread of making an error of judgment is the greatest obstacle to your work.

I am delighted that our understanding of the peripheral origin of hunger or craving for food and its influence upon behavior is quite similar because that seems to be followed by the next step, that all the affections and sentiments are hungers or cravings, and, as a stream of sensations, are produced by characteristic autonomic tensions.

I would like to say that I am inclined to regard the *neutralization* principle of the autonomic craving and the formulation of the law of the conservation of energy, in a philosophical and physiological, as well as a psychological sense, as the most important thing in my contribution. (I mean by *neutralization* of the autonomic striving, that the disturbed autonomic apparatus seeks for a stimulus that will, through counterstimulation, produce again a state of motor-sensory tension which will be comfortable.) Psychologists, etc., insofar as I am aware, have not offered a satisfactory explanation of emotions and the instincts to act in a characteristic manner except the naive theory of prearranged, concatenated reflexes.

I hope that we will be able to develop a thoroughgoing understanding of each other's interpretations of the personality, because now there seems

to be an unusually receptive attitude in the people for a biological understanding of human nature.

Adolf Meyer to Edward J. Kempf, January 16, 1919 (AMP, Series I).
I have indeed very little inclination to answer your characterization in kind.
Moreover, I abstain from a public criticism whenever I feel I would do
more to help the reactionaries than those who will find themselves in time,
and who only need come with specific questions to get answers.

As long as specific facts such as the great uncertainty of the direct autonomic control of striped muscles do not affect your formulation, why not
show in a few simple constructive instances of observation and interpretation and adjustment which of the accumulated mass of facts become necessary and what perspective they give us that would not be available with a
simpler scheme? The role of affects necessarily makes the *study* of affects
highly desirable and welcome; hence I ask for a simple and unencumbered
statement and if possible its pragmatic test in a concrete instance.

Your mode of reference to the "psychobiological level" makes me wonder what idea you have got of it and where? Have you ever given any evidence of digesting what you boil down as a record of unproductivity? It
ought to have at least the advantage of being quickly disposed of. Have you
ever asked a specific question concerning any of my writings which would
show one tenth of the penetration you ask from me with this long and to
my mind not very happily boiled down monograph? Where have I refused
to answer objections which would "object"? The silence of others has
made me more silent. Should I answer Abbot, Hamilton, and Southard
any more than I did? And where have the "other psychiatrists" (who are
they?) found me unwilling to express myself so as to be open to critical
examination? A charge of this type would indeed be worthy of a frank
statement with specific names and facts. In the meantime I shall hope not
to endanger the reputation of my staff. The most serious danger would be
the lack of a certain kind of loyalty on the part of some of the past members
with their lack of initiative in availing themselves of what *is* offered them
and in making it their duty to acquire the grasp on essentials which will
entitle them to figure as belonging to the group. I am not a schoolmaster
and I feel I have given free opportunities to the most heterogeneous types
of people without imposing myself on them. If that is wanted why not go
where it can be had?

As to the uniqueness of the position I hold there may be differences of opinion. I like to make it so, but the support available is not quite in harmony with the ambitions. That may change for the better.

Show me in one or more sufficiently simple and clear instances how you use your concept and you will not find me unresponsive.

Edward J. Kempf to Adolf Meyer, January 21, 1919 (AMP, Series I).
It does not seem to be appropriate to cite remarks and opinions that are casually made because in themselves they only show a general trend of reaction which is easily changed. In giving a frank statement of my impressions I do not regard myself as having been disloyal or unfriendly. I don't think such things constitute disloyalty. I gave my impressions which were forced upon me by the manner in which you dealt with my work and it is probably this noncommittal attitude that is causing disappointments in important centers.

I may say that I have read everything that you have written on the personality that I have been able to find and have tried to digest its generalities as well as the few places where you deal with clearly defined mechanisms. I have not been impressed by the term "reaction tendencies" or "reaction complex" because it savored too much of the old idea of instincts or habits as concatenated reflexes, and, similarly, the concept of constitutional inferiority underlying the psychosis begs the issues in the case and depresses scientific curiosity. The tendency to pass up the mind–body problem as not needing an explanation because it does not bother you is naturally discouraging because of its method of evading vital questions. One concept that you use has been valuable to me, that is [that] the organism acts as a "unit" or unity. This is selfevident, but you have not explained, that I know of, how it may or does produce consciousness of self, of delusions, hallucinations, etc. . . .

The expanding schism between psychiatry and psychology had become evident by the early 1920s. Growing tensions led the young but influential National Research Council to sponsor a conference in the spring of 1921 on the relations between the two specialties. Chaired by Clark Wissler, the meeting brought together a variety of people representing both. A number of issues were discussed: How could medical, psychological, social, and educational problems be differentiated from each other? What was the difference between psychology and psychia-

try? If psychologists dealt with the shaping of behavior, how could their activities be distinguished from those of psychiatrists? Should psychologists be licensed and permitted to practice for fees? Was the term clinical *appropriate as applied to psychology? Disagreements at the conference proved so pervasive and fundamental that the participants were unable to agree on a set of general resolutions. A few months later Professor Edwin G. Boring (1886–1968), a distinguished young psychologist at Clark University and secretary of the American Psychological Association, wrote to Adolf Meyer. Boring noted that the American Psychological Association, at its next meeting in December 1921, wanted to arrange a symposium "Psychology in Its Social Applications." The symposium would also include a discussion of the relationships between psychology and psychiatry. Boring hoped that Meyer, along with C. Macfie Campbell and Richard Cabot, would attend. His letter to Meyer on October 10 was followed by an illuminating correspondence on growing antagonisms between psychiatry and other related mental health professions.*

Adolf Meyer to Edwin G. Boring, October 15, 1921 (AMP, Series II).
Your letter of October 10 finds me in a somewhat questioning mood. Somehow there has been so much highly questionable discussion lately of the commercialization of psychology that the discussion of the relation of psychiatry and psychology has suffered a great deal. About ten years ago we had a symposium on the value of psychology to psychiatry, as far as I remember, absolutely free from these extraneous considerations, and I wish it might be possible to keep it so. Whether I have much to add to what was said then is, however, doubtful. My collaboration with Dr. Watson was too short and stopped before we could reach what would have interested me—partly because he was somewhat steeped in Freudian preconceptions and vocabulary, so that discussion was not always sufficiently to my taste discussion of fact as actually found and worked with. With his negativistic attitude toward any formulation of facts which I and many others would want to include in psychology, there was really little chance to get anywhere, and men who like yourself might be interested in a critical formulation of the facts as we find them and of psychological and psychobiological terminology were not within my reach; hence my reluctance. I do not shirk the obligation, but should be very glad to be somewhat clearer about the purpose.

I was sorry not to find you at Clark this summer and appreciate this occasion to get in touch with you again.

Edwin G. Boring to Adolf Meyer, October 19, 1921 (AMP, Series II).
The proposed symposium on psychology and social relations is a matter of compromise, as are all such things, I regret to say. The Program Committee wished primarily to do something that would direct interest from gossip in the halls to the content of the meetings. It sounded out various persons and compromised first the issue of practice versus science, and second the difference of opinion with regard to social psychology and psychiatry. You have in my letter the result. The interest in psychiatry, I think, was partly stimulated by a conference on that subject at the National Research Council last spring.

My own desire was especially keen for you to take part in order that the trend might not run unduly away from the fundamental problems toward the more practical issues. I still feel quite the same way, although I realize that we may be putting a burden upon you. Even if you feel that what you might say was a re-presentation of what you had said at other times, it seems to me that your personal urge for a greater synthesis among divergent points of view, combined with your seniority, would make your participation especially important.

A Program Committee of juniors can not very well dictate to seniors what they shall say, so that the exact nature of this symposium has to await acceptance from the participants. Cabot and Campbell have accepted. McDougall has indicated reluctant willingness, but urged us to leave him out and invite Paton. Boas has not yet replied.

It is a little unfortunate that there should be so much pressure for time. I got hold of Langfeld three days after he arrived from England and we started this thing at once. Perhaps the mistake lay in not beginning in the Spring.

More than this I can not tell you, and I fear the final decision will have to rest with you. I do assure you of my personal conviction that you will interest and that your participation will be of a great deal of value to the members of the Association.

Adolf Meyer to Edwin G. Boring, October 21, 1921 (AMP, Series II).
It looks to me as if the program were getting loaded too much with the medical and not especially psychiatrically trained friends of psychology. Your hesitancy about the "program committee of juniors" should, I think, be overcome. It is a very important thing that the younger men should give themselves the fullest possible expression, and as far as I myself am con-

cerned I feel very much in the junior ranks, if, at least, that means a feeling of still impending growth. The snag in this present situation is the diversity of issues. I do not see how the relation of psychology and psychiatry can fit into a question of psychology in its social applications, unless we discuss the social applications of psychiatry and the help derived from the psychological aspects of psychiatry. As a rule, I feel thoroughly sick of my having yielded for about two weeks preceding a performance, and as I have a public lecture on December 6 giving a version of what others think can be handled only under the head of psychoanalysis, I am inclined to say that if the Association has not at least two bona fide psychologists on the program of the symposium, I should consider myself excused because of the undesirability of giving an exclusively medical performance. I hope you consider this fair.

Edwin G. Boring to Adolf Meyer, October 24, 1921 (AMP, Series II).
You create a dilemma. If I am to sit back and make objective judgments, then I am inclined to think that the conference will be better with you in it and that you will be happier with yourself out of it. The Program Committee has let itself go in this direction at "the call of the people" and there is no use in our discussing the value of giving the people what they want, since we are already committed. Since you place the responsibility of advice upon me and give me *carte blanche* as a "junior," I should say that I should regard it as "fair" for you to consider your own comfort in the matter, and to refuse us on the ground that the conference will not be sufficiently worth while in your opinion.

You will certainly not hurt our feelings any more than fair criticism may always do, if you take this position; and I only hope that you realize that there is no lack of cordiality in my suggesting it. I have already told you why I was anxious that you should be included, but I am not anxious for you to be included against your judgment or to your embarrassment.

Adolf Meyer to Edwin G. Boring, October 26, 1921 (AMP, Series II).
Considering it all, I believe that your suggestion is the right one. It will be best to wait for a better definite opportunity more clearly in keeping with my actual interests and work.

As psychiatric social workers created a professional identity during and after the 1920s, conflicts with psychiatrists increased. Although psychiatric social workers attempted to differentiate themselves by emphasizing their concern with the family and community environment, they were never able to establish a clear-cut line. Indeed, when psychiatric social workers spoke about social adjustment, they seemed to be engaging in the kinds of therapeutic activities that transgressed upon psychiatric turf. The conflict between the two groups, moreover, transcended strictly professional issues. Before 1940 psychiatric social work was an overwhelmingly female occupation, whereas psychiatry, although it had a substantial female component, was dominated by men. Hence professional conflict was inseparable from conflict involving sex roles. The following correspondence reveals some of the difficulties of defining professional boundaries. The first letter, by Douglas A. Thom (1887–1951), a psychiatrist who held a number of important administrative and teaching positions, is an early effort to define psychiatric social work. The second letter, by Adolf Meyer, was a response to a request by Sybil Foster, a member of the Advisory Committee on Standards of the American Association of Psychiatric Social Workers, that he offer his own definition of psychiatric social work. The third letter, by Hester B. Crutcher, director of social work for the New York State Department of Mental Hygiene, concerns some of her discussions with a committee of the APA charged with fostering closer relations with the AAPSW.

Douglas A. Thom to Dr. F. F. Hutchins, December 7, 1922 (USVAP).
I think that it is hardly necessary to write you regarding the value of social service in connection with out-patient departments. We are both cognizant of the fact that it is absolutely impossible to render service to the great group of disabled soldiers that we are caring for through the out-patient departments here in Boston and in New York, and which service I understand you hope to develop elsewhere, without a well organized and well trained social service staff.

The psychiatric social worker should serve as an interpreter between the clinic and the community. She must make it possible for the physician to treat not only the medical condition under consideration, but as you know, it is frequently necessary to treat the environment in which the individual lives. To do this effectively, the type of skill is necessary which combines insight into individual and personal characteristics, with a knowledge of the dangers, influences and resources of the community. The interpretation of this environmental picture in such a way as to make the physician see plainly the social forces at work, and the development of a scheme of social adjustments, is the social worker's contribution. In other words, the physician depends upon the worker to broaden and amplify his knowledge and understanding of the social element in the situation. He should be informed, too, with regard to the community resources that may be utilized, such as opportunities for employment, schools, social agencies, etc., in order to have the initiative and judgment to work out a plan of social treatment which will fit in with what is being done for the patient medically.

It is essential to remember that the function of the social worker is to work in cooperation with the physician. She must be the type of individual who can take hold of a social situation and carry out the necessary social adjustments in an intelligent and forceful way. Her suggestions should be invaluable to the physician, and should be given freely. The social worker should come nearer to working with the physician than any other of his assistants.

It is quite obvious, I am sure, that the training and experience of the psychiatric nurse is not of a kind to make her valuable as a psychiatric worker; and unless she goes through exactly the same process of education that the social worker has found it necessary to do, there is nothing in common between the two professions.

This whole subject has been thrashed out so often by those who are most interested in the care of neuro-psychiatric cases, and their conclusions are so available, that it seems hardly necessary to go into it again. I am sure that such men as Dr. Campbell at the Psychopathic Hospital in Boston, Dr. Kirby of the Psychiatric Institute in New York, Dr. Salmon and Dr. Singer, and other leaders in the psychiatric field of medicine will agree with me heartily that social service is absolutely essential to the success of outpatient clinics, and that the neuro-psychiatric nurse cannot be substituted for the psychiatric social worker.

Adolf Meyer to Sybil Foster, January 17, 1930 (AMP, Series II).
I have asked the workers in our social service department to give their definition[s] and send them unchanged with my own introduction.

The characterization is what interests me. The definition will have to vary according to what the physicians and helpers work out together.

Questions may arise as to the extent to which the social worker will assume therapeutic authority in the handling of the patient.

The crux of the entire situation lies in the extent to which the problems and solutions can be and are socialized. On these points both physicians and social workers are not clear enough as a rule.

My feeling is in favor of using the socialized and socializable facts and arrangements and keep out of the social worker's sphere the matters which are too specialized or too questionable as social diet. The social worker had best be a practitioner of the accepted and acceptable resources of life, rather than a reformer or one dependent on concepts and assumptions which have not been adequately socialized themselves.

For this reason the psychiatric social worker requires training and judgment in matters of distinction between social and personal needs and views.

This training will have to be work rather than theory. The evaluation of both the work and the theory desirable for training will turn on the sense and judgment displayed by the centre and its leading spirits, and the type of community for which the balance has to be adjusted.

The psychiatric social worker has to cultivate the sphere of mediation between the social group and the psychiatrist, with a definite obligation to be specially concerned with the socialized and socializable sphere.

I herewith send you the notes jotted down. . . .

Psychiatric social work demands experience with cases and conditions and situations in which mental disorders and mental problems play a role: the insanities and the minor disorders and deficiencies in which the personalities cannot be treated as the average "normal."

The social worker in this case has to attend to all the problems required in social work generally, with special experience as to what not to do or presuppose and judgment as to what can and shall be done to bring about social and individual adjustments planned by the physician, or required by the common sense of the situation.

(1) The function of the Psychiatric Social Worker, as I see it, is to put into effect the recommendation of the examining psychiatrist. This may consist in gathering data for diagnostic study, planning for and carrying out treatment suggestions—in fact, taking any steps necessary to assure the patient's protection and promote his recovery.

(2) Psychiatric Social Service is that which deals with a study of the personality of the patient, the environment from which he comes, and that to which he will return, and that which assists a patient in adjusting himself and his environment.

(3) The function of the Psychiatric Social Worker is to carry out as far as possible the recommendation of the psychiatrist. This may include for aid in diagnosis and treatment, such duties as obtaining family history; description of home and work environment; personal history—including an account of the patient's activities in terms of what he says and does; securing for the patient suitable work, recreation, living arrangements, etc.; and interpreting his personality to his associates.

Family case work principles are employed and a recognition of the problems of mental hygiene is essential.

(4) Psychiatric Social Work is the re-integration of the personality problems of an individual so that the individual can function satisfactorily in the community, by bringing under control as far as possible the factors in the individual and in the environment that brought about the difficulties of the individual.

Hester B. Crutcher to Mildred C. Scoville, January 31, 1938 (AAPSWP).
I am very sorry indeed that we missed you on Saturday but you said so specifically that you would be at the hotel by 12 to 12:15, that when you did not come at a quarter to one, we assumed that you had been unavoidably detained.

In brief, the following covers my discussion with Dr. Hartwell. He feels that the A.A.P.S.W. is quite an important organization. He thinks that there is great need for the development of educational and training centers around hospitals and clinics for social workers. He thinks it is much more desirable to have the experience in psycho-therapy with a psychiatrist much closer at hand than he is in the average family welfare agency. If the A.A.P.S.W. could do nothing more than create some good training centers, he feels that it would more than justify its existence.

In discussing membership Dr. Hartwell said that as he understood it there were a great number of members who were no longer in a psychiatric settings. He felt that only those in a psychiatric setting should be active in the A.A.P.S.W. The rest might be associate or some other kind of member. He thinks the point of view of those people not in psychiatric centers is not particularly essential for the outlining of policies for workers in a psychiatric setting.

In discussing the general attitude of the A.P.A. about social workers in general and about the A.A.P.S.W. in particular, he said that he did not think the A.P.A. was nearly as interested in this problem as they should be. It is as important to them as it is to social workers to have good training centers in psychiatric settings, but as far as he knows, there has been no effort whatsoever to secure these. He says that his committee is only a very small group and, while they are interested in social work and its contributions in the personality of the adjustment of the individual, that they by no means represent the general attitude or interests of the A.P.A. In other words I glean that few members in the A.P.A. care whether school keeps or not.

There may be some other points that we covered in our discussion which escape me at the moment, but I think I have covered the important things.

In 1932 the Committee on Psychiatric Investigations of the National Research Council undertook a study of mental illness, which resulted in the publication of The Problem of Mental Disorder *in 1934. Edited by Madison Bentley, Sage Professor of Psychology at Cornell University, and E. V. Cowdry, professor of cytology at Washington University, the volume included papers by psychiatrists, related biological scientists, and social scientists. During the planning stage, tensions were clearly evident. In the following letter, Adolf Meyer (who contributed a paper entitled "The Psychobiological Point of View") expressed some of his concerns about the involvement of nonpsychiatric specialties in psychiatric problems.*

Adolf Meyer to John C. Whitehorn, February 12, 1932 (JCWP).

I am very glad to know that you will represent the Association in the National Research Council. Professor Bentley, Dr. Cowdry and others have evidently obtained a fund of $10,000 from the Carnegie Corporation of New York to make an investigation of putting the psychiatric house in order. As far as I can see the motives are all that can be desired but I am very keenly under the impression that it is a mistake to assume that psychiatry can be helped very much by those who do not appreciate what is actually being done and who think that only new methods brought in from the outside will be able to bring it salvation. This is what I feel was back of the recommendation. The petitioners spoke of the diagnoses of mental disorders being notoriously in a hopeless condition. This, I think, is uncorrect. It is more likely that the concept of diagnosis has to be adjusted to the facts. Just as I feel that the problem with pathology is the necessity of adapting it to such conditions as we are actually dealing with if it is going to be more useful than is realized by those who take it in the narrower sense—and the same holds also for psychology.

I hope it will be possible to lead the no doubt perfectly well meaning friends of psychiatry to see the worthwhileness of reenforcing what is actually being done rather than seek the salvation in more or less artificial synthesis. I cannot help feeling that we are confronted with a move resembling very much the one of Dr. Van Gieson's "Correlation of Sciences," where I should be all in favor of intensification of work that is already bringing us closer to the unavoidable realities.

These, I think, are points which the National Research Council ought to consider. I cannot help but feel that they have formed their policy largely without any actual contact with psychiatric workers.

I am delighted to hear that we may have your projected visit the fourth week of April. I should think that after my last Salmon lecture, April 22, I shall be very happy to turn to renewed freedom from the very binding sense of obligation towards a difficult task.

Even within medicine proper, boundaries between specialties were rarely clear and often overlapped. When neurology developed during the latter part of the nineteenth century, its jurisdictional claims conflicted with those of psychiatry. Indeed, during the 1920s and 1930s some people began to call themselves "neuro-psychiatrists," a term that created intellectual difficulties, given the differences that existed between psychiatry and neurology. In the following letter, Frankwood E. Williams recalled the peculiar origins of the term, thus revealing a humorous wrinkle in the practical difficulties of establishing clearly demarcated boundaries between medical specialties.

Frankwood E. Williams to Dr. Frank Norbury, November 14, 1935
(AFMHP, uncatalogued).

Miss Martin has told me of your letter in regard to the use of the word "neuro-psychiatry" in connection with the war work of the National Committee [for Mental Hygiene] and I have told her I would be glad to write you and give you what information I have.

Whether the word appears in the literature previous to the war, I do not know, although others have told me that they have seen it in pre-war literature. I have never checked up on the matter. I remember, however, quite well how the term was coined (so far as we knew at the time) and used in connection with the war work. The original war-work committee of the National Committee was called the Committee for Organizing Psychiatric Units for Base Hospitals. Notices of the work of the committee were sent out to all psychiatric and neurological societies, clinics and hospitals. The response from the psychiatrists was good, from the neurologists not so good. The neurologists objected to the name of the committee. They hesitated to take service in a unit the name of which did not accurately describe the work they themselves were prepared to do and presumably would do in the service. Many of them did not feel equipped as psychiatrists and did not feel that they could join a unit if the work was to be distinctly psychiatric. Others who had had some training as psychiatrists and felt competent in that field but later in their private practice were practicing as neurologists, did not wish to change their specialty to psychiatry. The suggestion was frequently made that the term neurological unit be used instead of psychiatric unit.

At first the matter did not seem an important one to Dr. Bailey and the rest of us in the office who were working very hard on the various aspects of the work of the committee, but as objections continued to increase and as it was quite evident that we were not getting the whole-hearted support of the neurologists, it became evident that we must give some attention to the matter. The problem became quite a troublesome one. Dr. Bailey and I discussed the matter day after day and racked our brains for a suitable name (Dr. Salmon, I think, was at that time in England. At least, I do not recall his taking part in these discussions). Dr. Bailey, a neurologist himself, as you know, did not feel that the name should be changed to neurological unit as that described the work proposed for the unit even more inaccurately than the term psychiatric. We discarded the term "neurological and psychiatric" unit as awkward. I do not know how many names we thought of and discarded for one reason or another, and then one morning as we returned to the discussion, the happy thought came to us (an inspiration, it seemed at the time) to call the unit neuro-psychiatric—"psychiatric" describing essentially the work of the unit and the prefix "neuro" adding the element of neurology that would, we thought, at least hoped, satisfy the neurologists. The name of the unit was then changed to "Neuro-psychiatric Unit." When the Division in the office of the Surgeon General was organized, it was called the Division of Neurology and Psychiatry, as you will remember, which was as it should be because in this Division, aside from Neuro-Surgery, both neurological and psychiatric problems were handled.

In renaming the unit neuro-psychiatric unit, it was neither Dr. Bailey's idea, I am sure, and not mine, nor Dr. Salmon's, when he was later consulted, nor anyone else's, so far as I know, that we were naming a specialty in medicine. The name grew not out of a medical need but a political one. The term had only political significance to those of us who used it first in the war work or in connection with the war work. I do not think that any of us felt that it represented anything that existed at the time in medicine or had any idea that its use would continue after the war or that men would come to call themselves "Neuro-psychiatrists" and I think that some of us were somewhat chagrined when after the war some comparatively few men did continue the use of the term in reference to their practice, for it did not seem to us then and it does not seem to me now that there is any justification for the use of the term medically. There were then and there are now the two specialties of neurology and psychiatry, each with an important and well-defined field. To be sure, there was then and there is still, although I think to a much lesser degree, a sort of no-man's land or anybody's land between the two specialties (the field of the neuroses) but this in no way united the two specialties, rather it separated them as the approach of each specialty to the neuroses was so distinctly different. The field remained anybody's land until the one specialty or the other could demonstrate that its approach, treatment and understanding of the neuroses was more nearly correct than that of the other. There were then and there are now excellent neurologists who have had inadequate training in psychiatry and who would not feel that they could call themselves psychiatrists. The same is true in psychiatry where there are excellent psychiatrists with inadequate neurological training, at least with neurological training sufficiently limited as to cause them to hesitate and to call themselves neuro-psychiatrists. There were then and there are now a few men who have been adequately trained in both fields. The number is so small, however, and in each instance perhaps the training and practice is so predominant in one field or the other that there would seem to be no reason to create even now the specialty of neuro-psychiatry. There was even less reason in 1917 and as I have said, our conception of the term and our use of it in connection with the war-work was political and not medical.

Miss Martin tells me that your letter raises the question as to whether or not Dr. Southard had not coined the word and you cite as a possibility his use of the word neuro-psychiatric nurse in connection with the training school at Smith College. I do not recall his having done so. So far as Dr. Bailey and I were concerned, the word was [a] new one at the time we settled upon it. It is quite possible, of course, that either he or I had previously heard the term or read the term somewhere else, but, if so, we were not aware of it at the time. If the word had come from Dr. Southard, I am sure we would have been aware of it, as we were constantly in touch with him at that time.

The term neuro-psychiatry was not used in connection with the Smith school. The Smith school was not for nurses but for social workers and they were from the inception of the school called psychiatric social workers. This was a term that I feel quite sure Dr. Southard did first use. There is still a question, I believe, as to whether the first "psychiatric" social worker was used at Dr. J. J. Putnam's neurological clinic at the Massachusetts General Hospital in Boston, or at one of the state hospitals in New York. At any rate, Miss Edith Burleigh, who was Dr. Putnam's first social worker was known merely as a social worker and the same is true of the first workers in the New York State hospital system. When Dr. Southard became director [of] the Boston Psychopathic Hospital, he laid much emphasis upon the importance of social work in connection with the hospital. He felt strongly also that social workers as then trained were not adequate for work in psychiatric hospitals but that in addition to their regular instruction, they should have special instruction in psychiatric work. Miss Mary E. Jarrett was the first director of social work at the Boston Psychopathic Hospital and she established instruction for the social workers who came to the hospital to work and for other social workers who were going to other hospitals. To differentiate these specially trained workers from those social workers coming from the schools of social work, Dr. Southard at that time coined the phrase "psychiatric social worker." This was shortly after the opening of the Boston Psychopathic Hospital in 1912, so that this term had been used, at least in Boston, five years before the war. Dr. Southard's proposal to Smith College in 1917, which was accepted, was to establish a school for the training of psychiatric social workers to be used in connection with the psychiatric units of the base hospitals. The graduates of this war-work school were utilized in the army and, as you know, the school continued after the war as an integral part of the work of Smith College and continues today. From that time on, the term psychiatric social worker came into common use and shortly after the war the training of psychiatric social workers began in the various schools of social work. The term neuro-psychiatry, I am sure, however, was not used in connection with the Smith school unless it may have been in connection with the unit, as, for example, the "training of psychiatric social workers for work in connection with the neuro-psychiatric unit of the base hospitals." If the word was so used, it was, of course, merely taken from the name of the units as given them by the National Committee and as approved by the Surgeon General.

It is pleasant to be writing a letter to you again. I remember so pleasantly our frequent contacts during those busy war years but these more peaceful years do not seem to have given us the same opportunities. I hope you are well and continuing to enjoy your work. As you no doubt know, I resigned from my position at the National Committee in 1931 and have been in private practice here in New York devoting my time practically entirely to psychoanalysis. I enjoyed my work with the National Committee but I think I have enjoyed life a bit more since I have been in private practice.

The concern with boundaries often reflected philosophical differences over the relationship between mind and body. In psychoanalysis, for example, there was a debate over whether a medical degree should be a requirement for practice. Some of the training institutes accepted people without a medical degree or medical training. In the following letter, however, Smith Ely Jelliffe, whose early training was in neurology, argued against lay analysts.

Smith Ely Jelliffe to Ernest Jones, February 10, 1927 (SEJP).
You have asked me to present, even if very briefly, my thoughts concerning the subject of "Lay analysis." My delay has been conditioned by a number of factors. Primarily I have been much in an ambivalent attitude; secondarily an excessive amount of professional and personal exigencies have interposed. The former have probably been the more compelling. I am not certain just where I can properly balance the whole problem.

If I cast the remarks I am to make in the form of a personal letter you will understand my reluctance to any dogmatic decision.

You may know, that of the New York men I have from the beginning espoused the cause of the necessity for a broader utilization of psychoanalytic assistants, medical, lay, or otherwise. This was as early as 1910 on my return to New York, after a broken three year interregnum spent in Europe, as I felt, that unless I cut myself from the slavish neuropsychiatric models that I had been forced into, nothing but a repetition compulsion of older attitudes of mind would be my lot. I made the break and flung myself into the newer movements for better or worse.

Through many discussions with Brill, I came to a clearer conception of the general psychoanalytic conceptions, towards which both White and myself in our many years of close personal contact, had been veering. Both of us, White and I, were dissatisfied with the Socratic static absolutisms, as were the reigning attitudes, and felt that a dynamic psychology was necessary. This I found in the Freudian conceptions, and the conflicts were resolved in a wholehearted desire to apply the principles and see where they led. Thus for me, the psychoanalytic method of investigation became of primary significance. It satisfied the urgings of research and gave adequate proof of its pragmatic values in therapeutic efforts.

As you know, I had translated Dubois, then Dejerine, and was ready to go further and we launched into the psychoanalytic movement.

Believing as I did, and do, that the psyche was as old as the soma (White's favorite phrasing), I arrived at a Neo-Hippocratic attitude and was not afraid to meet the issues.

You probably know how this, of necessity, precipitated a break, with the reigning attitudes in this, the U.S.A. neurological crystallizations. This is personal history and possibly of secondary importance.

So when I came to utilize psychoanalytic principles I soon found the necessity for accessory aid. Many problems came to my consultation room and I sought assistance where I could find it—not always wisely as later experience demonstrated. I developed a number of semi-trained and more fully trained assistants. These might be envisaged as "lay analysts."

My activities in this line naturally produced the reactions pro and con which are now under discussion. In actual relations these kept me out of our local psychoanalytic society which were more or less dogmatic contra, on the situation. Some of the members, it is unnecessary to mention their names, considered me anathema because I had lay assistants. And I watched and learned and, in short gradually swung to the opposite pole, and now rest, for the time being, in this attitude.

This seems to be reinforced from several angles. May I mention some?

Primarily, I believe that every maladjustment, which in our frame of activity may be called "disease," has a psychogenic component. Naturally I am not asinine enough to include therein the realm of pure "accident." A dislodged brick on a corner stone that hits a passer by, I do not include as of psychogenic importance. The infectious diseases, may also be excluded—although constitutional studies may show some psychogenic capacity for "dispositional" implication; these apart, psychogenesis cannot be a priorally excluded. Hence my studies in organic disease, coincident with and parallel to Groddeck's similar researches. Thus I handed over patients with epileptic manifestations, tuberculosis, tumor formation, diabetic situations and others to my assistants, as research problems.

Apart from a detailed recapitulation of these problems I finally arrived at disappointment, and why? These problems which I myself could envisage since I had a biological and medical background, could not be seen by my assistants in the necessary larger frame which would hope for solution.

So after 15 years of reality testing I have come to believe that only those thoroughly trained in biogenetic lines can adequately envisage the "proteus" of "medicine."

So long as the conception, "mens sana in corpore sane" remains regnant, I must acknowledge defeat. I do not really believe in this. I have come to believe that a healthy body—individual or social, can only come about when the opposite, a healthy body is dependent upon a healthy psyche, shall be the slogan. *But,* and this needs to be emphasized that only a student well versed in the *machine,* as well as its *functions,* can really deal with the situation. So long as the machine per se. is considered of paramount importance no advance can be made. Here is the dilemma of the structuralist as opposed to the functionalist.

When, as in caricatural picturing, flat feet were considered of more importance—as in recruit selection in our army testing than flat heads—I bow my head and with Puck, exclaim, "What fools these mortals be" so, so [*sic*] long as the masses consider physical fitness as superior to mental fitness, I cannot progress. When the social body gets to such an enlightened situation, as to consider mental capacity superior to physical capacity, then I feel I can begin to function openly. In other words when our "medical practice" acts shall consider that "treatment" of "mental" situations is infinitely more important than the giving of drugs, etc., and shall devise legislative restrictions as to who shall practice "medicine," then and only then, shall I dare to show my hand. This time has not yet arrived in our "moron" civilization. Reluctantly I grant, that personally I am still a part of this civilization.

This may seem a long way away from the focal point of our discussion, but in my feeble way, I would believe it is not im-pertinent.

If "Medical" problems are as subtle and as deep as my remarks would seem to indicate, how can the lay analyst deal with them; i.e. intensively. If mental situations are infinitely more complex and more important than physical situations, and as yet the lower aspects are as imperfectly grasped by doctors as they are, how can anyone not versed in the anatomical and physiological intricacies of the human body, deal with those superlative situations which are at present envisaged as "mental"? May not it be said that here, "Fools rush in where angels fear to tread"?

This is really the precipitate of my experience. Lay analysts have no business to enter in; even if medical analysts are still grossly inadequate. Our slogan should be then—educate, stimulate, force the physician to enter into the kingdom of his own, even if he has not appreciated the "Land of Jordan." *This is the ideal postulate.*

As for the so called "practical" issues, it is well recognized by those who see the many problems to be met that the "physician" is illy equipped to meet the situation. The many "cults" offer evidence of this "medical" unpreparedness. These never would have come into prominence—Christian Science, Mental Healing, Coueism, and innumerable other aspects of pseudo-medical practices, if the "doctor" had been *on the job*,—i.e., if he had really, sincerely and deeply appreciated the "human being as a whole" instead of the partitioning of the body into its "diseases."

The "psychoanalytic" formulations have turned the world of previous smug rationalizations "topsy turvey." They have been "revolutionary," I would rather say "evolutionarily" of importance. They threaten to "debunk" our smug complacent Victorian, Popeian formulae, that all is well with the world. "What ever is is right." Any one with a grain of sense knows to the contrary.

As psychiatrists confronted competing claims, their desire to integrate themselves into the mainstream of the medical profession grew correspondingly stronger. They often urged their medical brethren to become more familiar with the insights of psychiatry. In the following letter, James K. Hall expressed such sentiments in no uncertain manner.

James K. Hall to Winfred Overholser, September 7, 1938 (JKHP).
Both of your reprints—"The Mental Hospital of Yesterday and Today" and "The Role of Psychiatry in General Medicine"—have entertained and enlightened me.

I believe that those of us who live in the South are class conscious and it may constitute a handicap to think rather in terms of ourselves and that our thinking may be, on that account, geographically delimited. I am saying this to serve as somewhat of a vestibule to the statement that scientific psychiatry, if there be such a thing, occupies in the South a place near the tail end of the medical profession. I feel that we take splendid human care of our mentally sick folks who are patients in state hospitals when consideration is given to the small per capita fund that makes the care possible. But almost every time I have any professional communion with a doctor who is not engaged in dealing with mentally sick folks and certainly every time I attend a general medical meeting in the South I am impressed painfully by my own belief, at least, that the doctors still look upon mental sickness as belonging outside the wall of legitimate modern medicine. At a medical meeting every once in a while some doctor, who may not be himself far removed from the moronic state, slaps me on the back familiarly and interrogates me condescendingly, usually as follows: "Well, Hall, how are all the nuts?" I think I have some understanding of his poor cerebration and of his language that would be offensive if I did not give charitable consideration to the origin of it. The doctor who is now forty-odd or fifty-odd years of age and who is engaged in medical work in which he seldom sees a mentally sick person knows nothing about psychiatry. But he is encountering psychiatric contributions to medical literature. He can do one of two things: he can supply himself with some psychiatric primers, so to speak; or get a good recent medical dictionary and read and learn something about psychiatric language. If he is possessed of professional curiosity, he will learn enough about psychiatry to know that the problems of psychiatry belong to medicine. But not many doctors who have reached mid or late midlife have such intellectual curiosity. They have to deal with psychiatry, therefore, in a different way. They know nothing about it, but they do not feel willing to confess that they know nothing at all about mental sickness. What such doctors do by patting me on the back familiarly and by making the foolish interrogatory is to declare themselves that so-called mental sickness does not belong to medicine; that it ought to be dealt with by quacks and humbugs, by certain ministers of the Gospel and by Christian Scientists. If the doctor of this sort can continue to seem to believe that psychiatric problems do not belong to modern medicine, then he has to make no apology even to himself, or to another, for his psychiatric ignorance. But such a doctor as I have just been talking about will be made to feel badly, exceedingly, by hearing you talk about psychiatry, of the need of knowledge of it in the general practice of medicine, and of the need of knowledge of psychiatry in practically all the other domains of human activity.

I have been exceedingly favorably impressed by the content of both your reprints. I think one of the largest duties of those of us who are dealing with mentally sick folks is to awaken the interest of the members of the medical profession in general in this highly important branch of medicine. Although our progress is slow, I do feel that we are making some progress. The psychiatrist is nowadays listened to with more attention and with more respect than he was listened to only a few years ago.

Please continue to let me have your reprints.

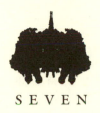

SEVEN

The Demand for Autonomy

During the 1920s and 1930s psychiatrists began to ponder the future of their specialty. Could psychiatric authority and legitimacy be preserved intact in view of the competing and overlapping claims of other mental health occupational groups, to say nothing about the activities of governmental regulatory agencies? Equally important, how could psychiatry reestablish its ties with medical science and thus restore the high status its members had enjoyed within medicine in the mid-nineteenth century? The unhappy state of affairs was evident in the findings of the Committee on the Costs of Medical Care (which conducted an extensive survey of American medical care between 1927 and 1932); its data revealed that neuropsychiatry was among the lowest paid of the medical specialties. Only three decades earlier, by way of contrast, the earnings of superintendents and psychiatrists employed in mental hospitals were well above the average of the medical profession as a whole. Moreover, many states, including leaders like New York, were finding it more and more difficult to attract new medical graduates to careers in institutional psychiatry.

Slowly but surely American psychiatrists began to search for new policies in an effort to arrest the decline in their status. Symbolic of the effort to break with the past were the name changes of their journal and professional organization in 1921. The following year the newly renamed APA created its Committee on Standards and Policies in emulation of the AMA's highly successful Council on Medical Education and Hospitals. The new committee sought to establish minimum standards for mental hospitals and urged that psychiatrists "be free from control by partisan politics."[1] Although the effort was frustrated by lack of adequate funds through the 1920s, it suggested that the specialty was receptive to novel innovations to

1. *American Journal of Psychiatry,* 81 (1924): 385ff.

enhance its legitimacy and define in more precise terms its authority. By the mid-1930s the APA was attempting to rate the manner in which states administered public mental hospitals. New York State, which had a strong Department of Mental Hygiene traditionally headed by a psychiatrist, was singled out as the ideal model for emulation.

The attempt to define mental hospital standards was matched by a growing preoccupation with the education of psychiatrists. Between 1870 and 1920 medical education had undergone a virtual revolution in the United States. Admission standards were raised; a graded curriculum was adopted; new standards for graduation were imposed; and the number of medical schools was sharply reduced to raise quality. The Johns Hopkins School of Medicine became the model institution; its example and commitment to scientific medicine were emulated by other institutions seeking to take advantage of the rising prestige of science generally.

Unlike other biologically based specialties, however, psychiatry did not gain a foothold in medical schools. Hopkins was an exception; the opening of the Henry Phipps Psychiatric Clinic in 1913 under the leadership of Adolf Meyer gave it a unique character. But a study by Ralph A. Noble nearly twenty years later noted that few medical schools provided students with an adequate introduction to psychiatry. In 80 percent of such schools psychiatric education amounted "to little more than a gesture"; confusion was the rule rather than the exception. About the same time, the influential Commission on Medical Education (organized in 1925 under the aegis of the Association of American Medical Colleges) noted that too many unqualified people dealt with nervous and mental disorders. "Probably in no other field of health work is there so much dangerous faddism."[2]

During the 1920s interest in psychiatric education mounted. The NCMH, with the financial assistance of the Rockefeller Foundation, developed a fellowship program for psychiatrists and other mental health professionals. Toward the end of the decade the APA's Committee on Medical Services undertook to define the qualifications necessary for the practice of psychiatry. About the same time, the NCMH established its Division of Psychiatric Education, which launched a major study of psychiatric education.

2. Ralph A. Noble, *Psychiatry in Medical Education: An Abridgement of a Report Submitted to the Advisory Committee of Psychiatric Education of the National Committee for Mental Hygiene* (New York, 1933), 80 *et passim; Final Report of the Commission on Medical Education* (New York, 1932), 214–16.

All of these developments contributed toward a movement that ultimately led to the establishment of the American Board of Psychiatry and Neurology in 1934, which certified people in both specialties.

The APA's interest in board certification, of course, was not in any sense unique. Since the early part of the century American medicine generally had been grappling with a series of problems revolving around structure, costs, and the relationships between the bulk of physicians who were generalists and the smaller number that had begun to specialize. The AMA might have been the institutional vehicle for organizing a comprehensive system for the delivery of medical services, but in practice it faced internal divisions and the demands of specialty organizations with their own distinct interests. Nevertheless, in 1933 the Advisory Board for Medical Specialties came into existence, and the following year it and the AMA's Council on Medical Education and Hospitals jointly adopted a compromise that defined common standards for new specialty boards so as to provide a role for both the AMA and the various national specialty organizations. Before 1934 only six specialties had established formal certification mechanisms. In 1934 alone, six new specialty boards came into existence, and in the succeeding six years, seven more were founded.

Just as the APA's movement to establish a specialty board gained momentum, the AMA created the potential for conflict with the APA. At its annual convention in 1930 the AMA had authorized its Council on Medical Education and Hospitals to launch a nationwide investigation of mental hospitals. This AMA venture into psychiatric turf immediately created considerable internal APA conflict and may have hastened the actual creation of a specialty board. Some feared a power play by the AMA that would be destructive of psychiatric interests; others urged cooperation with the investigation in order to retain influence on the outcome. Fearful that psychiatric legitimacy and authority were being threatened by both the AMA and other emerging mental health professions, James V. May used his presidential address at the APA convention in 1933 to denounce interlopers and to demand that qualifications for the practice of psychiatry remain under psychiatric jurisdiction. "The only question at issue," he insisted, was whether psychiatric "standards are to be left to the judgment of neurologists, psychologists, internists, general practitioners, sociologists, social workers, biologists, biochemists, laymen and amateurs not occupied for the time being with other fads, or whether they are to be established and maintained by The American Psychiatric

Association."[3] The harsh reaction probably led the AMA to ignore and bury its own study of mental hospitals.

The movement to establish a specialty board was also complicated by divisions between psychiatry and neurology. Although clear differences between the two specialties existed, there remained a large gray area where the two overlapped. Many psychiatrists, including Adolf Meyer, had been trained in neurology and insisted on the necessity of understanding the physiology and structure of the brain. Yet members of the American Neurological Association were not especially sympathetic toward their psychiatric colleagues, whom they regarded as scientific illiterates. Nevertheless, neurologists also feared the adverse consequences that might follow the growth of nonmedical specialties in the mental health field and were thus receptive to some form of cooperation.

By the end of 1933 neurologists and psychiatrists, despite their differences, had come to the conclusion that a specialty board should be established. Agreement on specifics quickly followed. The new board would have four representatives each from the APA, the American Neurological Association, and the AMA's Section on Nervous and Mental Diseases (two of whom would be psychiatrists and two, neurologists). Separate examinations would be given for certification in psychiatry and neurology, although anyone, if qualified, could take both. Thus both the APA and the American Neurological Association gained a measure of assurance that the definition of their specialty as well as control over education and certification would remain in their respective hands. In October 1934 the American Board of Psychiatry and Neurology was formally organized.

Psychiatrists were not concerned simply with maintaining their dominance over competing occupational groups. They also feared that the activities of public officials and agencies threatened their independence. Beginning in the 1860s most states began to create administrative structures designed to impose order and efficiency upon an increasingly complex system of public welfare. The creation of external agencies enhanced the possibilities of conflict with a specialty that before 1940 was concentrated in public mental hospitals. On the one hand, psychiatrists sought a measure of autonomy based on their presumed expertise; on the other hand, state governments emphasized their responsibility for establishing public policy and maintaining accountability.

3. James V. May, "The Establishment of Psychiatric Standards by the Association," *American Journal of Psychiatry*, 90 (1933): 9.

As early as 1875 the Association of Medical Superintendents of American Institutions for the Insane had gone on record about the dangers of unwarranted interference in the affairs of public mental hospitals. To endow "supernumerary functionaries" with the authority to scrutinize "the management of the hospital, even sitting in judgment on the conduct of attendants and the complaints of patients, and controlling the management, directly by the exercise of superior power or indirectly by stringent advice," the resolution noted, "can scarcely accomplish an amount of good sufficient to compensate for the harm that is sure to follow."[4]

The troubling issues posed by professional insistence upon the need for autonomy and the public demand for accountability persisted in subsequent decades. By the 1930s the APA's Committee on Standards and Policies had even developed a system that rated states in terms of their regulatory apparatus. The highest category was reserved for those states in which central agencies were staffed with qualified psychiatrists and lay people selected on the basis of ability. The Committee also recommended that such agencies be headed by a trained and reputable psychiatrist. Nevertheless, the underlying issues of professional autonomy and public accountability were never resolved. If psychiatrists gained independence from public control, by what standards would they be judged, and who would assume the role of judge? Could state governments, which were legally and financially responsible for the welfare of dependent groups, abrogate their responsibilities without providing some form of supervision and control?

During the early twentieth century there were mounting concerns over the inability to attract quality physicians into psychiatry. Attention focused on a variety of issues: working conditions in mental hospitals; salaries; opportunities for research; and the psychiatric training given to young medical graduates. The following documents illustrate some of the problems. The first two are an exchange between Dr. Leonard Stocking, superintendent of Agnews State Hospital in California, and William A. White. The third is a memoir of experiences as a psychiatric intern at Bellevue Hospital in New York City (a reception and referral institution) in 1933 and 1934 by Dr. Joseph Wortis (1906–   ), who subsequently studied with Freud, had a distinguished career in the specialty, and served as editor of Biological Psychiatry.

4. *American Journal of Insanity,* 32 (1876): 346–55.

Leonard Stocking to William A. White, July 9, 1928 (WAWP).
We are finding it difficult to maintain satisfactory medical staffs for our State Hospitals. Possibly you are having the same experience, or again possibly you are able to offer more inducement to medical men to enter the service, or have a source of supply which we have not. We feel we must do something, and I am one of a committee to report and advise what seems necessary to do to bring into our service better qualified and more earnest physicians. Will you kindly give me your opinion.

Must the salaries be better, the living conditions more satisfactory, and opportunities to properly raise and educate a family, leave of absence on salary for reasonable times and at reasonable intervals to attend centers of psychiatric instruction and make touch with others, etc. etc.? What do you think should be the minimum and the maximum salary and how graded?

I will be very glad indeed to know your view.

William A. White to Leonard Stocking, July 14, 1928 (WAWP).
I have your letter of the 9th instant, which I shall try to answer in accordance with my experience.

In the first place, I have maintained for a long time that it is impossible to hire physicians, by which I mean, of course, that it is impossible to hire physicians of the kind that you want. One can not go out into the market and for so much money per annum gather in the type of physician that he wants in his hospital, no matter what he may offer; and such things as you mention in your letter, as living conditions, leaves of absence, and I might add retirement features, and the like, are nothing in the world but portions of salary in a disguised form. My belief is thoroughly grounded that there is only one way to get the kind of physician that you wish in your State Hospitals, and that is to offer the physician a career in his profession, or at least the opportunity to equip himself for such a career. This means that more important than living conditions and salary is the scientific equipment of the hospital and the opportunity for doing medical and scientific work. With a complete medical equipment I think it would be better not to consider the question of living conditions if it can be avoided. We find that we get along very nicely by no longer furnishing living conditions at all for physicians. They can then go outside, have their own homes, their own menages, and run them to suit themselves, whereas, as you know, if they stay in the institution the way in which the institution houses and feeds them seems to be a continuous source of irritation, a continuous object upon which all their discontent is projected.

Added to the above, my experience teaches me that the only way to maintain a Staff that is at all adequate is to appeal to the recent graduate. I practically appoint no one on my Staff except young men just out of college, and the higher positions are filled by promotion. Most of the young men come in, spend one, two or three years, they get their professional equipment and they go out on their own. A certain number of them who are institutional types and who are in this respect valuable in the institution remain and are promoted to higher administrative positions. A certain other few who are interested in research problems above everything else prefer to remain where these problems can be pursued under such favorable circumstances.

These are in general the principles which I think should govern. They need to be carried out under the stimulus of a directing head who is himself primarily interested in medical problems and who can stimulate the interest and coordinate the endeavors of the different members of his Staff, each necessarily differently equipped and each with different tendencies, interests and objectives. This does not mean, of course, that salaries are unimportant, but in my opinion they are less important in such a scheme than they are ordinarily considered because by far the larger proportion of men who come to the hospital stay only a short time. For the more stable administrative positions, of course, adequate salaries should be paid. This goes without question. The thing that I am arguing against is to think that doctors can be attracted by salary alone.

Joseph Wortis, "Observations of a Psychiatric Interne,"
June 25, 1934 (copy in AMP, Series I).

My work started on the disturbed ward where the violent patients are kept. I looked around when I came in. Half the patients were tied to the bed in "camisoles"—the name we use for strait-jackets—where they lay quietly, or squirming helplessly about. Some were in separate rooms where they kept yelling all sorts of things, mostly empty repetitions. A number of patients, especially on the women's side, were allowed the run of the hall, where they walked up and down, talking to themselves or to each other, or—very frequently—to me, the doctor in the white uniform. They all wanted sympathy, or special favors, or news of when they were going to go home. Every psychiatrist has his favorite phrase to quiet patients with. I soon learned to say "I'll see you later," or "We'll see what we can do for you." I rarely could do anything.

Most of the patients could be spoken to. Patients who were stark mad and assaultive—the lay idea of a madman—were not common. They were on the whole irritable, maudlin, sometimes sullen and bewildered. If they were noisy they were given sedatives.

The doctor in charge, Smith, was a stout sleepy-eyed young man, intelligent but lazy, who would dictate a few words rapidly on each patient when he made the rounds. He sized up his patients quickly, and made his diagnoses, as such things go, with fair accuracy—it was really not important. The main thing was to get papers signed and get the patients off as soon as possible to a State Hospital. Many of the patients were simply senile, others had some other disease: blood-poisoning or meningitis, or a fractured skull. Still others had syphilis, and it was important to discover this. But many of the patients simply went as "manics," which is a form of excitement of unknown origin which cures itself, but cannot be cured. Where no gross physical signs were found, it was assumed the patient had no bodily disease. It was not our habit to make thorough medical examinations: routine urine or blood examination, for example, there was in fact little provision for such work. In any single case we were free to call a medical consultant—usually an interne.

The fixed period of observation was ten days, but many of the alcoholics (who made up half of the 18,000 admissions last year) were discharged on the following morning after a night's sleep. Other patients were kept longer when necessary, that is when there was delay in getting papers signed, difficulty in finding friends or relatives, legal red-tape, or because some curative measures were undertaken—psychotherapy, for example, or medical care.

I have not investigated the legal status of this period of observation, because I know that whatever the law may provide, in point of fact, the psychiatrist in charge has complete power over the fate of the patient, and patients who are fresh or disagreeable are sometimes told that they will be kept until they behave, as a disciplinary measure, even though they are psychiatrically normal, or reasonably so. The concept of "insanity" is so loose, that anybody who is a nuisance or is thought to be one, is committable. Since most of the patients at our hospital were poor and ignorant, they had no legal redress. Though they are legally entitled to protest their commitment before a court and are indeed actually given notice that this commitment will come up before a court on such and such a day, actually they are kept under lock and key, are given no hint of their legal privileges, and are allowed to appear before the court only when the matter is otherwise likely to have a disagreeable issue for the psychiatrists in charge. (The cases come up before judges—not a jury—and the recommendation of our psychiatrist is almost invariably followed.) Of course, it must not be pretended that the psychiatrists have any special interest in committing a large number of patients; it is my belief however that something less than justice is done for the numerous borderline cases which require close and extended study and very much fair play. The natural tendency of psychiatrists is to see psychiatric symptoms everywhere. Commitment is a very simple solution from everybody's point of view, except the patient's, and the alternatives of treatment or discharge are seldom very attractive, because treatment is likely to be ineffective, and because discharge usually means discharge into the same environment, into the same problems, with the likelihood of readmission soon again.

There was always the comforting feeling too, that if the patient behaved nicely in a state hospital, he would be discharged later anyway. The principle of shifting responsibility, or passing the buck, which was a prominent principle in our psychiatric hospital, was thus religiously observed. Many psychiatrists had the feeling or conviction that a "rest in the country," as they liked to call it, would be a good thing too. This was no doubt true for those cases which would profit from a change of scene, away from a complex situation, where they could think things over,—as when a young girl attempts suicide following a love affair,—but for many cases this was not true at all, and it seemed that a term in a state hospital would only diminish the chance for normal adjustment in the outside world later on.

A frequent type of commitment was that of disagreeable patients from other hospitals, who talked back, or fought with the nurses, would complain of neglect, and would finally be sent to us in an ambulance. They were often chronic invalids who had grown disagreeable from general impatience and physical weakness—they were of no particular medical interest to the internes in other hospitals, who were usually glad to have them go, and when they came to us they were usually transferred to state hospitals as soon as possible. Many of them were simply old and neglected people, with generalised arteriosclerosis and failing hearts. We would find they had memory defects, as old people have, and were "uncooperative and irritable." Nobody wanted to take care of them, and they were sent to state hospitals to die.

Where did our patients come from? There was an important difference between our part of the hospital and the others. A medically sick person usually knew when he was sick, and came of his own free will: our patients were mostly brought to us. The one big exception were the drunken bums who flocked to our admitting office by the dozen, mostly because they could get a bath, free food, and lodging. Our treatment of the drunks was on the whole the noblest aspect of our psychiatric service—nowhere else, I was told, were they accorded so convivial a welcome. But times have changed: they became too great a drain on the hospital's resources and were no longer admitted unless obviously sick. The law requiring the arrest of drunks began to be enforced, and alcoholic cases became much less frequent.*

Sometimes patients came in for help themselves. These were often young and trustful people who felt there was something wrong with them and who came to us for advice or help. One boy hitch-hiked all the way in from the Middle West and arrived past midnight with a little bundle and a dirty note from a doctor. He was suffering from an obsessional wish to kill his father. He was ultimately sent back to his home state under custody.

Occasionally I was able to discover a malingerer (which is not always easy) who was penniless and homeless, and preferred a psychiatric hospital to the street. Many patients were brought in by friends or relatives, or by the police, often by an ambulance in answer to a call, or from another hospital. Private doctors sometimes referred patients to us, social workers sometimes recommended them. All attempted suicides were referable to us. Cases were frequently sent to us by the courts—a considerable number of the cases were prisoners. It will be observed that most of the people responsible for the reference of a case to us are laymen, or doctors with no special psychiatric knowledge or experience, for the average doctor has learnt little psychiatry in school (though nowadays much more is being taught) and has never worked in a psychiatric ward. There is probably no branch of medicine in which lay attitudes become so important. Conduct, for example, which in a group of Bohemian artists or foreign students would pass as perfectly normal, becomes obviously "crazy" in another group. The innocent expression "you're crazy" becomes important, and the more strait laced and intolerant a community or group may be, the

---

*This of course did not help the great problem of drunkenness, for intoxicated people are certainly medically insane and often dangerously sick,—fractured skulls were particularly common among them and may be easily overlooked. The differential diagnosis between a 'dead drunk' and some other kind of coma may at first be difficult.

more frequently will it be used. It is therefore not surprising to find over and over again a type of patient whose chief symptom is behaviour which is not understood or liked by the group they happen to be in; a young negress for example who dyes her hair red, takes sun baths, and is interested in spiritualism, or a young Jewess who writes poetry, hates her parents, and falls passionately in love with her teacher. Psychiatrists for the most part carry their lay ideas with them into psychiatry. They tend on the one hand to overlook qualities which they have in common with their patients and to overemphasize qualities which are strange to them.*

What is done with the patients? The purpose of the admitting office is to pass on the suitability of the case and to send him to the proper ward. Patients are almost invariably accepted, on the assumption that there must be something wrong, or they wouldn't be there. Refusing to admit a patient after a very brief interview is a responsibility which the admitting officer may afterwards regret, so he plays safe, and very properly lets the doctor upstairs dispose of the case, after more detailed examination. If the patient is brought in by an ambulance surgeon, a note is written by him in the record to say why, together with any other helpful information. Short statements from other informants are added. A brief statement from the patient is written down, to indicate the main symptoms, and a brief description of his general appearance and behaviour is added. The patient is given a quick superficial physical examination to see if emergency surgical or medical care is needed. A surgical and medical interne is always available. A sedative may be prescribed. If the physical symptoms are especially prominent,—if the patient for example is in coma and cannot be aroused,—he is sent to another part of the hospital.

There are separate wards for men and women, for the violent, for the semi-disturbed, and the quiet, for the bed ridden, for prisoners, for children, and for alcoholics. After the patients are bathed, and put into grey hospital pajamas and kimonas, they are sent upstairs where they are more thoroughly examined by the psychiatrists in charge. Additional notes and observations are made from daily interviews; the nurses make frequent notes on their behaviour, their temperature is taken, they are fed simple fare and

*It is of fundamental importance in psychiatry to have a wide knowledge and experience all kinds of human beings, to say nothing of animals, and to interpret symptoms, like dreams, only from a knowledge of the whole of the patient. An isolated symptom, torn from its moorings, need not be given too much prominence.

are given simple reading matter, but most of their time is spent pacing the wards or talking to each other; as tawdry woebegone, disconsolate a group as ever I have seen. The chief wish of most of them is to get out.

On visiting days, relatives and friends are interviewed for additional information, for other versions of patients' stories, for life histories, etc., and are advised on the care of the patient if he is to be discharged, or are asked to sign papers if he is committable. In general it can be said that a friendly family with some insight into the patient's condition, is usually allowed to take care of the patient if they wish to, and can. Most of the patients however are poor and helpless, their families have neither insight nor patience, or are unwilling to help. Not seldom they are vindictive toward the patient and are glad of the riddance. There are times too when it is personally advantageous for a relative to send the patient away.

There are various ways of disposing of a case. He may be committed to one of several state hospitals, or on the other hand, may be let scot free, — "to his own custody," as we say, or to the custody of relatives. In almost all discharged cases, as a precaution, to prevent charges of negligence, the relatives are asked to sign a statement that they are taking the patient out on their own responsibility, and against the advice of the doctor. A hospital social worker is sometimes assigned to the case to keep an eye on the patient, to help him with advice, and to help him find a job. Their chief service is in providing contact with other organisations which may be helpful. There are any number of these: girls' clubs, reformatories, orphan asylums, religious institutions, for the aged, the homeless, the poor, employment agencies, relief organisations, Save-a-Life League for suicides and the like. None of them succeed very well in providing what the patients need most; money and congenial work, sympathetic friends, and sexual satisfaction. The patients themselves are usually hard to manage and difficult to satisfy. They frequently came back.

The treatment in our psychiatric hospital was most effective in two classes of cases: (1) cases of physical disability, e.g., heart disease or a fractured skull, or (2) mild neuroses that simply needed a talking to. All the vast field of psychoses in between; the chronically maladjusted, the vaguely sick, the periodically or chronically insane, had next to nothing done for them. It was almost a pleasure to diagnose syphilis of the brain or brain tumor, because you felt that could at least be treated. Other psychoses due to hardening of the arteries or high blood pressure were grateful material because we felt we could at least begin to understand them. But all these were in the minority. Before the vast bulk of our material we stood baffled, helpless and forlorn, for we had had power neither to help nor to cure, nor even very often to understand.*

During the 1920s interest in some means of certifying psychiatrists was on the rise. Concern with establishing minimum standards of competency obviously played a major role. Nevertheless, fear of the intrusion of nonmedical specialists in the mental health field was also present. Upon recommendation of its Committee on Medical services in 1929, the APA appointed another committee (which included Adolf Meyer, George H. Kirby, and Edward A. Strecker) to formulate a plan to define the qualifications and training necessary for psychiatric specialization and to specify common ground between psychiatry and neurology. In 1931 Meyer wrote to a number of people soliciting their suggestions. His letter, as well as replies by T. N. Weisenburg (1876–1934) an eminent neurologist who was also editor of the AMA's Archives of Neurology and Psychiatry; *Edward A. Strecker (1887–1959), director of the Pennsylvania Hospital Department of Nervous and Mental Diseases; and Louis Casamajor (1881–1962), an eminent figure in New York neurological and psychiatric circles, follow.*

Adolf Meyer to Louis Casamajor, May 11, 1931 (AMP, Series III).
To my regret the discussion of the report of the diploma committee has been delayed for various reasons, among others the strong leaning of the psychiatric group to consider an independent move. I still wish that we might work out a broader scheme, holding psychiatry and neurology and mental hygiene more closely together. The difficulty I see lies in the tendency to use lay-workers for psychoanalysis, the vigorous propaganda of the "clinical" psychologist, and the tendency of the neurologist to enter psychopathology without any breadth of psychiatric experience. That the psychiatrist should pass as neurologist is less apt to occur, although there might be instances.

The questions arising might be the following:

---

* It should be said that such were at least my feelings. I don't know how many psychiatrists would agree. It is a presumption of psychiatry (as of other sciences) that it explains things, when it is only offering the latest theories.

What would you ask for as an adequate neurological training for a psychiatrist to pass as neurologically intelligent, and what to be recognized as a neurologist?

What would you consider as an adequate psychiatric training for a neurologist to pass as psychiatrically intelligent, and to assume the responsibilities of psychiatric cases?

What would you demand in the way of general medical requirements to allow any person to claim the right to practice medicine as psychiatrist and neurologist?

What would you demand in the way of neurology and psychiatry to allow anyone to practice medicine and to assume responsibility of a patient? Is a degree in medicine necessary? And how shall the field be covered?

The next question would be: How can we expect to examine satisfactorily in the various branches?

Dr. Ebaugh has given his ideas in the last number of the *American Journal of Psychiatry*.

Dr. Strecker's first report, and the various discussions, among them your formulation, give valuable data. Would you be good enough to formulate the considerations and recommendation for a report to the two associations? Should we try to get an understanding with the analysts? Or shall we proceed so as to let the various branches make their own rules (the ortho-psychiatrists, etc.)?

I wish we could recommend more common ground. What would be your recommendations?

T.N. Weisenburg to Adolf Meyer, May 12, 1931 (AMP, Series III).
I am sorry that the Committee has been unable to get together in the matter under discussion. After the meeting which you, Strecker and myself attended in Philadelphia, I had a discussion with Miss Scoville of the Commonwealth Fund and told her what we proposed to do. She was very enthusiastic about it and from what she said I am quite sure that we can get the Commonwealth Fund to finance such a meeting, which now more than ever is necessary so as to clear up the whole matter of the education of neurologists, psychiatrists, psychologists, mental hygienists, psychoanalysts and so forth.

To illustrate the need for such a thing, my attention has been called to a paper submitted to the *American Journal of the Diseases of Children,* which is an A.M.A. publication similar to the *Archives.* The title of this paper which

I believe has been accepted by this journal, is "The Menace of the Psychiatrist," and it is a protest against the kind of education which parents are now receiving through books, radios, pamphlets and so on. From my observation and what I know about the matter I am quite certain that there is now a well defined reaction against ill-timed and over-emphasized mental hygiene stuff, and unless we look out and take our bearings the cause of psychiatry will suffer.

Anyone who is at all alive to the situation is well aware of the attempt on the part of psychologists, analysts, particularly lay analysts, and many psychiatrists to popularize not so much their subject as themselves. The number of popular books which have come out in the last year or two for the benefit of the public is staggering. I have received so many that I am unable to get sufficient individuals to review them. As you know I have been sending you a great many. I have now about forty books still to review. Not all of them of course have been written in this country.

Besides that this business of popularizing mental hygiene in radio addresses and editorial pages in women's magazines would be perhaps worth while if it could be done in such a way as to educate the public, but has any attempt ever been made to educate the public which has been successful, especially by such means?

I feel from the standpoint of the editors of the *Archives of Neurology and Psychiatry* that we should take a very definite stand in this matter for after all isn't it our function to lead psychiatric thought?

From my experience with psychologists, especially in the war, I feel certain that the one thing that they have done has been to try and sell themselves not only to the medical public but to the layman. As propagandists we neuropsychiatrists are not at all in their class. Only second to them are the psychoanalysts. I am convinced that commercialism is the background of their efforts.

From your letter you state that there is a strong leaning of the psychiatric group towards an independent move. If American psychiatry is to be judged by its scientific output it has certainly made a very sorry showing in the last few years. Most of it has been poor stuff. One reason for it is because psychiatrists themselves have had insufficient training. It seems to me from this angle that of all the different specialties they can least afford to stand on their own legs.

So far as the "tendency of the lay-workers for psychoanalysis and the vigorous propaganda of the 'clinical' psychologist" is concerned, we need pay little attention to it for their goal is entirely commercialism. Of course there are neurologists who enter psychopathology "without any breadth of psychiatric experience" and there are "psychiatrists who pass as neurologists," but then need we pay any attention to them? After all our objective is to state as vigorously as possible what training we wish to give neuropsychiatrists and I am quite certain that if we are right in the matter, as I know we are, that we will have no difficulty in establishing our ideas so that they will be universally accepted.

Feeling therefore as I do I think it is time for us to have such a meeting. Why could not a group be appointed of the American Psychiatric Association to meet with a similar group of the American Neurological Association, adding to these a sprinkling of psychoanalysts, a representative of the Mental Hygiene Committee and some representatives of Funds, such as the Commonwealth Fund. I am quite sure that if we lay out our program carefully that a one day discussion would be sufficient, for a selected group could be asked to present their ideas in concrete form and the meeting of this group should be asked to pass upon the ideas which are presented.

Edward A. Strecker to Adolf Meyer, May 14, 1931 (AMP, Series III).
Thank you so much for your letter and it was nice to hear from you again. The questions you raise are so interesting and important that they would seem to justify some sort of a meeting but I suppose that would be difficult to arrange. It seems to me that the trends of psychiatry have been of such a nature that the most we could expect of a psychiatrist along neurological lines would be that he be trained in the fundamentals of the anatomy of the nervous system and have a fairly good conception of neuropathology. It seems to me that when a psychiatrist goes further than this, he becomes neurologically minded which makes him inadequate in the problems of the neuroses. I may be wrong, but I think a neurologist needs psychiatric training more than a psychiatrist needs neurological training. I say this from my experience in practice where I have found that functional cases are so often badly treated by pure organic neurologists. I think the general medical training should include graduating from a good medical school and at least two years internship in a good hospital or the equivalent of this. In my mind the degree in medicine is absolutely necessary. I suppose we could not examine satisfactorily in the various branches until all of us, neurologists, psychiatrists and psychoanalysts and so forth had come to some minimum basis. This would mean that all would have to make concessions.

Louis Casamajor to Adolf Meyer, June 1, 1931 (AMP, Series III).
On my return from California last week I found your interesting letters in regard to the committee that was considering the question of a standardized training for men working in neurology and psychiatry. I was sorry not to have seen you in Boston as I would liked to have talked over many of the points that you raised. I did not get there in time to present any of the report that you sent me but I understand that Weisenburg turned in some kind of a report although I do not know just what it was.

It strikes me that the questions that you raise in your letter of May 11th are extremely to the point and so much so that I would not care to state now just what my answers to those questions would be. I feel I should want to talk over these matters with a number of men and at least try to get my own ideas clarified before endeavoring to put them on paper. Don't you think that the matter has gone far enough now so that the committee should get together for a long meeting and really exchange some ideas? I believe that more can be done that way than with individual letter writers. If you would care to call a meeting of the committee I should be willing to go almost anywhere to attend it provided I had about five or six days notice.

I was interested to learn from your letter of May 23rd that you were to meet Dr. Rodman of the National Board of Medical Examiners. That I think should be a most interesting meeting and I for one would be interested to know just what the attitude of the National Board was upon a neuro-psychiatric examination. I believe we could get a lot of help from a man like Rodman who has been working in the field of examinations now long enough to know something real about it. I sincerely hope you will be able to interest him in the problem of our committee for I am sure that we are going to need the help of the National Board in no matter what solution we propose.

As the debate over a specialty board in psychiatry intensified, new issues emerged. Would a joint board with neurology, or a board associated with the AMA, diminish the authority of psychiatry to regulate itself? Both Edward N. Brush (1852–1933), superintendent of the Sheppard and Enoch Pratt Hospital from 1891 to 1920 and editor of the American Journal of Psychiatry *from 1904 to*

1931, and William L. Russell (1863–1951), the psychiatric director of the So-
ciety of the New York Hospital and former president of the American Psychiatric
Association, expressed these fears in their private correspondence.

Edward N. Brush to Dr. Franklin G. Ebaugh (Colorado Psychiatric Hospital),
March 3, 1931 (AMP, Series II).

Your letter of the 24th was received on the 27th. As you appear to ask it, I
am taking the liberty of offering advice and asking a few questions. If I
appear to be offering advice where it is not required, you will I hope excuse
it as the blunderings of an old man.

As I recall the facts Dr. Meyer in his address as President in 1928 called
attention to the desirability of having some diploma or degree or title that
should distinguish the approved Psychiatry. In 1929 the subject was brought
up in the admirable report of Dr. Strecker. See Journal of September 1929.
And after after some discussion a committee consisting of Doctors Meyer,
Kirby and Strecker was appointed to take up the whole subject and report
and a tentative report was made at the meeting in 1930. Your paper as thus
far completed appears to be a report of the committee, of which *Dr. Meyer*
is Chairman. At the same time it appears to be with another matter pertaining to the Committee of which Dr. Barrett is Chairman, and of which
you are a member. You first propose a Board to carry out Dr. Meyer's suggestion and second to investigate and determine a proper list of medical
schools, hospitals and instructors competent to give the required training
in Psychiatry. Does not this second part have to do with the general matter
of psychiatric teaching, and therefore as I have intimated belong to Dr.
Barrett's committee [?] Your third sub-division proposes to arrange through
a suggested Board the qualifications of those who desire to practice psychia-
ry and to present a certificate to those who meet the established standard.
A phrase in this portion of your paper stating that it is the object "to test
physicians' fitness to practice psychiatry" may lead to some misunderstanding, especially among hospital appointees. No one familiar with the object
of Dr. Meyer's proposition would misunderstand this, but there are some
who might be misled into the belief that the association was endeavoring
to limit the practice of psychiatry to those upon whom the proposed Board
has placed the stamp of its approval. Should not your whole paper make it
much plainer that it outlines what will be proposed by the Committee [?]
As it now reads it would appear that the Board of Examiners is already in
existence, that it has established certain regulations. I feel that the tentative
scheme worked out at the meeting in December is excellent and that it will

be fully elaborated in Dr. Meyer's report and quite possibly in some degree by Dr. Barrett.

You say it is suggested that in forming the established board, four members should be chosen from the American Psychiatric Association, two from the section of mental and nervous diseases of the American Medical Association, and one from the American Ortho-Psychiatric Association. Personally I am adverse to any relations with any outside organizations, which would permit the naming by those organizations of a member or members of the Board. A board of this kind must be established under definite regulations, and those regulations can only be made without friction by a single body. Moreover after the Board has been appointed it would result [?] it may desire to establish certain rules and regulations subject to the approval of the appointing body and if there were two or three bodies joined in making the appointments to the Board, I feel that difficulties would arise. The American College of Physicians and the American College of Surgeons, both of which conduct examinations and inquiries into the fitness of applicants for membership of their individual bodies are entirely independent, they work out their own rules and regulations and as far as I can learn do this without consultation with or advice from other organizations.

As far as the section of the American Medical Association to which you refer is concerned, it has no autonomous power. Its actions upon any matter, except possibly its own program, are referred to the main organization, hence in [*sic*] the selection of a member or members of the Board by that section would necessarily be referred to the Council of the A.M.A., for approval, a body which had given no definite thought upon the matter nor which is in a position to express an informed opinion or make a wise selection. Our association is the oldest National body in the Country. It is the only one devoted to Psychiatry in all its relations, and [*in*] its hands alone, I feel should be left the consummation and regulation of this very laudable project. Pardon me for inflicting this lengthy communication upon you. You ask the latest possible time for getting your material in. If I can have it by the 12th of this month, I shall be under many obligations. I am endeavoring to get the March Journal out of the way, so that I can take up the May issue.

William L. Russell to Adolf Meyer, July 28, 1931 (AMP, Series II).
I think I shall have to try and take a little vacation. I am unable to get away before next week owing to a conference which I shall have to attend on

Tuesday next, but hope then to run up to Salisbury, Conn., and spend two or three weeks with Ernest. His wife and children are going to Maine to make a visit with some friends, and I am in hopes that he and I can have a real good loaf together. If it had not been for this, I should have tried to run down to see you. I hoped to go to Philadelphia to have a conference relating to the meeting of the American Psychiatric Association next year. This, however, is interfered with in one way or another, and will not come off until the first or second week in September.

The heat is so very great here that I hope you are not suffering greatly in Baltimore. If it is any worse than it is here, I feel pretty sure that you and Mrs. Meyer will feel it necessary to move to a cooler region. In any case, you will no doubt be back in September, and I hope then to have an opportunity to pay you a visit. I am not sure what Dr. Amsden's plans are, but he was hoping that he and I could go over some matters relating to your clinic together. Perhaps he will be able to wait until September.

You will recall that when we last met, we talked about your Committee on Psychiatry in Medical Education of the American Psychiatric Association. The present members, you will recall, are besides yourself, Dr. Kirby and Dr. Strecker. The Committee was enlarged by two at the last meeting of the Association, and in going over some names, you suggested that perhaps Dr. Ebaugh and Dr. Singer might be added. Since then, I have noticed in the *Journal of the American Medical Association* of June 20th, that Dr. Ebaugh introduced a resolution in the Section of Nervous and Mental Diseases of the American Medical Association, of which I enclose a copy. I have already received one letter drawing attention to this action on the part of Dr. Ebaugh, and suggesting that this perhaps was not altogether a suitable thing for him to do in view of our own Committee. Also it was suggested that he might very well have taken this matter up at the meeting of the Psychiatric Association which he had attended the week before. Dr. Ebaugh and Dr. Singer have both, as you know, been quite active in promoting psychiatric activity in the American Medical Association. This is, of course, entirely commendatory and not to be discouraged. On the other hand, it would be very desirable, would it not, if before making definite propositions of this kind, our own members might consult the officers or the proper Committee in our organization.

I know we must be broadminded about any developments that are in the right direction, whether they fit in exactly with our schemes or not. My own impression, however, amounts almost to a conviction that psychiatry can only feel secure if it maintains a fair degree of leadership in all developments that relate to it. I am afraid that we cannot feel at all safe in the hands of neurology. I enclose herewith a copy of a report recently presented to the New York Academy of Medicine which illustrates what I fear. You know, of course, that the Academy is laying down new qualifications for Fellows. It is proposed that in future all those who join the Academy will at first become members. To be a Fellow, it will be necessary to join a Section and then to meet certain requirements laid down by the Section, for Fellows of the Academy in the special field represented. The report which I enclose is a tentative draft of the qualifications for a Fellow of the Academy in Neurology and Psychiatry. You will note that the Committee itself is practically all neurological. You will also note that the qualifications are four fifths neurology and one fifth psychiatry.

I am wondering, therefore, whether we should not try to line up the American Psychiatric Association on a rather independent footing with reference to shaping the standards of psychiatry in medical education, in medical practice, and in institutional standards, etc. You must know, I am sure, that I am not trying to indicate to you what course you should follow with regard to your Committee. I am looking to you for guidance more than anything else. I feel, however, that Ebaugh is a man who proceeds without a great deal of reflection, or without feeling any great necessity for counselling with others. This type of man is sure to forge ahead and do something. On the other hand, such men often do something that it takes years to undo. I do not know Singer at all well and I am not sure whether he is a kindred spirit with Ebaugh in that respect or not. I do know, however, that he is not active in the American Psychiatric Association, and I think very rarely attends any of the meetings.

I hope you will give this matter considerable thought, because I feel myself as though there are developments pending that are of great importance, and a great deal will depend, I believe, on the extent to which they are shaped by men who really know the psychiatric field and issues and have sound judgment concerning the lines which should be followed. This subject can, of course, wait until we meet, though I shall be glad to hear from you about it. What I am aiming at now is really to bring to your attention the situation in regard to Ebaugh and his activities in the A.M.A., and the bearing on what will be the best course for us to follow in our Association.

I do hope that you and Mrs. Meyer are keeping well. Dr. Raynor underwent a severe operation yesterday for liver disturbance which had shown itself by repeated attacks of pain and occasional jaundice since last January.

The operation showed a chronic inflammation of the pancreas with apparently intermittent obstruction of the common duct. He is doing very well, I believe, thus far, but just what the effect will be on his future health is hard to say. It is very unfortunate for the Society of the New York Hospital.

Mrs. Russell is continuing to do well but is still confined to bed and in the hands of a nurse.

In 1930 the delegates at the convention of the AMA authorized its Council on Medical Education and Hospitals "to make a thorough investigation of all hospitals caring for mental patients." Shortly thereafter the council hired John M. Grimes, a young physician with no training in psychiatry, to undertake a study of American mental hospitals. The initial reaction of psychiatrists was muted, but during 1931 and 1932 a number of leading figures began to voice misgivings. Some expressed concern about the right of an external organization to establish standards and policies for mental hospitals. Although the AMA eventually buried the Grimes study, the investigation stimulated the movement to establish a specialty board under psychiatric control. In the first three letters, William L. Russell explained his reservations about the activities of the AMA. William A. White, on the other hand, felt that cooperation rather than rejection was a more appropriate strategy. In this respect he took a quite different position than George M. Kline (1878–1933), commissioner of the Massachusetts Department of Mental Diseases, and James V. May (1873–1947), superintendent of Boston State Hospital and soon to be elected president of the APA. The remaining four letters between White and Kline or May illustrate psychiatric concerns in the events leading up to the establishment of the American Board of Psychiatry and Neurology in 1934.

William L. Russell to Adolf Meyer, December 21, 1931 (AMP, Series II).
I have your letter relating to the next joint meeting of the Council on Medical Education and Hospitals and Federation of State Boards, in which you asked whether I would be disposed to attend the meeting as a representative of the American Psychiatric Association.

I have to confess that I feel quite insecure in regard to the course which it would be best for the American Psychiatric Association to follow. There will be a meeting of the Executive Committee of the Association on the 30th inst. when the project of the American Medical Association may be discussed. I assume that you will be in New York to attend the meeting of the Research Association on the 28th and 29th. If you can stay over until the next morning, I hope you will arrange to join us at the Executive Committee meeting.

I have received in today's mail a letter from Dr. Ebaugh in which he encloses a memorandum of a communication which has been drawn up by the Psychiatric Advisory Committee of the Council on Medical Education and Hospitals of the American Medical Association. Perhaps I am altogether too conservative, and if so, I am sure it is not my desire that anyone should follow my advice. I am, however, quite unable to feel secure in committing the American Psychiatric Association to seemingly approve of the program of the American Medical Association. I think we would be in a much better position if our own Association could continue as it has in the past to be the principal agency in shaping the standards and policies of the hospitals so far as this may be possible for any organization. This of course would necessitate the adoption of more precise and effective methods than in the past and expenditure of funds which are not at the present time available.

William L. Russell to Adolf Meyer, January 8, 1932 (AMP, Series II).
I return herewith the list of women physicians which you were kind enough to send me. Dr. Burdick, of course, I know very well, and had already presented her name.

I also enclose herewith copy of a letter which I have received from Dr. Singer and a draft of a reply that I have written. I have not yet sent the reply. If you see anything objectionable in it, I shall be glad if you will advise me.

You may very well feel uncertain concerning the program of the A.M.A. I understand that Dr. Grimes has already stated that there will be quite a number of empty wards in the state hospitals, as a result of the investigations of the A.M.A., meaning, I judge, that many patients will be discharged. I presume that if we mobilized the psychiatric forces within the A.M.A., and brought to bear the resources of the A.P.A., a completely new program and setup might be brought about. I feel quite sure, however, that a merely advisory committee will not have sufficient control to shape the activities. In fact this has already been demonstrated.

On the other hand, I am wondering whether the American Psychiatric Association cannot strengthen its resources and proceed with a program of its own. I have been inclined myself to try making a cooperation scheme with the National Committee for Mental Hygiene. The trouble is that at the present time there is, it seems to me, a slipping of psychiatric control there. The new Scientific Administration Committee, which takes the place of the former Executive Committee, is composed of seven psychiatrists with Dr. Bernard Sachs counted as an eighth to constitute a majority of one to meet the requirements of the new Constitution, that a majority of this Committee should be psychiatrists. I note that at the first meeting which was held last night, and which unfortunately I was unable to attend, the notice I received showed that of eleven who said they would attend, only four were psychiatrists. The notice said that at this meeting the plans for the future of the National Committee would be discussed. However, it seems as though it may be possible to create within the National Committee a Division of, perhaps, Psychiatry, or Preventive Psychiatry and Hospitals (there is a Division of Hospitals now). Possibly it might be arranged that a Committee of the Psychiatric Association be appointed and then adopted by the National Committee, to have charge of the activities of this Division. A similar arrangement was entered into, you will recall, in some of the war work, and in the Division of Statistics when it was being organized. The American Psychiatric Association has an accumulated fund of about $26,000. If a permanent executive officer could be employed, about $800 could be saved on the cost of the Journal, and about $500 on the expenses of the secretary. It is quite likely also that an executive secretary could increase the number of subscribers to the Journal, and also the advertising, which would bring in additional revenue. An annual appropriation could then be made from our surplus to carry perhaps half the salary of our executive. The other half would be paid by the National Committee for services rendered to it. The National Committee would also furnish office space and perhaps some clerical help.

I am quite aware that this arrangement might not meet with the approval of a good many. On the other hand, it seems quite clear that the Association is not at the present time in a position to finance a project of this kind unaided, and I am unable to think of any other arrangement that might be made. Once a permanent office was established with a Committee to supervise its activities, it is possible that support might be obtained from the foundations and otherwise, for work in connection with the hospitals, which we have long wished to do, and which would be, I believe, of very much superior character than what could be expected from the American Medical Association.

I know that this is not quite in line with your particular interests and I am writing it simply that you may think about it in connection with the situation with the A.M.A.

I shall be very glad to send your name to the National Research Council, and to know that you will be on hand to represent psychiatry there. Unfortunately, Dr. Whitehorn's name has already been printed in the pamphlet of the Council, but Dr. Howell has written me that it will be perfectly all right for me to propose someone else when I get the official invitation to present a candidate.

I shall speak to Dr. Cheney about the Chicago trip, and if he is not able to go, will advise you again. There is, I think, no-one else on your Committee who would contribute anything more than Ebaugh. Drs. Strecker and Campbell are the other two who might be thought of. Dr. Kirby, I am sure, would not want to undertake such a task. The January 2, number of the *Journal of the American Medical Association,* on page 54 presents a program which will be part of the conference to be held in Chicago in February. I have been asked to attend this conference and to discuss Dr. Grimes' report. Of course I shall not accept.

William L. Russell to William A. White, January 27, 1932 (AMP, Series II).
I am glad to have your letter in which you express your views concerning the A.M.A. situation. Your viewpoint is broad and generous, and what you say with regard to the survey, "if it could be properly engineered," was what we all felt *a year ago*.

At that time you will recall the officers of the American Psychiatric Association, and later its Executive Committee volunteered to render every assistance possible, and they organized and furnished presiding officers and speakers for two or three sessions of the congress held in Chicago last February. Several of those who attended this conference met with the Advisory Committee of the A.M.A., and offered their views and advice freely and frankly. I do not think that anything they recommended was adopted.

It will, of course, readily be conceded that those who are managing the A.M.A. project do not consciously intend "to be vicious or destructive to the interests of the mental hospitals," and are acting in good faith. Good faith, however, is no substitute for sound knowledge and wise planning and execution. The leading psychiatrists of the country are members of the American Medical Association which has thus within its own organization the best psychiatric wisdom available. The American Psychiatric Association is not in a position to play the role of physician to the A.M.A., as patient. The hospitals and psychiatry seem rather to be the patient, with the A.M.A. undertaking to be the doctor. The American Psychiatric Association, on the other hand, may be looked upon as the old family doctor, who has been supplanted by someone whose standing and skill he is not quite sure of. The American Psychiatric Association is the organization of the hospitals, and has a place and responsibility which are quite special. After having made a brave effort to help the A.M.A. with its undertaking, and finding that its views and advice were ignored, would it not be better for the Association, like the old family doctor, to stand by in watchful waiting? This is what was decided upon at a meeting of the Executive Committee held on December 30th, and the officers of the Association must act in accordance. Dr. Cutter, Secretary of the A.M.A. Council, spen[t] an evening with Dr. Cheney and me recently. He seemed well disposed and desirous of entering into cooperative relations with the Association. What he asked was that representatives of the American Psychiatric Association be sent to confer with Dr. Singer's Committee. We reviewed with him just what had happened last year and since, and advised him that we did not think that official representatives could be sent without further action by the Executive Committee or Council of our Association. We also expressed as our own opinion that there seemed to be little reason to feel that anything more would come of such a conference than last year, and we hardly thought that the Association should go to the expense and effort.

We also suggested to him that if the A.M.A. wished to enter into really cooperative relations with the American Psychiatric Association, the Council on Medical Education and Hospitals should send a formal request asking that representatives be appointed to meet similarly appointed representatives of the Council of the A.M.A., in order to consider a plan of cooperation which would be mutually satisfactory. Like others whom we have met from the A.M.A., Dr. Cutter did not seem very clear as to what was aimed at by the A.M.A. Council, or what course had been planned. He was also non-committal in regard to entering into any arrangement with the American Psychiatric Association which would permit of any except advisory relations. I explained to him that the majority of the members of our Association were actively engaged in hospital work, and it was really the hospital organization. For that reason, it might not be advisable for it to permit itself to be placed in a position in which it might seem to be responsible for any activity relating to the hospitals, over which it had no control.

I am inclined to think that this whole question of official participation of the American Psychiatric Association will have to be left over until the meeting in May. My own feeling is that it will be a safeguard to the situation if the Association maintains its independent position, realizing that the A.M.A. is sure to proceed in its project, and has psychiatric resources within itself, which, if properly organized, will enable it to manage wisely and well. At the present time the disposition does not seem to be to proceed in that way, but that, it seems to me, is no reason why our Association should feel that it is necessary for it to become involved.

George M. Kline to William A. White, January 20, 1932 (WAWP).
In talking with Dr. May yesterday I noted that he is going to write you regarding the February meeting in Chicago of the Annual Congress on Medical Education, Licensure and Hospitals, at which you are to take part, especially in the preliminary report of the survey of mental hospitals by Dr. Grimes.

I am sorry that it was not possible for you to be present at the recent meeting of the Executive Committee of the American Psychiatric Association at which this project of the American Medical Association came up for free discussion. Perhaps you are already familiar with what took place at that Committee Meeting, as well as the views of many of us regarding the methods being pursued by the American Medical Association through the questionnaire method, and the manner in which the survey is being carried on. No doubt May will go into no little detail about the whole matter and quite possibly Dr. Russell has written you.

I am in hopes that you will be in possession of full information regarding this project of the American Medical Association, which is being pursued along lines that cannot meet with the approval of any of us, as well as officials of the American Psychiatric Association.

I am informed that Dr. Grimes, who is in charge of this survey, has had no experience in a mental hospital and is not even a member of the American Medical Association.

Pardon me for boring you with this long letter, inasmuch as others will go into detail regarding the matter, which does, and should, give us concern.

William A. White to George M. Kline, January 23, 1932 (WAWP).
I have your letter of recent date regarding the Chicago situation. I may say to start with that I do not think it is going to be possible for me to get to Chicago in any case, and I so stated in the first instance, when I was invited

to read a paper at this section, but in the hope that I might find my way there my name was put upon the program to discuss Dr. Grimes's paper. However that may be, I feel disposed to make the following comments for your delectation inasmuch as you have expressed yourself with equal frankness to me.

When the A.M.A. originally decided to make the survey of the mental hospitals I felt then, as I do now, that it was really a tremendously important moment in the history of the mental hospitals of these United States,—that such a survey, if it could be properly engineered might be of tremendous significance to these institutions in all sorts of ways which you can visualize quite as well as I. Shortly after this decision was reached and Dr. Grimes had been appointed to make this survey he called upon me. I realized from my talk with him that he did not have any special knowledge of institutions of this sort, and he was perfectly free to admit this. I learned, too, very shortly thereafter that he was not even a member of the A.M.A., but I must confess that my contact with him was a perfectly agreeable one; he seemed to be intent upon his job and interested, open-minded, willing to learn and to cooperate, and I said and felt at the time, whereas perhaps his selection might not be the most happy one that could be conceived, yet after all the selection had been made and it was up to us to make the best of it. I also had in mind the experiences which come to us once in a while, and of which a very outstanding illustration has occurred in my experience here in Washington, and that is that some times a man who comes into the field from outside can see certain things clearer than the man who is in the field himself. In other words, he comes open-minded to his task and without the prejudices that the average person who has spent many years perhaps in a rather narrow horizon working in the field, might have.

Now today, in spite of the strictures contained in your letter, I feel very much the same way. I cannot believe that the action of the A.M.A., or their Council on Medical Education and Hospitals or Dr. Grimes himself, or any of them, collectively or individually, indicates that they are pursuing a course in which they consciously intend to be vicious or destructive to the interests of the mental hospitals, and not being able to believe this, I have to believe that they are acting in good faith, and under these circumstances it seems to me that it is up to us to cooperate with them and wherever possible to join them in their councils in a spirit of friendship and cooperation,—to give them our advice when they ask it, and in all other ways show our willingness to do anything and everything which we can to the end of the best interests of the mental hospitals. I do not see how such an attitude on our part could possible do us any harm. If we are overruled in any of our contentions we can still bring in minority reports or express our individual opinions or our collective opinions as recorded by the Association. It does not estop us from any of these things and it gives us access to what is going on. Further than this, to withdraw from an effort which is conceived in a spirit of helpfulness, as I believe this was, is like standing aside at a time of need, and I do not see how a person observing such a condition of affairs from the outside could have any sympathy with it. If they are ignorant and misinformed it is up to us to impart to them the necessary knowledge. To get mad because they do not do what we think they ought to do when we know perfectly well that they do not know the things which we think they ought to know, is just precisely in my opinion on a par with a physician who gets mad with his patient because the patient does not get well. We ought to improve every opportunity for seeing that these people are exposed to information about these hospitals, and if we withdraw and refuse it, it seems to me we are in an indefensible position.

I may be entirely wrong in this whole business. I may not really understand the fundamental reasons for your feelings, but I give you this thought for what it is worth in response to your letter.

William A. White to James V. May, November 17, 1932 (WAWP).
I have your letter of the 16th instant. I was present at the meeting you referred to and heard the entire discussion. I have also had contact with the question from time to time for the past something like three years, I think, and while I understand your position and that of Dr. Russell fully, I am not altogether won over to your point of view. In fact I originally was of the opinion that the Psychiatric Association ought to go in with the A.M.A. in this survey on the general theory that if a thing is not being done well and you refuse to have anything to do with it you are pretty well stopped from any fault you have to find with it after it is done. In addition to this feeling of mine, this further situation developed at the New York meeting. Mr. Willoughby Wallin, of Chicago, was there. He has recently taken part in a survey of the State hospital system for the Governor in his capacity as Chairman of the Illinois Board of Public Welfare Commissioners. Now his position, with which it seems to me, we must have a good deal of sympathy, is practically this: He is in an important tactical situation. He wants to

do what he can best do for the State hospitals, and he is a layman. Now under these circumstances, if a survey comes out by the greatest medical organization in the world and that reaches certain conclusions, what is he, as a layman, going to do about it, except to agree with it? But if, on the other hand, there comes out perchance a minority report which points out the defects in this survey, shows up its weak points, indicates much more completely the actual state of affairs, that document is just as powerful a document for him to point to as the majority report. In other words, I felt that the strongest position we could be in was to be on the inside, know what was going on, offer our advice, and then if the whole thing went "fluey" be in a position to make a rousing minority report.

Now this attitude may be wrong, but it seems to me to have many strategic advantages. We are confronted by what Mr. Cleveland used to say is a condition and not a theory. The survey has not been organized as we would like to have it. The personnel that has been picked out to make it is not the personnel that we would have picked out. We are in a situation which is not of our choosing. How can we best deal with it? By passing out of the picture, or by getting into the game, doing what we can to make it right, and then when it is wrong, saying so in large capitals? We discussed the matter at great length and as you know from the vote, the majority, in fact everybody except I think Dr. Russell, voted for it in the form in which it has gone through. Hincks and Hamilton were both there and understand fully the spirit and the intention of the resolution as passed.

May I say in passing that I was talking with a well informed newspaper man last night, who told me in connection with my discussion of this subject that some of the best legislation that has come out of Congress has come as a result of minority reports. Think of it from this point of view and see how it strikes you. It seems to me that there is much to be said for it. We have to fight in this world with the weapons that are available, not the weapons we wish we had. It seems to me that the whole thing is a question of strategies and therefore a question of opinion as to what constitutes the best course. Of course no one will regret more than I the withdrawal of Dr. Russell from the councils of the National Committee. I don't suppose it is possible for everybody to agree, but I do wish we might present a united front.

I shall send the correspondence which you sent to me on to Dr. Hincks, together with a copy of this letter, immediately, so that he may have the advantages of the opinions therein included.

James V. May to William A. White, November 19, 1932 (WAWP).
I am sorry you take the position you do in regard to the various investigations, whatever they may be, which are being made by the A.M.A. of the mental hospitals of this country. Their whole survey, as you know, rests in the hands of the Council on Medical Education and Hospitals, which includes in its membership no psychiatrists and, as far as I know, no one who has had any experience whatever in our branch of medicine. There is, as you know full well, an Advisory Committee, whose recommendations have never received any consideration whatever by the Council, as far as I know.

The American Psychiatric Association has kept out of this matter officially because of the feeling that if we lent ourselves to such a movement we must assume some responsibility for a survey over which we have no control whatever and which should be made by psychiatrists, or at least by persons qualified to pass upon subjects pertaining to mental hospitals, even if they are not psychiatrists. This investigation should, in my opinion, have been placed in the hands of the American Psychiatric Association. If our organization lends itself to this movement and becomes a party to the actions taken by the Council on Medical Education and Hospitals, and assumes some responsibility for its findings, and, being a party to this movement, places itself in accord with their action, we may find ourselves in serious difficulties. Probably nothing of the sort will happen, but this is nevertheless a possibility.

In such an event, it will be a most unfortunate thing if the National Committee for Mental Hygiene has not left itself in a position of neutrality so that it could then take such action as might be deemed necessary from a partial and disinterested point of view. If it makes itself a party to the A.M.A. findings, that becomes an impossibility, should such a necessity arise.

While the A.M.A. investigation probably will not amount to anything, in view of the fact that their official records show that there are no mental hospitals in this country at all (all of the State institutions being covered as hospitals for nervous and mental diseases), there probably is nothing to fear. It is, however, in my opinion, a great mistake not to make some provision for the future, when persons who are as ignorant as the officials of the A.M.A. are about our mental hospitals propose to sit in judgment over our work and make what will be looked upon as an expert survey of the whole situation.

If this thing results disastrously, it will be because some of our psychiatrists have lent themselves to the A.M.A.'s activities and because of the fact that the National Committee for Mental Hygiene is doing the same thing. Not being able to control this situation ourselves, we should, in my opinion, have remained wholly on the outside, where we can attack their findings if it becomes necessary later, and present a united front.

You will note, from the preliminary review already made by Dr. Grimes, that they are taking full advantage of the fact that psychiatrists representing practically all of our fields have participated in their activities as members of the Advisory Committee. It is unfortunate that this should have ever happened.

The great majority of psychiatrists worked in public institutions. Like their brethren in private practice, however, they sought the right to establish standards and policies for their hospitals. Yet their autonomy was in part curtailed by virtue of their status as public employees. Consequently, tensions often arose between their demand for independence and the insistence of public officials for accountability. The institution psychiatrists often phrased the issue in terms of freedom from partisan political interference. The problem of reconciling autonomy and accountability was illustrated in an incident in Massachusetts. In 1936 the colorful Democratic boss and then Governor of Massachusetts James Michael Curley (1874–1958) refused to reappoint Dr. Winfred Overholser (1892–1964) as commissioner of the Department of Mental Diseases. As justification, Curley claimed that conditions in some state institutions, notably Boston State Hospital, were a disgrace. Curley then nominated a physician without prior experience in psychiatry as the new commissioner; next he removed from office Dr. James V. May, the superintendent of Boston State Hospital. The result was a clash that received national publicity. Although Curley left office in January 1937, the controversy persisted, and the APA became involved. The legislature eventually endorsed the new governor's recommendation that a special commission be created to investigate the care of the mentally ill in the state, but its deliberations did not result in fundamental changes. Most psychiatrists claimed that Curley had been motivated solely by political considerations. Their private correspondence, however, revealed their concern with autonomy and independence. In the first letter, Dr. C. Macfie Campbell (1876–1943), superintendent of Boston Psychopathic Hospital, offered his own judgment. The following three letters by Overholser, who by this time had succeeded the recently deceased William A. White as super-

intendent at the prestigious St. Elizabeths Hospital in Washington, D.C. (an appointment widely perceived as a vindication), and the final letter of Ross M. Chapman (1881–1948), president of the APA, are revealing of psychiatric perceptions.

C. Macfie Campbell to Clarence B. Farrar (editor of the American Journal of Psychiatry*), February 19, 1937 (CBFP).*

I return the proof of your editorial on the situation in Massachusetts. It seems to me to present the facts, which are familiar to me, in a very clear form, and gives additional data which I had not previously known.

At the Boston Psychopathic Hospital we live a life somewhat detached from the political currents of the times and are not always aware of what is going on in political circles.

You may have had sent to you recent newspaper articles dealing with the situation in the state hospitals, articles which are bound to be profoundly disturbing to the relatives of patients and to the community in general, and which do not reflect much credit on modern journalism. The final outcome, however, of all this activity may possibly lead to a greater interest in and fuller knowledge of the needs and difficulties and limitations of the state hospitals by the average citizen and the assurance of practical steps to give the hospitals the necessary support and stability. Your editorial may prove useful as a contribution to this consummation, which is so devoutly to be desired.

I have taken up your other article with Dr. Wells.

Winfred Overholser to Clarence B. Farrar, February 19, 1937 (CBFP).

On my return to the office yesterday, I found your charming note of February 12 regarding the "comic opera." The situation has been decidedly hectic since my last letter, although yesterday for the first time I have been able to look at a Boston paper without finding the affairs of the Boston State Hospital smeared over the front page. Dr. Norton has been vying with the gentlemen of the press in attempting to prove that his is probably the worst institution in the United States, if not in the world. The high professional level of his action may be gathered from the fact that he has taken an obvious delight in showing newspaper reporters and cameramen through the institution, pointing out particularly mattresses which were said to be torn and sheets which were dirty, although some of my informants who visited the institution were thoroughly impressed with the fact that Dr. Norton seemed to know exactly which bed to go to and that the whole affair savored very strongly of a staged show.

The latest touch of humor was a recent surprise visit by the Governor, escorted by the Commissioner of Public Safety and several state police officers, to the Wrentham State School to ascertain whether charges of "immorality" were founded. In this "investigation" the Department of Mental Diseases was entirely ignored, but later on, His Excellency condescended to have the Commissioner of Public Health investigate the alleged existence of a few cases of gonorrheal proctitis. Fortunately, the Commissioner of Public Health is an extremely high-grade person and his statement has, I think, put the quietus on the outrageous charges and implications. It now appears likely that the Governor's proposal for a Commission of Investigation to be appointed by him will be favorably acted upon by the legislature. I am informed, too, that it is likely that such a commission will, thanks to the good offices of such few (?) decent-minded people as are still left in Massachusetts, recommend that a survey be made by Dr. Hamilton and his Committee. Perhaps eventually some of the mess can be straightened out, but at the moment, Norton is vindicated, or at least put on a sixty-day trial, and Commissioner Williams is still, as usual, I am informed, in a state of mental fog.

Winfred Overholser to Clarence B. Farrar, January 13, 1938 (CBFP).
The enclosed item may be of some interest to you. There are of course many more things that might be said—things that might undoubtedly occur to you as you read the report of the Commission which I mailed to you yesterday. The animus, of course, is obvious as one reads the report. There are aspersions even upon Dr. Kline, as well as upon Dr. May and myself, and upon Dr. Barrett, and an apparent attempt is made to discredit everything that has gone before in order to emphasize the need of giving the Governor a free hand in organizing matters. No credit whatever is given for the good things which have gone before, and apparently no attempt was made to ascertain them. Neither Dr. May nor I was asked any questions, and apparently all the information that the Commission has received from Dr. Perkins, who is partisan in the affair, is distinctly disloyal and unethical. It is of some interest to note that with regard to the Governor's statements on page 7 I left the large figure in for consideration, at his own specific direction. I had prepared an alternative figure and was prepared to submit it when I received word from him that the larger figure was to stand.

The Legislative Committee has just reported a resolution to continue the commission for another year, and as one of my friends in Massachusetts writes me "nobody can do his best when there is snooping." The whole situation is a mess and the commission seems to be doing everything in its power to make matters worse. It is interesting to note that there are on the Commission, besides Dr. Briggs, a physician—Otis Kelley—who is also a priest, and who has not been in institutional work for 10 years or more; the Chairman is Judge of the Boston Juvenile Court; and another member is a very close personal friend of the Governor—a judge of the Probate Court; one member is a particularly obnoxious Irish politician from Cambridge—a member of the Legislature—who, during my service as Commissioner, was constantly pressing for favors; another is a former president of the Senate, who takes the matter extremely lightly and is a very vacillating individual; and still another member—an architect—is a close personal friend of Mr. Curley, in fact drew the plans for Mr. Curley's residence. I think you can see why not a great deal, except politics, can be expected from the Commission.

Winfred Overholser to Clarence B. Farrar, April 12, 1938 (CBFP).
Hell continues to pop in Massachusetts. The situation has come to the stage now that the Governor is being forced into the position of defending the State hospitals against the onslaught of Auditor Buckley. It has even gone so far that after Buckley had made his charges about Westboro the Chairman of the Commission on Administration and Finance, one of Hurley's appointees, employed a private firm of auditors to check on the State Auditor, all of which reminds me of the song entitled "Who Takes Care of the Care-taker's Daughter," et cetera? Numerous accusations have been made by the Auditor regarding Boston State and Medfield. It looks as if there may be a little fire with all the smoke at Medfield, because, according to the latest report, the Board of Trustees have put Dr. Holt on probation for a year. Both the investigations there are said to have shown laxity in discipline and purchasing.

I enclose a few clippings which may interest you. The latest atrocity is that Hurley is trying to replace the Commissioner of Public Health—an outstanding man—Dr. Henry Chadwick, with a Lithuanian pediatrician, who submits as his chief qualification for public health work the fact that he was once a lieutenant in the Volunteer Militia before the War!! You can well imagine that the mental state of the superintendents is not being improved by any of these antics.

I have been hoping from day to day to hear from you as to the final decision concerning the introduction of pre-frontal lobotomy in the provincial hospital system.

I am looking forward to seeing you in San Francisco.

Ross M. Chapman to Henry R. Atkinson (president, Massachusetts Civic League), February 7, 1938 (CBFP).

I have been slow to reply to your letter of January 22 which came to me accompanied by the "Report of the Special Commission Established to Study the Whole Matter of the Mentally Diseased in Their Relation to the Commonwealth, Including All Phases of Work of the Department of Mental Diseases." The reason therefor lies in the difficulty I have had in finding a mood in which I might write with sufficient restraint. I hold that fine body of physicians now administering the affairs of most of the various individual mental hospitals of Massachusetts in high regard. I have known them for years. The Commonwealth and the country at large are greatly in their debt. I fear that the Report will not add to their feeling of security in the faithful pursuit of their duties.

Massachusetts, long a model for the other states of our country in the effective administration of its state hospitals for mental diseases, arrived at its high standing in this respect under the guidance of Dr. George Kline. It is a painful experience to see the splendid services of Dr. Kline over a long period of years referred to so casually and critically. Dr. Kline was succeeded by a nationally known psychiatrist, highly regarded as an administrator and clinician, Dr. James V. May, Superintendent of the Boston State Hospital, who against his own wish stepped into the breach until such time as a permanent successor to Dr. Kline might be named. A temporary appointee, he could not properly inaugurate new policies nor plan extensive changes in the administration of the state hospitals in accordance with his own ideas.

Dr. Winfred Overholser, trained by Dr. Kline, finally took his place, administered the affairs of the high office of Commissioner of Mental Diseases with distinction and then when he was beginning to work out his plans he failed of re-appointment at the end of his term. That, in the light of the events that have followed, was unfortunate for the Commonwealth. To neither Dr. May nor Dr. Overholser does the report of the commission do justice.

State care of the mentally ill is one of the most complicated of the whole range of activities carried on for the benefit of the public health. It presents highly technical medical and nursing problems and broad educational re-sponsibilities. From the body of the report one may conclude that the commissioners did not appreciate the scope of the field they were studying nor did they show reasonable grasp of any phase of their subject. There is nothing to indicate that the commission has among its membership any-one with state hospital administrative experience, or that the commission was exposed to the influence of anyone with such experience, yet the ad-ministration of the state hospitals for the mentally diseased is the subject of study. I wonder what the reaction would be if a commission of one lawyer and six laymen were appointed to study the whole matter of the courts in their relation to the Commonwealth. Dr. L. Vernon Briggs has rendered in related affairs great service to the state and to the country but it would seem that on this special commission he must be at a disadvantage.

The body of the report is superficial, unconvincing and at times be-wilderingly unclear. For instance note Section C, page 25, "Other Condi-tions and Policies in the Care of the Mentally Ill." Almost equally puzzling is the next Section on "Education, Research and Prevention."

I do not wish to comment at this time on the plan for reorganization or the proposed Act abolishing the Department of Mental Diseases in creat-ing the Department of Mental Health save to call attention to the manifest risk involved in giving to the "Commissioner of Mental Health," with one associate Commissioner, power to appoint and remove superintendents, even with the suggested safeguards. With a politically-minded, unsym-pathetic and ruthless Governor and a subservient Commissioner the effec-tiveness of the state hospitals could be destroyed almost overnight.

From the deplorable country-wide publicity one would think that Mas-sachusetts in this important public health matter had gone completely out of control. I, of course, do not believe it. Do you not think, however, that the Governor and Legislature might not be persuaded to call on the Na-tional Committee for Mental Hygiene, which in the past twenty-five years has acted as advisor to almost all of our states, to act in a similar capacity to Massachusetts?

I am writing this letter not as President of the American Psychiatric Association but as an individual.

Psychiatry and Society

Psychiatrists, like physicians generally, preferred to perceive themselves as impartial scientists untouched by nonmedical influences. They did not justify their claim for autonomy on the grounds of self-interest. On the contrary, they insisted that their legitimacy flowed from their role as knowledgeable and objective scientists as well as from their commitment to the welfare of their patients in particular and society in general.

Yet psychiatry, like virtually all other professions, functioned in an interdependent world that precluded isolation. In spite of their perceptions of themselves as impartial and objective scientists, psychiatrists were influenced by a variety of external forces that molded their outlook. The tendency to expand psychiatric theory beyond the boundaries of mental illness was evident in the thought of the founders of the specialty in the early nineteenth century. In dealing with some of the specific moral (i.e., psychological) causes of insanity, for example, they ranged far afield. So broad was their analysis that few institutions remained exempt from their critique. Religious and political institutions in particular were singled out as causal elements in bringing on insanity. Psychiatrists were especially fond of emphasizing the defects of American education, which allegedly failed to provide children with a proper and healthful environment. Some condemned existing educational institutions as too permissive; others attacked them for their rigidity; still others argued that schools raised the expectations of children to unattainable levels and thus failed to prepare them for the reality of later life. Nor was it unusual for psychiatrists to relate a vague and amorphous social structure to insanity. "In this country," a well known psychiatrist noted in 1851,

> where no son is necessarily confined to the work or employment of his
> father, but all the fields of labor, of profit and of honor are open to

whomsoever will put on the harness and enter therein, and all are invited to join the strife for that which may be gained in each, many are in a transition state, from the lower and less desirable to the higher and more desirable conditions. They are struggling for that which costs them mental labor and anxiety and pain. The mistake or the ambition of some leads them to aim at that which they cannot reach, to strive for more than they can grasp, and their mental powers are strained to their utmost tension; they labor in agitation; and they end in frequent disappointment.[1]

In their voluminous writings, mid-nineteenth century psychiatrists attempted to persuade their fellow citizens to behave in accordance with certain norms. While the behavioral norms of psychiatrists were no different from those of most Protestant Americans, they were clothed with a religious and scientific mantle—a fact made possible by the vagueness of contemporary etiological theory and the ardent desire to prevent disease and promote health. Few aspects of life were omitted. Psychiatrists told educators how to educate children; the ministry how to observe true religion; husbands and wives how to behave toward each other and how to raise children. During the Civil War northern psychiatrists emphasized the nobility of a conflict that diverted attention from the pursuit of material goals and strengthened the national character.

By 1900 the moral and religious content integral to mid-nineteenth-century psychiatric thought had diminished and the commitment to science had intensified. Nevertheless, the faith in science created in turn, an illusion of knowledge and power; psychiatrists began to argue, implicitly if not explicitly, that their specialty had a vital role to play in human affairs generally. Claims on behalf of psychiatry therefore went beyond the issues of mental disease and began to include social and political concerns as well.

Reality, of course, was quite different. Psychiatrists may have perceived themselves as disinterested and objective scientists, but in practice they were influenced by the same racial, sexual, religious, and professional differences as the larger society. Consider, for example, the status of female physicians in psychiatry. Before 1870 psychiatry was an all-male specialty. After that date some mental hospitals began to employ female physicians to deal with female patients. By the turn of the century as many as two

1. Edward Jarvis, "Causes of Insanity," *Boston Medical and Surgical Journal,* 45 (1851): 303–05.

hundred women had worked in mental institutions. In 1900 thirty-eight hospitals employed female physicians, although twenty-three were concentrated in Pennsylvania, New York, and Massachusetts. Social rather than medical forces were largely responsible for the growing number of female physicians in mental hospitals. The differentiation of sex roles in the early nineteenth century had created a semiautonomous "woman's sphere" that presupposed a world in which women could offer each other a kind of intimate friendship and companionship unavailable in a male-dominated society. Related to this attitude was the belief that female patients might be more open and receptive to physicians of the same sex.

Opposition to the employment of female physicians in mental hospitals on the whole was not intense, in part because hospitals were already structured along sex lines. Moreover, male physicians were receptive to the idea that female patients might be more responsive to physicians of their own sex. Those psychiatrists who rejected the intellectual equality of the sexes were also prone to accept the moral and emotional superiority of women— a belief that helped to open hitherto closed doors.

The employment of female physicians in mental hospitals, however, did not imply equality. Men received higher salaries, and the chance of a woman being promoted to a superintendency was nil. In 1919, 16.7 percent of the medical staffs in mental hospitals were women, but none had attained a superintendency. Female physicians also encountered hostility from many (but not all) of their male counterparts, who believed that women in general lacked the traits necessary for the practice of psychiatry or the administration of hospitals. After delivering a paper on the status of female physicians in mental hospitals, Dr. Mary M. Wolfe of the Department for Women at the Norristown State Hospital in Pennsylvania observed that a woman must have "a tremendous amount of native ambition before she can be ambitious for the reason that there are no material rewards for her" in terms of advancement. Like many other women, Wolfe retreated into a defensive position by denying the relevancy of sex: "The whole matter," she concluded in ambiguous terms susceptible to a variety of meanings, "resolves itself into a question of individual ability, attainment and character and not into a question of sex."[2] Louise G. Rabino-

2. Mary M. Wolfe, "The Present Status of Women Physicians in Hospitals for the Insane," American Medico-Psychological Association, *Proceedings*, 16 (1909): 349–56.

vitch, the first female physician to own and publish a psychiatric journal, never received a hearing because her militant criticisms of American psychiatry, which reflected her European training (and perhaps her Jewish background), appeared so alien. Those women who made a career in psychiatry had a far more difficult time than their male counterparts, few of whom were able to overcome sexual stereotypes.

Nor was psychiatry immune from the racial and ethnic divisions of the larger society. Many believed that susceptibility toward mental illness was in part determined by race. Even though the work of Edward Jarvis in the 1840s had completely discredited data from the federal census purportedly proving that free blacks had far higher rates of mental illness than black slaves, southern psychiatrists all but ignored these findings. They argued that the abolition of slavery *had* led to a general increase in mental illness among blacks. Because the black personality was overwhelmingly emotional and passionate (as compared with the rational and intellectual character of whites), they maintained, the removal of the constraints of bondage had led to debauchery and disease. In mental hospitals, segregation was the norm rather than the exception. Similarly, some psychiatrists shared with native-born Protestant Americans antipathies toward minority religious and ethnic groups.

Psychiatrists were not content to limit their activities to the care and treatment of the mentally ill. Their faith in the redemptive powers of science and rationality also led them to pass judgment on and become involved in a variety of current issues and problems. Their faith in scientific psychiatry led them to offer advice on the rearing of children, the rehabilitation of criminals, the prevention of mental disease, the adjustment of workers in industry, and even war and peace. Although an occasional voice was raised in protest, the thrust of the specialty in the decades preceding World War II was to expand sharply its jurisdictional limits.

The effort to expand psychiatric authority, of course, would ultimately meet with resistance from a variety of other groups in the postwar decades. Critics would eventually call into doubt the very basis of psychiatric legitimacy. In so doing they would raise a number of fundamental questions, the answers to which have yet to be given.

In the early twentieth century there were virtually no black psychiatrists. Concerned with introducing psychiatry into the medical curriculum and thus to sensitize all physicians to its significance, William A. White decided in 1910 to offer regular clinics in psychiatry for all medical students in the District of Columbia. He immediately encountered strong racial antipathies. At one of his clinics, white students refused to take part because of the presence of black medical students from Howard University. Unlike many of his psychiatric colleagues (whose racial views differed but little from those of white Americans generally), White was sensitive to black feelings and attempted to resolve the issue by offering separate clinics even though such a compromise was personally distasteful. His behavior brought him the thanks of both the dean and the medical students of Howard. White continued to cultivate cordial relations with Howard students in later decades as well. The following correspondence illustrates the intrusion of racial concerns into medical and psychiatric education in this era.

Wilbur P. Thirkfield (president, Howard University) to William A. White, September 30, 1910 (WAWP).

Permit me to express to you my deep satisfaction over the fact that through your generous kindness, we are to have your regular clinics in psychiatry open to the students of Howard University, as I am informed through our mutual friend, Dr. William L. Robbins. I have laid the matter before Dean Balloch, and we count it a great addition to the course we are able to offer these students.

I am sure you will find them eager and earnest students, and you will have the satisfaction of building something of your life and thought into men who are to go forth as the leaders and teachers of their people, and who will largely determine not only the physical future of the oncoming millions of the colored people in our land, but also safeguard the millions of white people with whom they are so closely and inevitably identified. . . .

William A. White to Dean Edward A. Balloch (Medical Department, Howard University), January 14, 1911 (WAWP).

Because of the recent unpleasantness in connection with my clinics in psychiatry, based upon the attendance of the negro students, I have concluded to discontinue them, at least until some satisfactory understanding can be reached among the several medical colleges.

I am writing this same letter to the other two colleges.

William C. Borden (dean, George Washington Medical School) to William A. White, January 16, 1911 (WAWP).

Referring to my telephonic communication with you in regard to the attendance of our students at your lectures, I sincerely hope that you will be able to give our students this instruction separate from the students of Howard University.

The Faculty and students of our school greatly appreciate the work which you have done and realize that it will be impossible to adequately fill your place in any way. Unfortunately the terms of contract which we have with our students are such that we cannot require them to attend mixed classes and I hope this fact will not prevent them from having your most valuable instruction. I will instruct them to report to Dr. Blackburn and to the clinics as before and sincerely hope that before Thursday the matter can be so arranged that they can attend your lectures also. . . .

William A. White to William C. Borden, January 19, 1911 (WAWP).

I have your letter of the 16th instant. In regard to the recent unpleasantness I wrote you a letter yesterday stating that I could not give any more clinics until the matter had reached some sort of a solution. I really believe that a solution will issue, though it may not occur soon enough for tomorrow's clinic. I think, however, that it will be possible to make some arrangement that will be satisfactory. I at least hope so, as my relations with the University have always been very pleasant and I should hate to have them interfered with in any way. . . .

Edward A. Balloch to William A. White, January 19, 1911 (WAWP).

Your letter of 14th instant, notifying us of the discontinuance of your clinics in psychiatry received, and in reply permit me to state that we regret exceedingly that you have felt it necessary to take such a step.

Your kindness in giving this instruction to our students was highly appreciated by us and by them and we desire to express our thanks for your courtesy in this matter.

Dr. Lucy E. Moten (principal) to William A. White, January 20, 1911 (WAWP).

Your action of recent date in refusing to draw distinction between the students of a profession, on the superficial basis of color, must meet with the hearty approval of all fair-minded people.

In behalf of the faculty of Normal School No. 2, I wish to congratulate you upon your manly and professional stand.

James C. Waters, Jr. (president, Upper Classmen of Howard University), to William A. White, January 21, 1911 (WAWP).

At the meeting of the Council of Upper Classmen of Howard University, held Thursday evening, Jan. 19th, it was considered and accordingly ordered that the President of the Council do express to Dr. White the thanks of the Council of Upper Classmen for the whole-souled, dignified, and manly stand taken by him upon the recent exhibition of race prejudice by certain alleged students who, like the men from Howard, had accepted an invitation to be present at Dr. White['s] lectures on mental diseases.

We have nothing to do with the motive which led to your assuming this fine attitude. It may be one of many, or indeed all of many considerations that underlies your position. What we care for, and what we so heartily appreciate is that when a situation arose calling for character and dignity, you experienced no difficulty whatever in meeting the situation, in a manner which is a credit to you, and a source of such gratification to us.

My dear Sir, you have carved out a warm place in the hearts of the scores of fine young men who compose the Council of Upper Classmen of Howard University.

William A. White to William C. Borden, February 1, 1911 (WAWP).

I have just written to the Dean of the Howard University Medical School offering to make arrangements for one of my staff to give separate clinics to the students with colored patients. This is the only solution I see of the difficulty and I think ought to be a satisfactory one. I would be glad, therefore, to have your students return to the clinics.

William C. Borden to William A. White, April 7, 1911 (WAWP).

As you have decided not to give any more lectures in Psychiatry, will you please let me know if the clinics are to be continued.

Your examination has been scheduled for the 25th of April and this would allow our students to have two more periods before that time.

William A. White to William C. Borden, April 8, 1911 (WAWP).

I have your note of the 7th instant. I do not believe I shall feel equal to giving any more clinics or lectures this year. I was unable to lecture last

Thursday because I did not feel well enough, and I do not think I want to take up the work again this season. I am pretty well tired out.

Edward A. Balloch to William A. White, September 20, 1923 (WAWP).
I desire again to think you for your courtesy in extending to our students the privileges of St. Elizabeth's Hospital and also for allowing Dr. Karpman to act as their Instructor in Psychiatry. He has proved to be a splendid teacher and has succeeded in the very difficult task of inspiring these students with a genuine love for Psychiatry.

Your cooperation in this matter has been of distinct benefit to the school and has afforded an opportunity to our students which otherwise they could not get.

Again thanking you for your cooperation and assuring you of my high appreciation of your courtesy, believe me . . . .

William A. White to Edward A. Balloch, September 22, 1923 (WAWP).
I have your very good letter of the 20th instant, which I need hardly tell you is most gratifying and deeply appreciated. I have been more than glad to cooperate with the several medical schools of the city, as far as lay in my power, for I firmly believe that one of the functions of an institution of this sort is the dissemination of such knowledge as may be possessed within its confines as far abroad as its influence extends. I have tried to do this consistently through the years, but in the past year or two have succeeded much more fully than formerly, so that I think today that there are more students who get their first contacts with psychiatry in this hospital than in any other place in the country certainly, and I must say I know no place anywhere where so many are taught. The privilege of doing the work is itself sufficient reward and when in addition to this we receive the graceful appreciation of the recipients of our efforts we are doubly paid.

During the early twentieth century psychiatry became more heterogenous. By the 1930s Jewish physicians were beginning to become prominent in psychiatry (although they had had a very heavy representation in psychoanalysis beginning with Freud). The exodus from Nazi Germany after 1933 brought additional Jewish psychiatrists to the United States. Like medicine generally, psychiatry was not immune from social and cultural anti-semitism; Jewish college graduates were often discriminated against by medical schools that imposed entrance quotas. In their private correspondence Jewish psychiatrists often complained about their treatment by non-Jewish colleagues. In the following letter, Gregory Zilboorg (1890 – 1959), a psychiatrist and psychoanalyst who migrated from Russia to the United States in 1891, complained bitterly about the anti-semitism allegedly manifested by Dr. George Henry. Zilboorg and Henry were then collaborating on a book (A History of Medical Psychology), *which was finally published in 1941, although the former was responsible for more than 90 percent of the text.*

Gregory Zilboorg to Smith Ely Jelliffe, November 7, 1938 (SEJP).
Your letter reached me this morning, and by the time you return to New York I shall be ready to send you a brief memorandum in regard to the Massachusetts situation.

I am glad you asked me about my History of Psychiatry. It is a very painful subject to me, and I do hope that you will permit me to talk the matter over with you and seek your advice.

It is now almost five to six years since the History was ready, and the reason for it not being published is quite simple. Dr. Henry, as you probably know, is neither a historian nor even an intellectual. At the time I asked him to collaborate with me I did not need his help, but he was going through a severe period in his life; was profoundly depressed and withdrawn and in order to divert him, and to give him a sort of push, I suggested that he look up some material on the history of mental hospitals, as well as organic psychoses. This he did rather poorly and very unscientifically. It turned out—his statement to the contrary—that he neither spoke nor read any languages outside English, and all the data that he compiled were from second, third and fourth-hand sources in various American journals. The result was naturally deplorable, because the information proved to be extremely inaccurate and, of course, lacked any perspective and synthesis. In addition, Henry is a very stubborn, frightfully impatient, narcissistic person. While I have been working, looking up sources and collecting material so as to correct (actually to supplant) the poor information he presented to me—which information by the way is not more than 5 or 10 per cent of the book, Henry became impatient and talked to everybody he could get hold of, saying that I am holding up the publication of the book; that the Jews are frightful people and that I being a Jew he could expect nothing from me but laziness and dawdling. Henry has two hates—the Roman Catholic Church and the Jews. These hates in him are combined, even in a lesser degree than the average man, with no thinking.

Henry is essentially an illiterate man from the cultural point of view, and his is a brain that gets easily exercised, but is never exerted with heavy thinking.

After one of his particularly vicious anti-Semitic outbursts, of which I learned, I finally confronted him with the facts. He, as is characteristic of such people, crawled. He at first stated that I tried to re-write, throw out, or not use at all any of the notes he wrote, and second; he began to say that there were Jews and Jews. He did not deny his anti-Semitism, but tried to qualify it in the manner of a great many anti-Semites who are also conscious cowards. In such matters I prefer a Hitler; with the latter I always know where I stand.

I was in Bloomingdale hospital at the time. I told Dr. Russell frankly why, under the circumstances, I stood ready not to publish the thing at all rather than to have Henry's and my name associated under the same title. Dr. Russell has always been very anti-Semitic, but his anti-Semitism was always covered with a suave quietness. He was careful and knew to whom to talk and not to talk, and to whom to express his views freely—although free expression has never been his forte. Russell never forgave me the fact that he accepted me on Thomas W. Salmon's insistence as a member of the staff of Bloomingdale hospital, only to discover later that I was a Jew, and thus by becoming the first Jewish member of the staff in the history of Bloomingdale hospital, I broke the precedent. Since that time Hitler came, and the question of anti-Semitism naturally became a more important issue to me. Added to this was the fact that with the death of Raynor, who was a dear friend and who planned an academic future for me, I had to give up all hope of such a career—a career which was always dearer to me than sitting and making money, and studying and reading at nights, instead of doing my research work at leisure.

Henry, in the meantime, was promoted to Associate professor, and to the difficulties which I have mentioned, was added another one. I did not feel like publishing a book with my name bearing no authoritative title, and Henry designated as Associate Professor of Psychiatry.

I want very much to publish the book; two or three publishers are after me to get the book out and I wish I were able to find a decent way of publishing it without Henry. Perhaps you will be good enough to help me with your advice? As a matter of fact, there is something fatal about the situation. I was to discuss the matter with Raynor and he promised me that he would suggest a way out. We were to talk the matter over on the very Saturday morning that he died.

So there I stand, with almost twelve years of serious research work all over Europe locked up in my drawer. And uncomfortably so.

Please get in touch with me upon your return to New York. With my very best wishes and regards.

As the number of women in psychiatry increased, so did the possibility of conflicts complicated by gender differences. The position of Clara M. Thompson (1893– 1958), who had a distinguished career in psychoanalysis, was by no means unique. Thompson had received her M.D. from Hopkins in 1920 and then held several positions at the Henry Phipps Clinic, where she had also served her intern- ship. In 1925 a series of events led to her resignation from Hopkins, although she continued to reside in Baltimore. Four years later she attempted a reconciliation with Meyer. The ensuing correspondence between them illustrates how theoretical differences became intertwined with sexual factors.

Clara M. Thompson to Adolf Meyer, October 23, 1925 (AMP, Series I).
Dear Sir:—I wish to hereby tender my resignation from the various posi- tions I hold in the Phipps Clinic—this resignation to take place at once.

Adolf Meyer to Clara M. Thompson, October 31, 1925 (AMP, Series I).
Your resignation is accepted. I am afraid it might be difficult for you, even if you desired to do so, to convince one of any reestablishment of a frank and whole-hearted relation to the Clinic. I cannot help feeling that, besides your own neglect of open discussion, a misleading influence kept you from a course of frank and direct inquiry and dealings. It may be the type and standard of psychoanalysis you have espoused, to venture on interpreta- tions where it would be easy to get the facts directly.

I do not ask for evidence of gratitude for what I have attempted to do at various times, although I should have appreciated some practical demon- stration of responsibility. It was deplorable that you could disregard as you did the spirit with which you always [were] dealt with. I regret especially that it does not become possible in this way to wipe out a record of actual and tacit misrepresentations and misjudgments that undermined your rela- tions with the Clinic. A method of hasty interpretation which you tended to endorse has created much trouble for Dr. Harken (who finally straight- ened it out) and has proven disastrous to your using a wide range of oppor- tunities to which I was willing to give my sincere support, although not an uncritical support. I appreciated your work, but deplored the influence of your associations.

Adolf Meyer to Dr. Warfield T. Longcope (Johns Hopkins Hospital), May 19, 1926 (AMP, Series I).

Dr. Clara Thompson resigned from the Clinic last October or November, and I allowed the resignation to pass because at the time I did not actually know that, in addition to matters which would have made continuation of service impossible, she had since June treated one of several patients of the Clinic for a fee of $100 a month at the offices of a clever but unsavory psychoanalyst, a Navy recruiting officer who was a U.S. spy in the Orient during the War. If any other facts were needed to settle the question of further connections with the Johns Hopkins Hospital, I should let you have them. It was only by accident that I heard of her working in the Neurological Dispensary. Had her name come up before the Board, I could not have allowed it to pass, and I am sure you would have concurred with my suggestion that the application should be turned down.

I suppose Dr. Ford did not know the details of the situation when he took her in. But even so, I do not consider it a very thoughtful and even a very friendly step on his part. He must have known something of the situation and also how she neglected the neurological aspect of the cases to a remarkable extent. She is bright, but unduly free of some traits we would like to consider obligatory. I wanted to speak to Dr. Ford but was taken ill before I could reach him. I hope to be on deck again in a few days and shall try to see him then.

Clara M. Thompson to Adolf Meyer, November 12, 1929 (AMP, Series I).

Four years is too long a period for a misunderstanding to exist without at least an attempt at understanding. I realize that it is largely my fault that no such attempt has been made, and it is in order to correct that fault that I am writing this letter.

I do not, of course, know whether you desire to re-establish any contact with me, and if you do not you may simply ignore this letter. For my part it would be a satisfaction to me to explain to you the real facts of my mistakes in the situation and those which seemed to me to be yours and to give you a similar opportunity. Then I feel that, even should we not wish to be friends, we can respect each other.

Should this wish be similar to yours I shall be glad to come over and talk with you sometime. It would be necessary to let me know about four days in advance so that I may arrange my appointments. Between 1.15 and 3.15 are the hours most satisfactory to me with the exception of next Tuesday.

Adolf Meyer to Clara M. Thompson, November 23, 1929 (AMP, Series I).
Your letter of Nov. 16 [*sic*] came just as I had to leave for a conference. Welcome as it was it leaves me still somewhat in doubt and with the wish that I might have had an answer to the letters I remember I wrote you without any other intention than to obtain a basis for a fruitful under-standing. You suggest if an opportunity to explain "the real facts of our mistakes" makes me shrink because I was not thinking of the situation in terms of mistakes but more of the condition of security & basic principles of human relations. At any rate a reply to my letter would have been a better basis for a meeting on common ground than that of meeting to ex-plain & excuse mistakes and appearances of mistakes; [a] quick reply might have made it possible to keep apart mistakes & mishaps, & to focus more on the basic attitudes and reactions. . . . This is not meant to be a rebuff of your welcome impulse, but an expression of what might well be the basis of future contacts.

Clara M. Thompson to Adolf Meyer, December 7, 1929 (AMP, Series I).
I was glad to receive *your letter.* I was surprised that you seem to have ex-pected an answer to the one you wrote me four years ago. I have not the letter at hand so can not quote exactly, but I remember quite distinctly one sentence to the effect that—it *would be difficult* even if I wished *to re-establish relations of confidence* with you & the clinic. It seems to me that such a sentence might discourage even a more aggressive person than my-self. However since you now suggest that I might begin by answering that letter, & since some one must start the ball rolling if it is to roll I have no objections to your suggestion & will in general reply to what I can recall.

I suppose our real difficulty, stripped of all the misunderstandings & tensions which developed later amounted to this—that you were *hurt that I turned to psychoanalysis,* adopting a method of therapy not advocated or taught in the clinic, and that in addition I *chose an analyst* of whom *you did not approve. I in turn was distressed at your disapproval* but unwilling to alter my course. The reasonable thing for me to have done under the circum-stances would have been to have left the clinic as soon as possible—and that is what I would have done if it had not been for my *attachment to you* (transference) growing out of the fact that I had *told my problems to you pre-viously* and, as in your method of treatment *the transference is not analyzed, my attachment had continued* to exist for several years. I was therefore confronted by two attachments & to individuals not friendly to each other & I did not manage that situation very well. In my attempts to make a compromise adjustment to you both I did you both an injustice, & suppose that the later situation between you & me was the direct result of the emotional tension which accumulated & made it impossible for us to talk frankly to each other—with the result that I possibly did unwise things & *you were content to get indirect information about me* rather than taking the matter up with me directly. In your letter you regretted the influence of my associates, meaning I suppose my analyst. I am quite willing to grant that his judgment was not always the best, certainly partly due to the accumulated tension from which we were all suffering. I would criticize him as well as you & myself in the situation. I feel that if any one of the three of us had been able to view the matter unemotionally many of the developments might have been prevented. This in general sums up my attitude toward the situation at the present time.

But to stop here would mean to leave certain things not clear. Therefore I should like to mention specifically two or three things.

You said that I had caused Dr. Harken trouble. This reference & an interview I had with Dr. Wertheimer on the day before I left the clinic are not clear to me. Dr. Wertheimer in his conversation with me said that he had talked with Harken & now he "knew all." I asked him what he meant & he would only reply that I knew perfectly well. The situation has always puzzled me & I would be grateful for an explanation. From what I know of Dr. Harken's past history I can not believe that even if I did something unwise in my treatment of him, I could have been greatly responsible for his behavior. But *you & Dr. Wertheimer must have had something rather definite in mind.*

The next matter has to do with a *piece of gossip* which I heard two years after I left Phipps. It was reported to me thus—that you said that you had asked me to resign because I was my analyst's mistress. I am not holding you accountable for a rumor. Of course I suppose something was said by some member of your staff which formed the basis for it. But when I heard it I realized that it was a natural inference to have drawn from some of my behavior & that you probably believed it. A more sophisticated woman & one less secure in her innocence would have been more discreet. It happens that I have never been his mistress at any time. I do not know whether you can believe that and I do not know that it matters anyway, but since I am telling you facts that is one of them.

There is only one other thing that I want to mention & that is your *having me removed from the neurology dispensary*. You may have thought you were justified in the step but it is very hard for me to take a natural history attitude towards this. The position was not of my seeking. Dr. Taneyhill invited me & made the arrangements. It seemed to me that either you feared I would do you some harm or it was merely an act of retaliation. The former idea seemed too ridiculous to entertain seriously, considering our relative positions, but when I think it was the latter it is very hard for me to keep an open minded objective attitude. Still I have tried to do so in this letter & I hope you will reciprocate in the same spirit.

Adolf Meyer to Clara M. Thompson, December 10, 1929 (AMP, Series I).
Your letter of December 7, 1929, brings out several points which undoubtedly deserve correction.

As to psychoanalysis, I was indeed distressed, not by the fact of your interesting yourself in it, but by your being unnecessarily blinded to important facts in some case not accessible to it. The choice of the analyst also had its share, and especially so because of the role you both, or at any rate the analyst, played in the Harken episode. The transference must have been ineffective on some essential points of allegiance—such as treating ward patients outside under conditions which the Hospital could not have tolerated. As to my being content to get indirect information about you, I am not aware that I acted in any essential point on hearsay. Some of the detail is not absolutely fixed in my mind although I could probably look up such items as the threat of a suit against the Hospital or University in behalf of Dr. Harken by the man whom you allowed to come to a lecture with a stenographer. As to the "gossip"—I neither asked you to resign nor does it quite ring true that I should have given any such "reason" for what anyhow I did not do, or that I should deal in gossip on any occasion. I connect your resignation with a conversation you had with a member of the staff instead of your coming to me after that lecture.

The neurological dispensary decision was based on the fact that you had left without any explanation or attempt at mutual understanding and had not been appointed again by the Hospital, and I did not consider it appropriate that any one leaving one department in that manner should enter another department without a question being raised. It was not retaliation, but a combination of provocations of an official and not merely personal character.

These are to the best of my knowledge the facts and the motives of whatever I had a share in with regard to a frankly distressing experience, but not one governed by "emotional tension" at least on my part. My reaction to it was and is very much more objective than seems to have appeared to you. You can, I think, readily see that any getting together can only be on ground[s] of a frank objectivity.

I no doubt have often said and felt that I have had bad experience with a number of devotees of psychoanalysis. Why should I not look for a less seductive type of formulation? I have always had and have now a deeply rooted confidence in the supremacy of the wholesome tendencies in many patients too exclusively viewed for what is "wrong with them." There are more socializable ways of helping than "psychoanalysis" and I like to further them. In your own case you stopped on ground of some superficial help you may have sought and obtained, and you prefer to work with conceptions handed out in a system too one-sidedly conceived and very effective at times, but only one of many reasonably effective methods.

I appreciate your letter as an attempt to eliminate emotionally tinged misconceptions. I trust that the objective facts I recall may put the entire issue on a more matter-of-fact ground.

Clara M. Thompson to Adolf Meyer, December 15, 1929 (AMP, Series I).
Thank you for your letter of Dec. 10. I have tried to see the matter from your point of view. It seems hardly worth while now to go into any more detail, since no facts can be undone anyway. I feel fairly certain that should it be conceivable that a similar situation could arise now I would handle it very differently, although even so I should not altogether agree with you. But I also feel fairly certain that I would be incapable of creating such a complex Driven situation.

As to psychoanalysis—I am convinced (and I think I have given other methods a fair trial) that in the hands of a well trained person who also has his own problems well understood it can do more therapeutically than any other method, so I have tried to become well trained & well analyzed & I think to the improvement of both myself & my efficiency. But I would go further & say that I think all psychiatrists would be more effective in any therapeutic method if they were themselves analyzed and had their own personality difficulties smoothed out.

As to Phipps—I am not sorry for the time I spent with you. I learned a great deal there. It has furnished me with a perspective which has no doubt helped me to evaluate my specialty in its true proportion. That statement may seem strange to you since you have not known me since my very-poorly analyzed days.

Psychiatric attitudes toward women often mirrored broader social perceptions even when phrased in medical terms. In early 1946 Edward L. Bernays undertook to make a comprehensive evaluation of women for McCall's Magazine, which had a circulation of nearly 3.5 million. Bernays surveyed a large number of people. He then hoped to use the data as a means of offering a series of recommendations about the "better integration of women into society." Among those included in the survey was Dr. William D. Partlow, superintendent of the Alabama State Hospitals and the Partlow State School. Partlow's response was phrased in terms of an older ideal, even though the position of women in the work force and in American life generally had changed dramatically in the twentieth century.

William D. Partlow to Edward L. Bernays, February 18, 1946 (WDPP).
You have requested some statement from me on the subject of "The present status of women's relationship to the desired ideal in a democratic society."

Briefly, from my long study of humanity from the various angles of woman's relationship to society, it is my positive conviction that woman's prime purpose is motherhood and that carried along with this as we observe all other animal life in its bed-making and house-making preparation, instinctively, in preparation for motherhood, that woman also is basically the homemaker and homekeeper. Any other function of womanhood is contrary to these basic ideas and purposes for which she was created if in any way such functions, occupations, or employment interfere with or conflict in any way with her basic purpose for which the Creator intended her, of mother and homemaker.

Of course, to better prepare woman for mature womanhood, motherhood and homemaking, all education should be properly adjusted and planned. She must have proper physical development, proper social environment and social experience as a part of her education.

The place woman may fill or occupy as regards business, industry, labor or any other occupation connected with the family economy or general economy of the country should be a secondary consideration and never permitted to conflict with the primary purpose for which woman was placed in the world by the Creator, motherhood, womanhood and homemaking and family relationship, if we shall expect one generation to transmit to its posterity, strength and stability. The influence of an ideal mother in every home in America would in my opinion, largely solve the problem of juvenile delinquency and juvenile crime.

During the early twentieth century, psychiatry began to move beyond the walls of mental hospitals. Increasingly its members began to affirm that their specialty had a vital role to play in resolving many social problems. William A. White was among the leading exponents of this view. Beginning in 1911 and continuing until his death in 1937, he became involved in an effort to reform prevailing legal tests of insanity in criminal trials. White believed that penal policy ought to rest on a "scientific" base; he rejected the traditional claim that the American legal system could not be divorced from the concept of personal responsibility. White was involved with the APA's Committee on the Legal Aspects of Psychiatry, which during the 1920s was beginning an effort to medicalize the disposition of criminals. The following correspondence, which involved such figures as Karl A. Menninger (1893–   ), then launching his long and distinguished career, and Felix Frankfurter (1882–1965), then a Harvard Law School professor and subsequently an associate justice of the U.S. Supreme Court, illuminates the growing belief that psychiatry had a vital role in dealing with social issues.

William A. White to Karl A. Menninger, April 19, 1926 (WAWP). The draft to which White alluded was prepared by the Committee on the Legal Aspects of Psychiatry. The second part of the draft statement, "The Credo of Psychiatrists in Re Crime," is reprinted immediately following White's letter. The copy is from the WAWP.

I have your letter, which I have read perhaps rather hurriedly because you seem to be in a great hurry to have it back. I can not go into details in correcting it because that is not the way I work. I can only say in general that I like it very much indeed. I think it gets the spirit of the situation very splendidly. As I read over the credos I rather liked the longer one the better. Let me add a few thoughts.

In the first place, the suggestion that all criminal behavior should be regarded as falling within the province of psychiatry. Such a bold statement can only be received with incredulity and misgivings by most people. To call every wrongdoer sick sounds silly. My attitude about it, however, is much like the attitude which you have so splendidly summed up *in re* responsibility. The idea of responsibility as related to the criminal is a fiction. Of course all things come to be fictions sooner or later. Concepts are only true as long as they serve a useful purpose, and the idea of criminal responsibility nowadays serves only to precipitate a metaphysical quarrel which is never decided every time anybody commits an anti-social act, whereas if all of them were considered psychotic they would all immediately be removed from the danger of further anti-social conduct by being properly segregated and then they would come to be let out only when there was a reasonable prospect that they had changed their method of reacting sufficiently to be a social asset instead of a social liability precisely as we now take care of the mentally ill. In other words, to do away with the whole idea of responsibility would have the practical result of taking a long step forward in the efficiency with which we attack the crime problem, so called. . . .

THE CREDO OF PSYCHIATRISTS IN RE CRIME
We believe

1. *That* the psychiatrist's chief concern is with the facilitation of human life adaptations, and with understanding and evaluating the social and individual factors entering into failure in this adaptation.

2. *That* crime is a designation for one kind of such adaptation failures, and hence falls definitely within the focus of psychiatry.

3. *That* crime as well as other behavior and characterologic aberrances can be scientifically studied, interpreted and controlled.

4. *That* this study includes a consideration of the hereditary, physical, chemical, social and psychological factors entering into the personality concerned throughout his life as well as (merely) in the specific "criminal" situation.

5. *That* from the study of such data we are enabled in many cases to direct an attack upon one or more of the factors found to be active in a specific case to effect an alteration of the behavior in a propitious direction; while in other cases where this is not possible we are able in the light of past experience and discovered laws to foresee the probabilities to a degree sufficient to make possible proper provision against subsequent (further) injuries to society. By the same experience and laws we are enabled in still other cases to detect and endeavor to prevent the development of potential criminality.

6. *That* these studies can be made with proficiency only by those properly qualified, i.e., scientists who have made it their life interest and study

to understand and treat behavior disorders. Such men will have had the psychiatric training and point of view of the members (membership) of the American Psychiatric Association.

7. *That* such studies and such procedure, and none other, would provide an efficient and scientific solution to the three problems of crime, viz;

1. The protection of society.
2. The rehabilitation of the "criminal" if possible; the safe disposition of detention of him if rehabilitation is impossible.
3. The prevention of crime by potential "criminals."

We believe that psychiatrists should never be obliged to answer partisanly with "yes" and "no" to questions pertaining to such complex questions as commitability ("insanity"), responsibility, punishability and curability.

We believe that psychiatrists testifying in legal cases should be employed by the court and report to the court after opportunity has been provided for a thorough psychiatric examination, with such aids as psychiatrists habitually use in clinics, offices and hospitals.

We believe in the development of any machinery that will assist in the carrying out of this program, including court clinics and resident psychiatrists in all penal institutions.

We believe in the permanent detention of the inadequate, incompetent, and incurably antisocial, irrespective of the existing legal punishment for the particular single offense committed.

We believe the use of hypothetical questions in legal cases and the use of the words "insane" and "insanity" should be abandoned.

We believe in systematic psychiatric preventive medicine in the form of child guidance clinics, mental hygiene clinics, and similar institutions and efforts.

William A. White to Felix Frankfurter, December 17, 1927 (WAWP).
Mr. Glueck will undoubtedly by the time you receive this letter have given you an account of our meeting in New York. I am only writing to supplement in certain details perhaps what he has already told you.

We felt that after all most of the results which would flow from a routine survey of prisoners from a psychiatric point of view that would be practical has already been done several times. It has particularly been done in Massachusetts, so that the kind of material from this descriptive angle is already reasonably well known. It would seem, therefore, that for the purposes of this survey it would be eminently desirable to push our work to another stage of development which has not been heretofore covered and thus advance the whole matter by so much. With the prestige of Harvard University back of such an advance we could at least expect that it would receive wide attention.

Taking as a point of departure the recent suggestion of Governor Smith that sentencing power be taken from the judiciary, the Judges merely presiding, as I understand it, for the purpose of conducting a trial the outcome of which is to either prove the defendant guilty or innocent. If the defendant is proved guilty then the Governor's suggestion is that his sentencing be handed over to a board, which among its personnel should include criminologists and psychiatrists. This suggestion, you know perhaps, has been made before specifically in the Cleveland Survey, where the suggestion by an eminent lawyer was made that the prisoner be committed to the care of the Public Welfare Department to be assigned by them to the most appropriate institution; and the legal member of our group stated also that this same suggestion had received consideration in one other quarter. In discussing this matter, particularly with Dr. Glueck, who is familiar with the New York prison system, it appeared to us that while this step was in the right direction it would probably, unless supplemented, fail of any real accomplishment, for after all there are only four or five different types of institutions and it would soon become rather a routine matter as to which institution the offender would be sent to. This despite the fact that it was the Governor's idea, I believe, that before sentencing the prisoner should go to the clearing house at Sing Sing, where he would be adequately studied so that his needs would really figure in this final disposition. We are quite in accord with this general proposition, for it would involve the utilization much more intelligently of the indeterminate sentence, suspension of sentence, parole, and probably commutation and pardon under conditions very much better than they are today.

The difficulty of the above program, however, is that aside from questions of suspended sentence, parole and indeterminate sentence the prisons would be just as badly filled as they are now without any provision for extending intelligent therapeutic aid to the prisoner along any consistently worked-out plan for his social rehabilitation, remembering all the time that the responsibility for the crime, if I may use the word "responsibility," is at least two-fold, namely, personal and social, that crime is essentially a social phenomenon and that society, while in the first instance it has a perfect right to protect itself from the depredations of the criminal, has a duty toward the criminal to endeavor to get him well from a social point of view so that he may come back into the community and function to his own as well as the community's advantage.

We therefore felt that the next logical step would be a therapeutic program addressed to the prisoner and that in order that a proper presentation of such a program might be made it would be very advantageous if we could present a number of cases, say ten or fifteen, that had been dealt with in accordance with such a program, together with the results obtained. Such a program might ultimately be a rather elaborate one and would surely include the whole matter of prison management as directed to the rehabilitation objective but would necessarily be founded upon intensive individual studies and therapeutic efforts. Such work could hardly be undertaken by Dr. Glueck or anyone else that I have been able to contact with who can only give a small amount of time to such problems and would require intensive study over a number of months by someone who did very little else. It was suggested, therefore, that we endeavor to get a properly equipped man for this work. The name of Dr. Alexander, of Berlin, came under discussion. Dr. Alexander is a very able analyst who has contributed a great deal to the knowledge of human behavior as a result of his work. He speaks English very well and it is conceivable that for a reasonable consideration his services might be secured. Another peculiar qualification of Dr. Alexander is the fact that he has done a great deal of work on what the psychoanalysts call "the neurotic's need of punishment." It has seemed to me for some time that our penal system, conducted as it is upon the theory that crime should be punished, ought to have some information about the meaning of punishment in the general scheme of things. Despite the fact that the Christian Religion for two thousand years has been talking about this problem, with a different terminology, however, it would seem that the penal system is on the whole pretty blind to its significance. To have as our research man, therefore, one who is particularly keen-minded on this special aspect of the delinquent's make-up would be a very definite asset. Incidentally, he would attract students who are in training in various places with the object of practicing extra-mural psychiatry, and there possibly would gather about him quite a group of enthusiastic student psychiatrists who would supplement the work that he might be able to do personally. It was thought that probably a fund of something like $15,000 might accomplish this purpose.

As you will see, such a program as above outlined would require more than we had originally planned; but I understand from Mr. Glueck that the time element is not so vital inasmuch as some other portions of the survey are not to be completed in schedule so that if this suggestion of ours is carried out we would not be materially behindhand, provided particularly we could undertake to take this matter up promptly, and if, of course, Dr. Alexander would accept, or not accepting, would be able to name some acceptable person in his place.

I was very sorry indeed not to see you, as was also Miss Sergeant, who would have liked very much to have had you present on the occasion of a little social gathering at her house that evening.

Felix Frankfurter to William A. White, December 20, 1927 (WAWP).
I am immensely grateful to you for all the time and thought you have put on that vital portion of our survey crudely and briefly called the psychiatric aspects. Of course, the elements to which you will give guidance concern *the* essential problem of what to do about crime.

Dr. Glueck had already reported to me in some detail the course of the discussion of the New York meeting, and I am happy to have you state the whole matter so clearly in your letter. It gives it precisely the authoritative formulation that I want as a means of raising the necessary funds. Personally I agree entirely with the objectives which you indicate and the methods for reaching them.

I shall use your letter as a fund-raising instrument. In view of the remarks made both by you and by Dr. Bernard Glueck about the hostility in some quarters to the terms "psychoanalyst" and "psychoanalysis," I ask your leave to change your characterization of Dr. Alexander as a "very able analyst" to read "a very able psychiatrist." And perhaps you will also allow me to change the phraseology "on what the psychoanalysts call the 'neurotic's need of punishment.'" I am aware that these are childish euphemisms, and I would not have thought of it but for the caution conveyed by Dr. Bernard Glueck against arousing the ignorant hostility of those we will have to turn to for money. I hope we may raise the money very promptly and begin the undertaking which you have so admirably outlined.

It was a personal as well as professional source of regret to have missed seeing you in New York. As Sheldon Glueck doubtless told you, my mother is in a failing condition and, of course, I cannot leave her.

With warm regards to Mrs. White and yourself for us both and with all good wishes. . . .

William A. White to Felix Frankfurter, December 27, 1927 (WAWP).
I have your letter of the 20th instant. By all means make the changes you suggest. I quite agree with you that they are desirable.

The compliments of the season to you.

As neutrality threatened to break down after the rise of the Nazis to power, a group of Dutch psychiatrists prepared a statement entitled "The Insanity of War." Endorsed by many European psychiatrists, the statement was also sent to Clifford W. Beers, who in turn forwarded it to a number of prominent American psychiatrists and others active in the mental health field. Their responses illustrated the range of views. Some clearly believed that psychiatry had an indispensable role to play in the prevention of war; others questioned the claim that psychiatrists possessed special qualifications compared to those of interested and concerned citizens. As a whole, the correspondence suggests that by the 1930s psychiatrists were well on their way to expanding their jurisdictional claims.

"The Insanity of War," November 4, 1935 (AFMHP, uncatalogued).

THE INSANITY OF WAR

Explanatory: The following statement, recently issued under the auspices of The Netherlands Medical Society, which has formed a Committee on War Prophylaxis, has been signed by 339 psychiatrists of 30 countries, and is being used as a warning against the surrender of our civilization to the insanity of war.

Statement

We psychiatrists, whose duty it is to investigate the normal and diseased mind, and to serve mankind with our knowledge, feel impelled to address a serious word to you in our quality of physicians.

It seems to us that there is in the world a mentality which entails grave dangers to mankind, leading, as it may, to an evident war-psychosis.

War means that all destructive forces are set loose by mankind against itself.

War means the annihilation of mankind by technical science.

As in all things human, psychological factors play a very important part in the complicated problem of war.

If war is to be prevented the nations and their leaders must understand their own attitude towards war.

By self-knowledge a world calamity may be prevented.

Therefore we draw your attention to the following:

1. There is a seeming contradiction between the conscious individual aversion to war and the collective preparedness to wage war. This is explained by the fact that the behaviour, the feelings, the thoughts of an independent individual are quite different from those of a man who forms part of a collective whole. Civilized twentieth century man still possesses strong, fierce and destructive instincts, which have not been sublimated, or only partly so, and which break loose as soon as the community to which he belongs feels itself threatened by danger.

The unconscious desire to give rein to the primitive instinct not only without punishment but even with reward, furthers in a great measure the preparedness for war.

It should be realised that the fighting-instinct, if well directed, gives energy for much that is good and beautiful. But the same instinct may create chaos if it breaks loose from all restraint, making use of the greatest discoveries of the human intellect.

2. It is appalling to see how little the peoples are alive to reality.

The popular ideas of war as they find expression in fulldress uniforms, military display, etc., are no longer in keeping with the realities of war itself.

The apathy, with regard to the actions and intrigues of the international traffic in arms is surprising to anyone who realises the dangers into which this traffic threatens to lead them. It should be realised that it is foolish to suffer certain groups of persons to derive personal profit from the death of millions of men.

We come to you with the urgent advice to arouse the nations to the realisation of fact and the sense of collective self-preservation, these powerful instincts being the strongest allies for the elimination of war.

The heightening of the moral and religious sense in your people tends to the same end.

3. From the utterances of well-known statesmen it has repeatedly been evident that many of them have conceptions of war that are identical with those of the average man. Arguments such as "War is the supreme Court of Appeal" and "War is the necessary outcome of Darwin's theory" are erroneous and dangerous, in view of the realities of modern warfare. They

camouflage a primitive craving for power and are meant to stimulate the preparedness for war among the speaker's countrymen.

The suggestive force of speeches made by leading statesmen is enormous and may be dangerous. The warlike spirit, as easily aroused by the cry that the country is in danger, is not to be bridled, as was evident in 1914.

Peoples, as well as individuals, under the influence of suggestions like these, may become neurotic. They may be carried away by hallucinations and delusions, thus involving themselves in adventures perilous to their own and other nations' safety.

We psychiatrists declare that our science is sufficiently advanced for us to distinguish between real, pretended, and unconscious motives, even in statesmen. The desire to disguise national militarism by continual talk about peace will not protect political leaders from the judgment of history. The secret promoters of militarism are responsible for the boundless misery which a new war is sure to bring.

International organisation is now sufficiently advanced to enable statesmen to prevent war by concerted action.

Protestation of peace and the desire for peace, however sincere, do not guarantee the self-denying spirit necessary for the maintenance of peace, even at the cost of national sacrifice. If any statesman should think that the apparatus to ensure peace is, as yet, insufficiently organized, we advise them to devote to this purpose as much energy and as much money as is now being expended on the armaments of the various countries.

We cannot close without expressing our admiration of those statesmen who show by their actions that their culture and morality are so far advanced that they can lead peoples to a strong organisation of peace. In our opinion they alone are truly qualified to act as the leaders of nations.

Dr. Robert Woodman (superintendent, New York Middletown State Homeopathic Hospital) to Clifford W. Beers, November 5, 1935 (AFMHP, uncatalogued).

. . . I am quite in accord with the ideas expressed and agree in placing a great share of responsibility upon the leaders of public thought. We have had since the date this was issued an example before us of how militant leadership has inflamed the Italian nation and I am sure that other nations are not less subject to being carried away in the same manner. I am sure too that the world at large appreciates neither how far mass psychology is the product of its leadership nor to what irrational extremes it can go under aggressive leadership releasing instinctive drives. Every problem is half solved when it is defined and I believe that widespread endorsement by psychiatrists of the views of the Netherlands Society and ample publicity of their views might be of some held in clearing the matter in the popular mind. If the world could get the idea that war leadership is crazy leadership and that warlike patriotism is a form of insanity it might help.

William A. White to Clifford W. Beers, November 5, 1935 (AFMHP, uncatalogued).

I have just read rather hastily the statement of the Dutch psychiatrists, which I saw a notice of in the papers recently. I of course was interviewed promptly regarding the matter and I said for the newspapers that I thought the motives were eminently admirable but that as yet we did not know enough of the social mechanisms and their laws of operation to be able to accomplish a great deal, that we probably would have to develop not only additional information but new methods in order to deal with these large problems. I still believe this to be true but I think that such a statement as the Dutch psychiatrists have made is an excellent one to be made public, and that it contains a statement of objects and aims which are worth while considering not only seriously in themselves but they call attention to the enormous mass of false beliefs and disarming methods by which the aggressive tendencies express themselves. I think it would be very well worth while to attempt to popularize such information along the lines they suggest, and I think it would be worth while for some of the foundations to back research along social lines in connection with these problems. The Carnegie Foundation already has a set-up which is for the purpose of maintaining peace, and they have made considerable progress in the technical methods of international relations. These should be supplemented and backgrounded by studies such as are indicated by the Dutch psychiatrists.

Dr. Ira S. Wile to Clifford W. Beers, November 6, 1935 (AFMHP, uncatalogued).

With reference to the statement issued under the auspices of The Netherlands Medical Society, I can only say that I am thoroughly in sympathy with all the data therein contained, and believe it is a sound and rational approach to what appears to be human weakness, to make pretence of peace while preparing for war. I believe the resolution should be broadly publicized and forwarded to the President of the United States, Secretary of State and all the Members of the Senate and House of Representatives.

Dr. George Blumer to Clifford W. Beers, November 6, 1935 (AFMHP, uncatalogued).

I have your letter of November 4th with a notice of the annual meeting and also the very interesting report on the Insanity of War. There is one paragraph in this, that while it may be true, is only a half truth, namely, "International organization is now sufficiently advanced to enable statesmen to prevent war by concerted action." This may be academically true, but practically the difficulty is in finding statesmen. Most countries are ruled by politicians, not statesmen. The difference is that a politician puts things over and a statesman puts them through. The trouble is not with organizations but with human beings. I am just as much opposed to war as you are, but I don't know how far we are going to get talking about it.

Dr. E. Stanley Abbot to Clifford W. Beers, November 11, 1935 (AFMHP, uncatalogued).

No request for endorsement of the statement sponsored by the Netherlands Medical Society had come to me, though I had seen the statement in one of the daily newspapers; so I have not written any opinion about it.

I approve heartily the *intent* and *purpose* of the statement, but I so strongly disapprove of the wording in many places, or certain exaggerations, of one or two serious omissions, and of what seem to me the unscientific assumptions and statements, that I cannot, as a scientist, endorse or sign it as it stands. I won't burden you with the specific faults that lead me to this conclusion.

Dr. Helen P. Langner (Department of Health and Hygiene, Vassar College) to Clifford W. Beers, November 12, 1935 (AFMHP, uncatalogued).

The statement which you enclosed with the announcement of the Annual Meeting interests me very much. I am not one of those who signed it, and this is the first notice of it which has come to me. I heartily commend the spirit which prompts psychiatrists to undertake some professional action in favor of peace, but keep asking myself how this can be done.

As psychiatrists, we must recognize that peace can not be established by talking against war. Peace, which can come about only through a willingness to understand and act upon the other fellows point of view in the direction of goals of mutual benefit, can not come about while the security of the participants is threatened. Talk of armament and disarmament emphasizes and intensifies the sense of insecurity. If we could act on the principle that cooperative attacks on mutual enemies of human kind, ill health, poverty, ignorance, etc., can be brought about by frequent discussion of these problems in international conferences, our efforts would be much more surely directed toward world peace.

The League of Nations through its international committees on health, education, and other fields of scientific research, is working in the right direction. Such international congresses as those of the physiologists, neurologists and mental hygienists, discussing their particular fields of research in relation to mankind in general, are to my mind the most effective agents in working toward peace.

Dr. Benjamin W. Baker (superintendent, Laconia State School, New Hampshire) to Clifford W. Beers, November 12, 1935 (AFMHP, uncatalogued).

As to this matter of war—war in my opinion will never be stopped by talk. It has been estimated that if all the people in London should shout at once it would not amount to more than one horse power.

When a small, productive nation can be persuaded not to reproduce faster than its territorial capacity will permit of, that will remove one cause of war. Certainly the active removal of the causes of war is one line of attack on this subject. With urgent reasons for fighting it is difficult to persuade contestants in the field not to fight—for the inclination will exist as long as the cause remains. Remove the cause and the inclination can perhaps be calmed down.

Dr. Forrest N. Anderson (director, Child Guidance Clinic, Los Angeles) to Clifford W. Beers, November 14, 1935 (AFMHP, uncatalogued).

In response to your "N.B." of the November 4th letter—in reference to the "Statement on the Insanity of War," let me state that I had no previous knowledge of the Statement. However, in my opinion psychiatrists have a somewhat special responsibility in matters so charged with "rationalized" emotion as war and war propaganda. We arrogate to ourselves some knowledge concerning the motives of human conduct—individual and collective. It would seem to me that we cannot avoid some more responsibility than has the layman for insight into our own motives, whether these have to do with our everyday personal lives or in more important social matters. I do not see how we can avoid some looking beneath surface rationalizations. I agree with the import of the Statement. If the aggressive instincts are to be canalized into more social valued uses psychiatrists do have an oblication as teachers and as self-questioning individuals.

Winfred Overholser to Clifford W. Beers, November 12, 1935 (AFMHP, uncatalogued).

Like most war veterans, I hope sincerely that the world will never see another war. I am, however, somewhat doubtful of the wisdom of making a psychiatric issue out of any war propaganda. One of the difficulties in the past has been that some psychiatrists were too ready to speak with dogmatism on a large variety of domestic and world affairs, and this tendency has done much to weaken the respect with which the opinions of psychiatrists are accepted by the general public. From such information as has come to me directly, it would appear that very few American psychiatrists have signed this statement and it seems to me that psychiatrists should be hesitant about signing it *as psychiatrists*.

Dr. Glenn Myers to Clifford W. Beers, November 12, 1935 (AFMHP, uncatalogued).

I have read the statement with interest, emanating from the Netherlands Medical Society.

It seems to me that the institution of the movement implied in this statement may eventuate far reaching effects. I remember a physician, who was at the same time a psychiatrist, saying that, if the influence of all the physicians in the country were united, the physicians of the country could elect him President of the United States. He did not wish to be President, but made his point that physicians collectively have great potential political power.

Dr. Charles F. Read (superintendent, Elgin State Hospital, Illinois) to Clifford W. Beers, November 13, 1935 (AFMHP, uncatalogued).

. . . I have been requested to express my opinion of a statement made by certain psychiatrists of Amsterdam concerning the insanity of war. Of course, had this statement been submitted to me, I would not have hesitated to sign it. However, I must confess that aside from paragraph I, it seems to me there is little in this statement which might not have emanated from any lay group of peace-minded, good people. It is our privilege and our right to protest against the madness of war, but giving utterance to well-worn phrases will not produce results. In fact, there occurs to me the simile of a group of learned men perched upon the rim of a volcano, blowing across its crater to cool the hot lava beneath and thus avert further eruption.

Dr. Karl A. Menninger to Committee on War Prophylaxis, The Netherlands Medical Society, Amsterdam, no date, copy sent to Clifford W. Beers (AFMHP, uncatalogued).

I have read your statement on the insanity of war with a great deal of satisfaction. I feel it is something we psychiatrists should have done long ago but perhaps now is the most timely moment that could possibly have been chosen to issue such a statement.

From a theoretical standpoint I think the interpretation of war as a mass form of self-destruction, cloaked by many conventional illusions, is entirely correct. From a practical standpoint, I think the dissemination of our view of the matter in the light of our technical knowledge and experience is one of the few remaining hopes of a suicidally bent world.

I shall do everything I can to diffuse this proclamation among my friends and both I and my colleagues of the Menninger Clinic and the Menninger Sanitarium and the Southard School wish you to know of our complete and enthusiastic endorsement of it.

Dr. Foster Kennedy to Clifford W. Beers, November 25, 1935 (AFMHP, uncatalogued).

I have been most interested in the manifesto of The Netherlands Medical Society. . . .

The only possible conclusion to be drawn from these assertions is that every nation must subscribe to the Covenant of the League of Nations and robustly and worthily sustain that Covenant. It is necessary too as far as possible by Economic Conference to effect a considerable redistribution of raw materials so that the friction which precedes War may be made as small as possible. People who cry "Peace, Peace, when there is no Peace" are promoters of War, as much as are Christian Scientists promoters of diptheria.

INDEX

Abbot, E. Stanley, 108, 210, 293. *Correspondence*: with C.W. Beers, 293; with W.A. White, 108
Addams, Jane, 159
Adler, Herman M., 181
Advisory Board for Medical Specialties, 231
affective personality, 24
aftercare of mentally ill, 144, 177
aged patients in mental hospitals. *See* mental hospitals, aged and senile patients in
Alabama Insane Hospitals, 100–101, 171
Albany Hospital, Pavilion F, 80
alcoholic hallucinations, 22
alcoholic psychosis, 15
alcoholism, 10, 15, 182, 238
Alexander, Franz, 287–88
allopsychic disorders, 23
almshouses, 12–13
alpha-ray, 136
Altegeld, John P., 60
American Association of Psychiatric Social Workers, 10, 215, 218
American Board of Psychiatry and Neurology, 10, 231, 245, 250–60
American College of Physicians, 247
American College of Surgeons, 247
American Journal of the Diseases of Children, 242
American Journal of Psychiatry, 245
American Journal of Psychology, 27
American Medical Association, 185, 231–32, 245, 247, 250–60; and

Association of Medical Superintendents of American Institutions for the Insane, 185; conflict with American Psychiatric Association, 231–32, 250–60; Council on Medical Education and Hospitals, 229, 250–51, 254, 256, 259; Council on Medical Education and Hospitals, Psychiatric Advisory Committee, 251; Section on Nervous and Mental Diseases, 248
American Medico-Psychological Association, 7, 56, 186; and classification of mental illness, 27–34. *See also* American Psychiatric Association *and* Association of Medical Superintendents of American Institutions for the Insane
American Neurological Association, 232, 244
American Occupational Therapy Association, 10
American Ortho-Psychiatric Association, 247
American Psychiatric Association, 7, 10–11, 215, 218, 229–31, 244, 246–48, 250–60, 283–85; and classification of mental illness, 30–34; Committee on Legal Aspects of Psychiatry, 283–85; Committee on Medical Services, 230, 241; Committee on Psychiatry in Medical Education, 248; Committee on Standards and Policies, 229, 233; Committee on Statistics, 29; conflict

APA (*continued*)
with American Medical Association, 231–32, 250–60; and political controversy over Massachusetts mental hospitals, 260–65; ratings of state regulation of mental hospitals, 233. *See also* American Medico-Psychological Association *and* Association of Medical Superintendents of American Institutions for the Insane
American Psychoanalytic Association, 175
American Psychological Association, 212–14
Amsden, Dr., 248
Anderson, Albert, 41–42, 95, 109–12. *Correspondence* with J.K. Hall, 41–42, 109–12
Anderson, Forrest N., 294. *Correspondence* with C.W. Beers, 294
Anthonisen, Dr., 116
anticatholicism, 274
Anti-Saloon League, 182
antisemitism, 273–76
anxiety neurosis, 28, 205
aphasia, 176
apraxias, 176
Archives of Neurology and Psychiatry, 241, 243
Aristotle, 134
Army, U.S., and World War I psychiatry, 220–22
arteriosclerosis, 237
Association for Improving the Condition of the Poor (N.Y.), 166–67, 169
Association of Medical Superintendents of American Institutions for the Insane, 7, 87, 233; and American Medical Association, 185; qualifications for membership, 186. *See also* American Medico-Psychological Association *and* American Psychiatric Association
Atkinson, Henry R., 264–65. *Correspondence* with R. Chapman, 264–65

attendants, in mental hospitals, 89–94, 150, 153
autonomic functions, 199–211
The Autonomic Functions and the Personality (Kempf), 198

Bailey, Pearce, 221
Baker, Benjamin W., 294. *Correspondence* with C.W. Beers, 294
Balloch, Edward A., 270–71, 273. *Correspondence* with W.A. White, 270–71, 273
Bancroft, Wilder D., 35
Barker, Lewellys F., 192
Barrett, Albert M., 27, 29–34, 158–59, 246–47. *Correspondence* with A. Meyer, 29–34
Barrett, Joseph E., 262
Bassett, 191
Beers, Clifford W., 138–63, 177, 289, 291–95. *Correspondence*: with F.N. Anderson, 294; with B.W. Baker, 294; with G. Blumer, 293; with W. James, 141–47; with F. Kennedy, 296; with W. McDonald, Jr., 147–56; with A. Meyer, 162–63; with G. Myers, 295; with W. Overholser, 295; with C.S. Read, 295; with W.A. White, 292; with I. Wile, 292; with R. Woodman, 291–92
behavior, organic vs. psychological explanation, 46–47
behaviorism, 177, 188–98
Bellevue Hospital (N.Y.C.), 235–41
Bernays, Edward L., 282–83. *Correspondence* with W.D. Partlow, 282–83
Bettman, B., 60
bilateral ovariectomy, 103
Billings, Frank, 159
Biological Psychiatry, 233
Blackburn, I.W., 70, 271
blacks: and incidence of mental illness, 269; in mental hospitals, 89; and

psychiatry, 270–73
Bloomingdale Hospital, 275
Blumer, G. Alder, 142
Blumer, George, 160–61, 181, 293. *Correspondence*: with C.W. Beers, 293; with C.P. Emerson, 160–61
board certification in psychiatry and neurology, 231, 245–60
boarding-out system of care for mentally ill, 87
Boas, Franz, 213
Book of Job, 134
Borden, William C., 271–73. *Correspondence* with W.A. White, 271–73
Boring, Edwin G., 212–15. *Correspondence* with A. Meyer, 212–15
Boston Psychopathic Hospital, 27, 48–54, 103, 130, 187, 223, 260–61
Boston Society of Psychiatry, 76
Boston State Hospital, 75, 260–63
Brackin, H.B., 94–96. *Correspondence* with J.K. Hall, 94–96
Briggs, L. Vernon, 71–76, 171, 263, 265
Brill, Abraham, 128–29, 224. *Correspondence* with W.A. White, 128–29
Brown, Lucille Field, 38
Brumbaugh, M.G., 86
Brush, Edward N., 76, 245–47. *Correspondence* with F.G. Ebaugh, 246–47
Buckley, Thomas H., 263
Burdick, Dorothy S., 251
Burleigh, Edith, 223
Burrow, Trigant, 191
Butler Hospital for the Insane, 147

Cabot, Richard, 212–13
calcium therapy, 121
Caldwell, J.P., 110
California, 171
California Insane Asylum, 12
calomel, 103
Campbell, C. Macfie, 48–55, 212–13, 216, 253, 260–61. *Correspondence*: with C.B. Farrar, 261; with C.M. Hincks, 48–55
Cameron, Ewen, 129
camisole, 151–52, 235
Cannon, Walter B., 200
Carlson, Anton J., 200
Carnegie, Andrew, 142
Carnegie Foundation, 173, 292
Carnegie Institution of Washington, 38
Casamajor, Louis, 128, 241–42, 245. *Correspondence* with A. Meyer, 241–42, 245
catatonic phenomena, 22
Catholics, 170
Census Bureau (U.S.), and statistics of insanity, 31–32
Census of 1840 (U.S.), 269
cerebral arteriosclerosis, 15
Chadwick, Henry, 263
Channing, Walter, 72
Chapin, John B., 74
Chapman, Ross M., 261, 264–65. *Correspondence* with H.R. Atkinson, 264–65
chemical restraint, 72
Cheney, Clarence O., 112–13, 253–54
Chittenden, Russell H., 161–63, 181
Christian Science, 181, 227–28
Civil War, 267
Clark, Charles H., 70–71. *Correspondence* with W.A. White, 70–71
Clark University, 130, 191
classification of disease, 185
classification of mental illness, 20, 27–34, 42–44, 185
Claude, Henri, 137
Cleveland, Grover, 258
Clevenger, S.V., 193
clinical psychology, 241
Cobb, Stanley, 180, 202–203, 207, 209
colectomy, 104, 120
colony system of caring for mentally ill, 87
Commission on Medical Education, 230

commitment of mentally ill, 80–82, 84, 100, 236–37
Committee on the Costs of Medical Care, 229
Committee for Organizing Psychiatric Units for Base Hospitals (National Committee for Mental Hygiene), 220–21
Committee on Psychiatric Investigations (National Research Council), 219
Commonwealth Fund, 181, 242, 244
community care of mentally ill, 84–87
Community Chest, 165
conditioned reflex, 198
Congress on Medical Education, Licensure and Hospitals, 255
Connecticut Society for Mental Hygiene, 139, 159
Connecticut State Hospital for the Insane, 138
Copp, Owen, 72, 75–76
Cotton, Henry, 76, 104, 108–23
Coueism, 227
Cowles, Edward, 59, 62, 186
Craddock, French H., 100–101. *Correspondence* with W.D. Partlow, 100–101
crime and psychiatry, 283–89
criminal responsibility, 283–89
Crutcher, Hester B., 215, 218–19. *Correspondence* with M. Scoville, 218–19
Curley, James Michael, 260, 263
Cutter, William B., 254

Darwin, Charles, 135, 203–205, 290
Darwinism, 21
Davenport, Charles B., 38
DeForest, Robert W., 142
Dejerine, Joseph J., 225
delerium, 22, 24, 164
d'Elseaux, Frank C., 51–52
delusions, 149
dementia, 22
dementia praecox, 15, 21–22, 24–26,

29, 41, 107–108, 113, 205. *See also* schizophrenia
dependency, psychopathology of, 165–70
de Saussure, R., 137
Diethelm, Oskar, 44, 106
digitalis, 103
dissociation, 22–25, 205
Dix, Dorothea L., 157
doctor-patient relationship, 8
Dodge, Cleveland H., 142
dreams, 22
Dripps, Robert D., 86
drug addiction, 15
dualism, 45
Dubois, Paul, 225
Dunlap, Knight, 191, 198
Dutch psychiatrists and antiwar statement (1935), 289–96

Eastman, Barnard, 68
Eaton, Dorman B., 56
Ebaugh, Franklin G., 242, 246–49, 253. *Correspondence* with E.N. Brush, 246–47
Eder, M.D., 47
Education: of physicians, 230; of psychiatrists, 230–33, 241–45, 248–60
Eldridge, Watson W., 124–25. *Correspondence* with W.A. White, 124–25
electrical treatment, 103
electroshock therapy, 105
Embree, Edwin R., 165–70. *Correspondence* with F.E. Williams, 165–70
Emerson, Charles P., 79–81, 160–61. *Correspondence*: with G. Blumer, 160–61; with A. Meyer, 79–81
Emerson, Ralph Waldo, 134
epilepsy, 15, 38–41
eugenics, 10
Eugenics Record Office, 38

Farrar, Clarence B., 261–64. *Corre-*

spondence: with C.M. Campbell, 261; with W. Overholser, 261–64

Father Matthew movement, 164

Favill, Henry B., 161–62. *Correspondence* with A. Meyer, 161–62

Federation of State Boards, 250

feebleminded, 10, 170–71

Fergus Falls State Hospital (Minn.), 98

Ferguson, R.G., 87–89. *Correspondence* with W.A. White, 87–89

Ferris, Albert, 74

fever therapy, 104–105. *See also* malaria therapy

Fischer's solution, 121

Fisher, Dr., 172–74. *Correspondence* with W.A. White, 172–74

Fisher, James T., 136–37. *Correspondence* with S.E. Jelliffe, 136–37

Flexner, Abraham, 175–81. *Correspondence* with A. Meyer, 175–81

Flexner, Simon, 20

focal infection theory of mental illness, 104, 108–23

Ford, Frank R., 277

Forel, O.L., 129

forensic psychiatry, 283–89

Foster, Sybil, 215–18. *Correspondence* with A. Meyer, 216–18

Frankfurter, Felix, 283, 285–89. *Correspondence* with W.A. White, 285–89

Freeman, Walter, 105

French, Lois M., 187

Freud, Sigmund, 28, 106–107, 129, 133, 135, 191, 198, 233, 273

Fuller, Raymond G., 16–17

General Education Board, 146

general paresis. *See* paresis

germ theory of disease, 185

Getchel, Albert C., 77–79. *Correspondence* with A. Meyer, 77–79

Gieson, Ira Van, 207, 219

Gilman, Daniel C., 142

Gitelson, Maxwell, 175, 183–84. *Correspondence* with E. Saxe, 183–84

Gjessing, R., 115–16. *Correspondence* with A. Meyer, 115–16

Glenn, John M., 142

Glover, E., 47

Glueck, Bernard, 128, 286–88

Glueck, Sheldon, 285, 288

glycothymoline, 76

Gordon, Miss, 66

Gosney, E.S., 174–75. *Correspondence* with W.D. Partlow, 174–75

Gothenburg system, 164

Gould, Helen, 142

Graves, William C., 158

Green, E.M., 25–27. *Correspondence* with A. Meyer, 25–27

Greenacre, Phyllis, 108, 116

Greene, James L., 158

Gregg, Donald, 103

Gregory, Menas S., 128

Grimes, John M., 250–51, 253, 255–56, 260

Groddeck, Georg, 225

Gross Anatomy of the Brain in the Insane (Blackburn), 70

Guy's Hospital, 64

habit disorder, 23–24

Hall, G. Stanley, 59–64, 179. *Correspondence* with A. Meyer, 59–64

Hall, James King, 1, 41–42, 94–96, 109–12, 130, 134–35, 227–28. *Correspondence*: with A. Anderson, 41–42, 109–12; with H.B. Brackin, 94–96; with W. Overholser, 227–28

hallucinations, 22–23

Hamilton, Allan McLane, 210

Hamilton, Samuel W., 128, 258, 262

Harken, Dr., 276, 279–80

Harlem Valley State Hospital (N.Y.), 128

Harpers Magazine, 183

Harriman, Mrs. E.H., 38

Hartford Retreat (Conn.), 138

Hartwell, Samuel W., 218
Harvard University, 286
Harvey, William, 135
Haviland, C. Floyd, 29, 84–87, 112
Henry, George, 274–76
Henry, Patrick, 134
Henry Phipps Psychiatric Clinic (Johns Hopkins), 21, 82–83, 230, 276–81
heredity, 38–41, 63–64, 140, 170–75; and mental illness, 45–46
Hering, Arthur P., 171–72. *Correspondence* with W.A. White, 171–72
Hincks, Clarence M., 48–55, 126–28, 258. *Correspondence*: with C.M. Campbell, 48–55; with H. Maier, 126–28; with W. Overholser, 128; with W.A. White, 128
Hinsie, Leland, 128
A History of Medical Psychology (Zilboorg and Henry), 274–76
Hitler, Adolf, 275
Hobbs, A.T., 112–15. *Correspondence* with W.A. White, 112–15
Hoch, August, 21–25, 164. *Correspondence* with A. Meyer, 21–25
Holt, Earl K., 263
Holt, Edwin B., 195
Hoskins, Roy G., 45–47. *Correspondence* with S.E. Jelliffe, 45–47
hospital, creation of modern, 9
hospitals, general: mentally ill in, 79; outpatient departments, 186; psychiatric wards, 186
Howard, Herbert B., 77
Howard University, 270–73
Howe, Samuel Gridley, 100
Howell, William H., 253
Huey, Edmund B., 191
human behavior, basis of, 34–37
Huntington's chorea, 15
Hurley, Charles F., 263
Hutchins, F.F., 215–16. *Correspondence* with D.A. Thom, 215–16
hydrotherapy, 103, 164
hyoscyamin, 103
hysteria, 22–24, 137

Illinois, 13
Illinois Board of Public Welfare Commissioners, 257
Illinois Eastern Hospital for the Insane. *See* Kankakee Hospital for the Insane (Ill.)
immigration restriction, 140, 163, 170
Indiana, 79–81, 171
infective-exhaustive psychoses, 25
insanity. *See* mental illness
"The Insanity of War," 289–91
insulin shock treatment, 105, 126–29
integration, 36

James, William, 139, 141–47, 193, 198. *Correspondence* with C.W. Beers, 141–47.
Janet, Pierre, 23, 25
Jarrett, Mary E., 223
Jarvis, Edward, 266–67, 269
Jefferson, Thomas, 135
Jelliffe, Smith Ely, 1, 34–35, 45–47, 96–100, 106–107, 125–26, 129, 136–37, 174, 224–27, 274–76. *Correspondence*: with J.T. Fisher, 136–37; with R.G. Hoskins, 45–47; with E. Jones, 224–27; with L. Kerschbaumer, 96–100, 137; with W.A. White, 125–26; with G. Zilboorg, 274–76
Jennings, Herbert S., 177, 189
Jews, 170; in psychiatry, 273–76
Johns Hopkins University, 181; Medical School, 21, 230, 276–82; School of Hygiene, 177. *See also* Henry Phipps Psychiatric Clinic (Johns Hopkins)
Johnson, Buford J., 191
Johnston, Mary, 16–17
Jones, Ernest, 191–92, 224–27. *Correspondence* with S.E. Jelliffe, 224–27
Jones, L.M., 109. *Correspondence* with W.A. White, 109
Jones, Lyman A., 66
Jung, Carl, 36, 191–92

Kankakee Hospital for the Insane (Ill.), 58–64
Kansas, 171, 183
Karpman, Benjamin, 273
Katzenelbogen, Solomon, 108, 116–23
Kelley, Otis, 263
Kelly, Fred C., 183
Kempf, Edward J., 84, 198–211. *Correspondence* with A. Meyer, 198–211
Kennedy, Foster, 296. *Correspondence* with C.W. Beers, 296.
Kentucky, 145
Kerschbaumer, Luisa, 96–100, 137. *Correspondence* with S.E. Jelliffe, 96–100, 137
Kesler, M.L., 110
Kirby, George H., 27, 94, 216, 241, 246, 248, 253
Kirkbride, Thomas S., 5
Kline, George M., 250, 255–57, 262, 264. *Correspondence* with W.A. White, 255–57
Kopeloff, Nicholas, 112–13
Kraepelin, Emil, 22, 28, 60, 64, 178

Laforgue, Rene, 137
Lambert, Charles I., 128
Lange [J?], 45
Langfeld, H.S., 213
Langner, Helen P., 293–94. *Correspondence* with C.W. Beers, 293–94
laparotomy, 116–17, 120
Lathrop, Julia C., 158–60. *Correspondence* with A. Meyer, 158–60
law and psychiatry, 283–89
lay psychoanalysts, 224–27
League of Nations, 294, 296
Le Chatelier, 35
Lecky, W.E.H., 134
Lee, Robert E., 134
Lewis, Nolan D.C., 114
Lichty, John A., 86
Lincoln, Abraham, 110, 134
Lind, Dr., 93
lobotomy, 105, 125–26, 264

Loeb, Jacques, 197
Logie, H.B., 42–44. *Correspondence* with A. Meyer, 42–44
Longcope, Warfield T., 277. *Correspondence* with A. Meyer, 277
Lovejoy, Arthur O., 191, 195–98
Luxenburger, H., 46

Mabon, William, 86
MacNider, William, 41
Maier, Hans, 126–28. *Correspondence* with C.M. Hincks, 126–28
malaria therapy, 121. *See also* fever therapy
Malzberg, Benjamin, 17
manic-depressive psychosis, 15, 25–26, 28, 43, 113
marriage regulation, 140
Martin, Miss, 220
Maryland Lunacy Commission, 171
Maryland State Conference of Charities and Correction, 171
Massachusetts, 4, 11–13, 87; politics and mental hospitals, 260–65; restraint controversy, 71–74
Massachusetts Department of Public Welfare, 165
Massachusetts General Hospital, 223
Massachusetts State Board of Insanity, 75–76, 78, 142
Maudsley, Henry, 47
May, James V., 231, 250, 255, 257–60, 262, 264. *Correspondence* with W.A. White, 257–60
McCall's Magazine, 282
McDonald, William, Jr., 147–56. *Correspondence* with C.W. Beers, 147–56
McDougall, William, 213
McKey, Miss, 97
McNairy, Dr., 109–110
medical education, 230; psychiatry in, 249
medicine, scientific, 8–9
Meduna, Ladislas von, 105
melancholia, 24

melancholic states, 22
Memorial Foundation for Neuro-
    Endocrine Research, 45
Mendelian theory, 172
Menninger, Karl A., 283–85, 296.
    Correspondence: with Committee on
    War Prophylaxis, Netherlands Medi-
    cal Society, 296; with W.A. White,
    283–85
Menninger Clinic, 183–84, 296
mental deficiency, 15. *See also* feeble-
    minded
mental health professions, rise of,
    187–88
mental hospitals: aged and senile pa-
    tients in, 12–14; American Medical
    Association investigation of, 250–
    60; attendants in, 89–94; blacks in,
    89; chiropractor in, 97; conditions
    in, 96–100, 233–41; criticisms of,
    56, 110–12; custodial role, 5–6;
    debate over size, 87–89; develop-
    ment and functions of, 2; diet at,
    70; financing of, 100–101; ideal,
    78; length of patient stay, 12, 16–
    17; in Massachusetts, 12; medical
    staffs of, 234–41; A. Meyer experi-
    ences at in 1890s, 58–64; mortality
    rates in, 15; nature of, 17–18, 57;
    number of, 2; organization of, 239–
    40; patient population, 11–17,
    239–40; patient rights, 109; patient
    testimony in, 90–94; and politics,
    57, 260–65; and psychiatry, 17–18;
    psychoanalysis in, 106–107, 130,
    136; restraint in, 71–74, 235–36;
    separation of curable and incurable,
    154; shaped by patient behavior, 57;
    social service departments, 187,
    215–16; in South, 94–96; state
    regulation of, 232–33; superinten-
    dents' frustrations in, 69–71; trans-
    formation of, 5–6, 11–17; women
    psychiatrists in, 267–69
mental hygiene, 9–10, 138–84,
    186, 243

mental illness: classification of, 20,
    25–34, 42–44, 185; community
    care, 84–87; curability claims, 4;
    definition of, 225–27, 236–37;
    etiology of, 3, 14–15, 20–21, 43,
    104, 108–23, 266–67; expansion
    of definition, 266–69; focal infec-
    tion theory of, 104, 108–23; mid-
    nineteenth century concepts of, 3–
    4; nature of, 20–21; pellagrous
    insanity, 25–27; prevention of,
    138, 163–64; public policy toward,
    6, 12–13; and race, 269; recovery
    from, 149; sex role, 53–54; state
    versus community care, 85–87;
    statistics of, 31–33, 44; treatment
    of, 3–6, 186. *See also* mental hy-
    giene; state welfare policy; therapy,
    psychiatric
mentally ill: aftercare of, 144, 177; in
    almshouses, 13; chronic, 5–6, 11–
    17; commitment of, 80–82, 84,
    100, 236–37; in general hospitals,
    79; hospital admission rates, 14; in
    jails, 79–83; mortality rates, 16–
    17; sterilization of, 140, 171–75
metrazol, 105
Meyer, Adolf, 1, 21–34, 42–44,
    59–69, 77–87, 104, 115–16,
    129–34, 156–64, 175–83, 198–
    220, 230, 241–57, 276–82; and
    C.W. Beers, 139–40, 156–63; and
    classification of mental illness, 26–
    34, 42–44; focal infection theory of
    mental illness, 108–23; human be-
    havior, 34–37; ideal mental hospi-
    tal, 78; insulin shock treatment,
    129; at Kankakee Hospital, 58–64;
    and E.J. Kempf and psychoanalysis,
    198–211; and Massachusetts policy
    toward mentally ill, 75–79; and
    mental hygiene, 175–83; preven-
    tion of mental illness, 163–64; and
    psychoanalysis, 130–34, 176, 189–
    90, 198–211; psychobiology, 19–20,
    106–107, 129–37, 176, 189–92,

198–211, 213, 219–20, 224–27, 241, 243–44, 273, 276, 278–81, 287–88; psychology, 212–15; state versus local care of mentally ill, 86; training in psychiatry, 241–45; at Worcester State Lunatic Hospital, 58–69, 156–58. *Correspondence*: with A.M. Barrett, 29–34; with C.W. Beers, 162–63; with E.G. Boring, 212–15; with L. Casamajor, 241–42, 245; with C.P. Emerson, 79–81; with H.B. Favill, 161–62; with A. Flexner, 175–81; with S. Foster, 216–18; with A.C. Getchel, 77–79; with R. Gjessing, 115–16; with E.M. Green, 25–27; with G.S. Hall, 59–64; with A. Hoch, 21–25; with E.J. Kempf, 198–211; with G.M. Kline, 255–57; with J.C. Lathrop, 158–60; with H.B. Logie, 42–44; with W.T. Longcope, 277; with W.G. Morgan, 181–83; with A. Myerson, 130–34; with H.S. Noble, 156–58; with H.M. Quinby, 64–69; with W.L. Russell, 247–55; with T.W. Salmon, 85–87, 163–64; with E.E. Southard, 27–29; with E.A. Strecker, 244; with C.M. Thompson, 276–82; with J.B. Watson, 188–98; with T.N. Weisenburg, 242–44; with W.A. White, 34–37, 129; with J.C. Whitehorn, 219–20
Meynert, Theodore, 186
Michigan, Psychopathic Hospital at the University of Michigan, 27
migraine headache, 39–40
A Mind That Found Itself (Beers), 138, 141–56, 177
mind-body relationship, 113
Mitchell, S. Weir, 56
Moniz, Egas, 105, 125
Mooers, Emma M., 66–67
Moose Lake State Hospital (Minn.), 98
moral management. *See* moral treatment

moral treatment, 4, 102
Morgan, William Gerry, 181–83. *Correspondence* with A. Meyer, 181–83
morphine, 103
Moss, Louise, 95
Moten, Lucy E., 271–72. *Correspondence* with W.A. White, 271–72
Mott, Frederick, 114, 174
Muller, M., 129
Muller, Max, 127
Myers, Glenn, 295. *Correspondence* with C.W. Beers, 295
Myerson, Abraham, 130–35. *Correspondence*: with J.K. Hall, 134–35; with A. Meyer; 130–34

narcosis, 127
National Board of Medical Examiners, 245
National Committee for Mental Hygiene, 84, 138, 165–70, 180, 220–21, 223–24, 230, 244, 251–52, 258–60, 265; application for grant to study psychopathology of dependency, 165–70; and classification of mental illness, 27–34; Committee for Organizing Psychiatric Units for Base Hospitals, 220–21; origins of, 139–63
National Conference on Nomenclature of Disease, 42
National Information Bureau, 165
National Research Council, 211, 213, 220, 253; Committee on Psychiatric Investigations, 219
Netherlands Medical Society, 289–91, 296. *Correspondence* with K.A. Menninger, 296
neurasthenia, 192, 195–97
Neurological Institute, 94
neurology, 175–76, 180, 241–45; and psychiatry, 220–24, 232, 241–45
neuropsychiatry, 220–24, 244–45
neuroses, 176
New York Academy of Medicine, 248

New York State, 14, 16–17, 87, 144; aged patients in state mental hospitals, 13; paretic patients, 14; recovery statistics, 16–17
New York State Charities Aid Association, 142–45
New York State Commission on Lunacy, 142
New York State Department of Mental Hygiene, 230
New York State Psychiatric Institute, 21, 44, 94, 128
Noble, Henry S., 156–58. *Correspondence* with A. Meyer, 156–58
Noble, Ralph A., 230
Norbury, Frank, 220–24. *Correspondence* with F.E. Williams, 220–24
North American Review, 56
North Carolina State Hospital (Raleigh), 95
Norton, Harold F., 261–62
nosology. *See* classification of mental illness
Noyes, Arthur P., 90, 93
nurses, psychiatric, 10, 95, 216

occupational therapy, 10, 88
O'Malley, Mary, 93
opium, 103
Osler, William, 62
Overholser, Winfred, 128, 227–28, 260–64, 295. *Correspondence*: with C.W. Beers, 295; with C.B. Farrar, 261–64; with J.K. Hall, 227–28

padded cell, 151
Page, Charles W., 75, 142
paramnesias, 22
paranoia, 24, 43, 64
paraphrenia, 28
paresis, 14–15, 20, 26, 104, 124–25, 185
Park, John G., 68
Parsons, Frederick W., 128
Partlow, William D., 100–101, 171, 174–75, 282–83. *Correspondence*:
with E.L. Bernays, 282–83; with F.H. Craddock, 100–101; with E.S. Gosney, 174–75
Pathological Institute of the New York State Hospitals. *See* New York State Psychiatric Institute
Paton, Stewart, 38, 146, 157, 213
pellagra, 15, 25–27
Pennsylvania, 13, 84–87
Pennsylvania Board of Commissioners of Public Charities, 84–85
Perkins, Dr., 262
Peterson, George, 137
Pinney, E.C., 89–94. *Correspondence* with W.A. White, 89–94
Plato, 134
politics, psychiatry and medicine, 57, 136, 260–65
Pollock, Horatio M., 31, 34
Presbyterian Hospital (N.Y.C.), 94
Prince, Morton, 191
The Problem of Mental Disorder (Bentley and Cowdry), 219
Psychiatric Institute of the State of New York. *See* New York State Psychiatric Institute
psychiatric social work, 10, 88, 169–70, 187, 214–19, 223
psychiatrists: and C.W. Beers, 147–63; compensation of, 229; criticisms of, 1, 6–7; debate over therapy, 102–37; disagreements among, 58; education of, 230–33; medical view of, 227–28; in mental hospitals, 57, 234–41; and mental hygiene, 138–84; migration of German psychiatrists in 1930s, 273; and psychoanalysis, 129–37; redefining their specialties, 7–11; and sterilization, 171–75; and women, 10, 96–100, 215–19, 267–69, 276–83
psychiatry: abandonment of mental hospital, 10–11; attitudes toward, 242–44; blacks in, 270; board certification, 231, 245–60; boundaries of, 185–228; as a career, 234–41;

and criminal behavior, 283–89; criticisms of, 56–57; demand for autonomy, 229–66; education in, 241–45, 248–60; faith in science, 267; heterogeneous nature of, 20; Jews in, 273–76; and law, 283–89; and medicine, 57, 139, 185–86; and mental health professions, 10, 187–88; and mental hospitals, 17–18; and mental hygiene, 175–83; and neurology, 180, 220–24, 232, 241–45; origins of, 2–7; political concerns of, 267; and psychiatric social work, 215–19; and psychology, 188–98, 211–14, 243–44; racial issues in, 270–73; research in, 20, 243; and social issues, 266–96; somaticism in, 19; and state regulation, 232–33; transformation of, 7–11, 17–18, 186–88; and war, 289–96; women in, 10, 96–100, 215–19, 267–69, 276–83; and World War I, 220–21
psychoanalysis, 19–20, 106–107, 129–37, 176, 189–92, 198–211, 213, 219–20, 224–27, 241, 243–44, 273, 276, 278–81, 287–88
Psychoanalytic Review, 34, 205
psychobiology, 21, 176–78, 180, 193–94, 197, 202, 204, 210, 219–20
Psychological Bulletin, 27, 194
Psychological Clinic, 164, 179
Psychological Review, 194
psychology, 169; clinical, 10, 187, 212; and psychiatry, 188–98, 211–14, 243–44
psychoneuroses, 176
psychopathic hospital, 9, 27–28, 146, 186. *See also* Boston Psychopathic Hospital; Henry Phipps Psychiatric Clinic (Johns Hopkins); New York State Psychiatric Institute; Psychopathic Hospital at the University of Michigan
Psychopathic Hospital at the University of Michigan, 27

psychopathic personality, 15
psychotherapy, 107–108, 129–37
Public Charities Association of Pennsylvania, 86
public poor relief, 165–66. *See also* state welfare policy
Putnam, James J., 223

Quinby, Hosea M., 59, 62–69, 78. *Correspondence* with A. Meyer, 64–69

Rabinovitch, Louise G., 268–69
Raynor, Mortimer W., 249, 275
reaction complexes, 28–29, 211
reaction tendencies, 211
Read, Charles F., 295–96. *Correspondence* with C.W. Beers, 296
Reader's Digest, 183
Reed, Charles A.L., 109–12
research institute in psychiatry, 9, 186
restraint in mental hospitals, 71–74, 150–52, 235–36
Rice, Mrs. William B., 142
Riggs, Austen Fox, 192, 197
Robbins, William L., 270
Robison, W.A., 107. *Correspondence* with W.A. White, 107
Rockefeller Foundation, 140, 165–70, 230
Rodman, John S., 245
Russell, William L., 87, 161–63, 247–55, 258. *Correspondence* with W.A. White, 247–55

Sachs, Bernard, 186, 252
Sage, Henry M., 87
Sage, Mrs. Russell (Margaret O.S.), 142
Sage Foundation, 142
Saint Elizabeths Hospital, 34, 89–94, 124–25, 173, 273
Saint Peter State Hospital (Minn.), 96–100
Sakel, Manfred, 105, 126–29
Salmon, Thomas W., 9–10, 84–87,

Salmon, Thomas W. (*continued*)
140, 163–65, 181, 216, 221, 275.
Correspondence with A. Meyer, 85–
87, 163–64
salpingectomy, 171
Sanborn, Agnes Goldman, 51
Sandy, William C., 87
Sanford, E.C., 77
Saturday Evening Post, 183
Savage, Mr., 91
Saxe, Earl, 183–84. *Correspondence*
with M. Gitelson, 183–84
Schilder, Paul, 128
Schiller, 35
schizophrenia, 15, 43, 45–46, 48–55,
105, 127–29. *See also* dementia
praecox
Schuyler, Louisa L., 142
scientific medicine, 185
Scoville, Mildred C., 218–19, 242.
Correspondence with H.B. Crutcher,
218–19
Scribner, Ernest V., 78
segregation of feebleminded, 170–71
Seguin, E.C., 6
Semon, Richard, 47
senility. *See* mental hospitals, aged and
senile patients in
Sergeant, Miss [A?], 288
Sermon on the Mount, 134
sex and mental illness, 53–54
sexual theory, 133
Sherrington, Charles S., 200
shock treatment, 105, 126–29
Sidis, Boris, 23, 25
Siemens, 46
Silk, Samuel A., 93
Sing Sing Prison, 169, 286
Singer, H. Douglas, 216, 248–49,
251, 254
Smith, Dr., 236
Smith, Alfred E., 286
Smith College Training School for So-
cial Workers, 222–23
social policy. *See* state welfare policy
social sciences and psychiatry, 187

social service in mental hospitals,
215–19, 240
social work, 187, 222–23
Solomon, Harry C., 33
somaticism in psychiatry, 19
South, mentally ill in, 41–42, 94–96,
227–28
Southard, E.E., 27–29, 75–77, 187,
210, 222–23. *Correspondence* with
A. Meyer, 27–29
Southard School of the Menninger
Clinic, 183, 296
Southern Medicine and Surgery, 41,109
Spencer, Herbert, 134
Springfield State Hospital (N.J.), 119
state board of control, 71
state welfare policy, 13, 57–58, 70–
71, 75–81, 84–87, 260–65
statistics of mental illness, 44
Stedman, Henry R., 71–74. *Corre-
spondence* with W.A. White, 71–74
Sterilization for Human Betterment
(Gosney), 174–75
sterilization of mentally ill, 140,
171–75
Stevenson, George M., 187
Stocking, Leonard, 233–35. *Correspondence* with W.A. White, 234–35
Stone, Robert G., 120
straightjacket, 152, 235
Stransky, Edwin L., 23
Strecker, Edward A., 241, 244–46,
248, 253. *Correspondence* with
A. Meyer, 244
substitutive process, 28
*Suggestions of Modern Science Concern-
ing Education* (Jennings, Watson,
Meyer, and Thomas), 177
suicide, 238
sulphonal, 103
symbolization, 35
syphilis. *See* paresis

Taneyhill, G. Lane, 191, 280
*Tentatives Operatoires dans le Traitment
de Certaines Psychoses* (Moniz), 125

therapy, psychiatric, 4, 20–21, 102–37, 186, 240; bilateral ovariectomy, 103; calcium, 121; colectomy, 104, 120; defocalization, 104, 108–23; drug, 103; electrical, 103; electroshock, 105; fever, 104–105; hydrotherapy, 80, 83, 103; insulin shock, 105, 126–29; laparotomy, 116–17, 120; lobotomy, 105, 125–26, 264; malaria, 124–25; psychological, 107–108; psychotherapy, 129–37; shock, 105

Thirkfield, Wilbur P., 270. *Correspondence* with W.A. White, 270

Thom, Douglas A., 215–16. *Correspondence* with F.F. Hutchins, 215–16

Thomas, William I., 177

Thompson, Clara M., 276–82. *Correspondence* with A. Meyer, 276–82

thyroid extract, 103

Timme, Walter, 36–37

Titchener, Edward B., 189–90, 198

Trenton State Hospital (N.J.), 104, 108–23

treponema pallidum, 124

trypasamide, 104

tumors, brain, 15

Tuttle, George T., 72

typhoid vaccine, 121

Vanderbilt Clinic (N.Y.C.), 94

vasectomy, 171

Veterans Administration, 11

Vincent, George E., 175

Virchow, Rudolf, 135

Virginia, 94–95, 171

Virginia General Hospital Board, 94

Virginia Western Lunatic Asylum, 12

Wagner, Charles G., 8

Wagner-Jauregg, Julius, 96, 104

Wallace, Alfred, 204

Wallin, Willoughby, 257–58

war, psychiatric attitude toward, 289–96

Waters, James C., Jr., 272. *Correspondence* with W.A. White, 272

Watson, John B., 177, 188–98, 212. *Correspondence* with A. Meyer, 188–98

Watts, James W., 105

Weeks, David Fairchild, 38–39

Weisenburg, T.N., 241–45. *Correspondence* with A. Meyer, 242–44

welfare, 6, 12, 165–66. *See also* state welfare policy

Wells, Dr., 261

Wells, F.L., 191

Wertham, Frederic. *See* Wertheimer, Frederick I.

Wertheimer, Frederick I., 279

White, William A., 1, 34, 38–41, 45, 70–74, 87–94, 107–109, 112–15, 124–26, 128–29, 172–74, 224, 233–35, 250, 255–60, 270–73, 283–89, 292; and focal infection theory of mental illness, 109, 112–15; heredity, 38–41; human behavior, 34–37; insulin shock therapy, 128–29; lobotomy, 125–26; malaria therapy, 124–25; mental hospital attendants, 89–94; psychoanalysis, 106, 130; restraint, 71–74; size of ideal hospital, 87–89; sterilization, 171–74; therapeutic optimism, 106–108. *Correspondence*: with E.S. Abbot, 108; with E.A. Balloch, 270–71, 273; with C.W. Beers, 292; with W.C. Borden, 271–73; with A.A. Brill, 128–29; with C.H. Clark, 70–71; with W.W. Eldridge, 124–25; with R.G. Ferguson, 87–89; with Dr. Fisher, 172–74; with F. Frankfurter, 285–89; with A.P. Hering, 171–72; with C.M. Hincks, 128; with A.T. Hobbs, 112–15; with S.E. Jelliffe, 125–26; with L.M. Jones, 109; with J.V. May, 257–60; with K.A. Menninger, 283–85; with A. Meyer, 129; with L.E. Moten, 271–72; with E.C.

White, William A. (*continued*)
Pinney, 89–94; with W.A. Robison, 107; with H.R. Stedman, 71–74; with L. Stocking, 234–35; with W.P. Thirkfield, 270; with J.C. Waters, Jr., 272; with J.G. Whiteside, 112; with R.S. Woodward, 38–41
Whitehorn, John C., 219–20, 253. *Correspondence* with A. Meyer, 219–20
Whiteside, J.G., 112. *Correspondence* with W.A. White, 112
Wile, Ira S., 292. *Correspondence* with C.W. Beers, 292
Williams, David L., 262
Williams, Frankwood E., 165–70, 220–24. *Correspondence*: with E.R. Embree, 165–70; with F. Norbury, 220–24
Wilmanns, Karl, 129
Wilmanns, Ruth, 129

Wisconsin, county care system, 84
Wissler, Clark, 211
Wolfe, Mary M., 268
Wolner, Oscar H., 99
women: and psychiatric social work, 215–19; in psychiatry, 10, 96–100, 215–19, 267–69, 276–83
Woodman, Robert, 291–92. *Correspondence* with C.W. Beers, 291–92
Woodward, R.S., 38–41. *Correspondence* with W.A. White, 38–41
Woolley, Herbert C., 93
Worcester State Lunatic Hospital (Mass.), 4, 11, 58–64, 77, 129
Wortis, Joseph, 129, 233, 235–41

Yale University, 181

Zilboorg, Gregory, 274–76. *Correspondence* with S.E. Jelliffe, 274–76